Therapist's Guide to Pediatric Affect and Behavior Regulation

Therapist's Guide to Pediatric Affect and Behavior Regulation

Sharon L. Johnson

AMSTERDAM • BOSTON • HEIDELBERG • LONDON
NEW YORK • OXFORD • PARIS • SAN DIEGO
SAN FRANCISCO • SINGAPORE • SYDNEY • TOKYO
Academic Press is an imprint of Elsevier

Academic Press is an imprint of Elsevier
32 Jamestown Road, London NW1 7BY, UK
225 Wyman Street, Waltham, MA 02451, USA
525 B Street, Suite 1800, San Diego, CA 92101-4495, USA

First edition 2013

Notice
No responsibility is assumed by the publisher for any injury and/or damage to persons or property as
a matter of products liability, negligence or otherwise, or from any use or operation of any methods,
products, instructions or ideas contained in the material herein. Because of rapid advances in the
medical sciences, in particular, independent verification of diagnoses and drug dosages should be made

British Library Cataloguing-in-Publication Data
A catalogue record for this book is available from the British Library

Library of Congress Cataloging-in-Publication Data
A catalog record for this book is available from the Library of Congress

ISBN: 978-0-12-386884-8

For information on all Academic Press publications
visit our website at elsevierdirect.com

Typeset by MPS Limited, Chennai, India
www.adi-mps.com

Printed and bound by CPI Group (UK) Ltd, Croydon, CR0 4YY
Transferred to digital print 2012

Working together to grow
libraries in developing countries

www.elsevier.com | www.bookaid.org | www.sabre.org

ELSEVIER   BOOK AID
International   Sabre Foundation

CONTENTS

v

CONTENTS

vi

CONTENTS

viii

CONTENTS

In an effort to improve the health and mental health of young children, physicians, mental health professionals, occupational therapists, educators, speech pathologists and others have diligently worked to understand the maladies and associated solutions to the constellation of difficulties which impact their optimal development. In much the same manner in which a pebble tossed into a body of water results in a ripple effect, each difficulty experienced by a young child has the potential of resulting in complicating consequences to their emotional and intellectual development. The realm of treatment is often multidisciplinary in scope, individualized and creative, recognizing there are many ways to treat and manage these issues. Thus, parents and professionals work together to develop a comprehensive plan for optimizing each child's learning potential and increased coping ability.

Central to the functioning of a young child is the concept of regulation. The development of regulation of mood, impulse, and an internal state of regulation is fundamental to the developmental process. The concept of regulation was fortunately recognized by a number of professionals who have dedicated their professional efforts to the understanding and treatment of the manifested difficulties experienced by young children. While the contribution of these practitioners and researchers is significant regarding regulation, their insight comprehensively encompassed the interrelationship of attachment, emotional regulation and internal regulation. Thus clarifying the complex relationship and interaction of numerous facets of development. As a result, those who specialize in working with young children acknowledge that, in addition to the diagnoses outlined in the Diagnostic and Statistical Manual and ICD-9, Regulatory Disorders of Sensory Processing (RDSP) characterize distinct responses and behavioral patterns, though dynamic and evolving over time, underlying many of the obstacles which interfere with the normal trajectory of development. Diagnostic acknowledgement of developmental process, such as RDSP, as it is intertwined with adjustment and pathology, is conceptualized in the DC:0–3R. The overlap of these three diagnostic frames can be found in the diagnostic "crosswalk" in Chapter 2 serving as a tool for the behavioral health provider in identifying the correct diagnosis describing the range of symptoms and developmental difficulties interfering with maximal developmental ability. Due to the inherent association between diagnosis and treatment planning, effective treatment requires an accurate diagnosis enhanced by a conceptual foundation of development and factors influencing enrichment versus pathology.

The far-reaching social consequences of the negative impact of developmental problems of young children reinforced the importance of early detection and intervention. The goal of early detection is to prevent more serious, long-term perceptual, language and sensory integrative and behavioral difficulties. The parameters or conceptualization of intervention may be impacted by the differing perspectives of "health" set forth by the variety of professionals on the treatment team. This may best be demonstrated in the regulations and requirements set forth by the structure of improving academic performance as outlined by the goals of the individualized family service plan (IFSP) and the individualized education plan (IEP). This text fully acknowledges the important focus of the IFSP and IEP, but is not limited to their scope or objective of outcome associated with academic performance of preschoolers and kindergarteners. Instead, the scope of intervention is comprehensive, including aspects of psychological and emotional functioning which may not be targeted for intervention with regards to improving academic performance but, indeed, are related to quality of life experience and relationship functioning in general as it pertains to the developmental and familial demands of the 0–5 year old.

Chapters 1 and 2 lay the foundation for conceptualizing the range of difficulties experienced by a young child (and, therefore, their family), how to identify and clarify symptom presentation, and accurate diagnosing with the aforementioned diagnostic nomenclature systems. The emphasis in Chapter 2 not only discusses thorough assessment procedures but also includes the type of processes used to conduct them without being a cookbook approach. Such flexibility in the assessment process is demanded by the stages of child development, individual needs, setting and circumstances. Thus, encompassing a multimethod and multi-informant approach with common assessment procedures. Chapter 3 provides a range of treatment possibilities for individualized treatment planning. Perhaps the most important aspect of the treatment-planning chapter is its representation as a balance between science and practice. Clinicians are always interested in the latest research. Unfortunately, the gap between research and practice, often due to financial limitations in the private sector, can be frustrating. Therefore, as much as possible, empirically-based procedures, "evidence based", and the vast clinical experience from the clinical practice of numerous practitioners with a history of providing services in a range of environments were gleaned with an emphasis on increased effectiveness and outcome oriented focus. Furthermore, the treatment section recognizes there may be an overlap between treatment planning from several different environments (i.e., individual/family treatment may share goals and interventions similar to those in the preschool/kindergarten environment), but that specific environmental demands also play a role in the unique selection of treatment goals and interventions and how they are operationalized.

The final chapter offers an array of beneficial forms from initial client information or patient information, additional business-related forms and interview question outline/format. The goal of interviews and other forms of documentation is to serve as a baseline, a clarification of the presenting problems, a thorough source of information to review and substantiate treatment progress, for work associated with collateral contacts and overall case management. The selection of forms is not an exhaustive collection but all were chosen for their potential utility and to meet a variety of needs in working with young children and their families.

CHAPTER 1

The Regulatory Disordered Infant and Child

"There is no such thing as a baby" – only a baby and someone.
Donald Winnicott (Finichel & Eggbeer, 1990)

To comprehend fully the implications of pediatric disorders of regulation in affect and behavior requires a fundamental background in child development, family systems theory and psychopathology. Such a clinical perspective provides the framework to utilize the following information as a basic review on normal or typical child development versus the development of psychopathology which is the foundation necessary for assessment, accurate diagnosis and effective treatment.

The regulation of affect and behavior are developmental processes extended through infancy and childhood, thus establishing the foundation of lifelong abilities and individual differences associated with self-control. The individual differences in emotional regulation underlie important differences in psychological well-being, social competency and, in some cases, evolving psychopathology. Therefore, this section will focus on the processes of development associated with emotion regulation, temperament, attachment, the role of emotion regulation being influenced by the child's conceptual growth and understanding, and social/environmental influences, thereby demonstrating a complex factorial interplay in normal and abnormal development.

It is nothing short of amazing that a human conception survives the journey to birth. Congenital abnormalities and the loss of embryos and fetuses prior to birth are caused both intrinsically and extrinsically. For those who survive, both parents and professionals are challenged by the presentation of early regulatory problems commonly exhibited by babies. Regulation is basically the sensory processing method used to recognize, organize, and make sense of incoming sensory information (hearing/auditory, vision/ocular, smell/olfactory, touch/tactile, taste/gustatory) and internal sensations (vestibular system which detects movement/tells us when we are surrounded by something that is moving or on something moving/tells us up from down/influences concept of outside space and proprioceptive system which is body awareness/tells us where the body parts are). An adaptive response is created by the external information being reviewed along with input from the body. When irregularities in regulation are present they are demonstrated by problems associated with sleep cycles, feeding, digestion, attention, arousal, mood regulation, and self-soothing. According to DeGangi (2000), these infants are often hyper- or hypo-sensitive to sensory stimulation. Most of these issues have been resolved by the time the infant is 6 months of age. However, some infants continue to demonstrate problems of regulation in these areas including mood regulation. For these infants, their development into toddlerhood is marked

1

by problems in regulation (Kostuik & Fouts, 2002; Fox & Calkins, 2003; Schore, 2005; Bell & Deater-Deckard, 2007):

- Difficulties with attention
- Sensory processing
- Intolerance for change
- Socially inappropriate behavior
- A hyper-alert state of arousal
- Severe separation anxiety.

As a result of the observation of infant to child difficulties with regulation in affect and behavior as well as increased emotional distress of the parents, these infants and children find their way into pediatric medical and psychological practices. The clinical presentations offer a unique opportunity to understand and to intervene early and proactively with young children and their families. Therefore, the understanding of *emotion* possesses important implications for revealing "normal" as well as "abnormal" development. This significant focal point is directed to the role and development of links between emotion, behavior and psychopathology. The clinical perspective seeks to clarify which category or parameters the infant/child demonstrates difficulty with, how much it interferes with their or others' lives and what the impact is to their level of functioning. There may be identified symptoms in one category and none in another or some symptoms in more than one category. The different types of regulatory disorders described by Diagnostic Classification: 0-3 (DC:0-3R) are utilized for the presentation of symptomology, disorders and subtypes.

NORMAL DEVELOPMENT OF REGULATORY PROCESSES IN INFANCY

Emotion regulation is a component of emotional activation in a network of multilevel processes consisting of internal and external processes responsible for monitoring, evaluating and modifying emotional reactions – specifically their timing and intensity in *meeting one's goals*. These processes are exemplified by the interaction and feedback between higher and lower systems, such as the mutual influence of multiple emotional related systems which sometimes contribute to maladaptive outcomes, especially in circumstances of environmental hardship (Thompson et al, 2008). This complex construct is an integration of behavior (including motor skills), genetic mechanisms, attention, cognition, environmental influences and emotional control (especially negative emotions). All of these factors contribute to the unique differences in self-regulation. Self-regulation is the ability to control inner states (responses) with regard to emotions, thoughts, attention, and function (performance) (Bell & Deater-Deckard, 2007). It is the development of competence in responding to life demands. The brain is continually sensing and responding to the needs of the body and the environment. An infant/toddler is able to maintain internal equilibrium by modulating sensory stimulation from their environment by altering or adjusting the intensity of arousal experienced while remaining engaged in an interaction or being able to disengage easily from an activity. Much of this regulation takes place automatically outside of conscious awareness. Therefore, an adaptive response is an appropriate action resulting from the synthesis of incoming sensory information received through the central nervous system. It can be conscious or unconscious (predominantly) and is the consequence of adequate sensory integration which, in turn, reinforces the improvement or continuing refinement of sensory integration. Therefore, normal regulation or modulation is not a straight trajectory, but rather a developmental process which takes place within a range of limits. Normal, healthy self-regulation is related to the capacity to tolerate the sensations of distress that accompany an unmet need through the repetition of the experience of a chain of associated stimulus response cues (Schore, 2001, 2005; Bell & Deater-Deckard, 2007; Thompson et al, 2008; Benson & Haith, 2009). For example:

$$hunger > discomfort > distress > tearful\,response$$
$$> satisfaction = learning$$

(this is a simple example of early learning that the feeling of distress will pass as a result of the intervention of an attuned adult. This leads to learning skills of self-management which includes increased tolerance and eliciting appropriate resources).

As the child learns to tolerate distress they become much less reactive and impulsive. This is a demonstration of the evolution of self-regulation. The responsiveness of the attuned adult facilitates the learning that allows the child to build the capacity to place a moment between the impulse and an action. Such a delay results in reinforcing success and increasing self-regulation. When the child is able to insert a moment between a feeling and an action they then have achieved the ability to take the time to think, plan, and develop a response to the challenge and demonstrate goal directedness. This scenario is a simplistic example of the multifaceted process of developing self-regulation. However, it does provide a useful display of the power of interplay between an infant/child and a positive effective caregiver. Additionally, it serves to demonstrate the emergent knowledge and skill development associated with self-regulation. The infant's success at regulation significantly depends on the caregiver's awareness, flexibility, and responsivity to the child's emotional expression and need for caregiver intervention. The toddler advances this theme with the ability to initiate a greater repertoire of self-regulating behaviors critical to developmental progression of independence, control and an identity separate from the caregiver. As the toddler makes the transition to preschool and subsequently to school there is a marked acquisition of an integrated set of domain-specific mechanisms or "self-regulation".

Over the course of development, initiated prenatally and evolving into sophisticated and self-initiated processes from toddler > preschool > school years, regulatory processes progress in association with the child's increasing capacity to regulate their motoric and effective behavior. This takes place first in the dyadic relationship (infant), progresses to guiding caregiver in toddlerhood, and later as a function of voluntary and effortful control. The transition from toddler to preschooler (age 2 to 3 years) is particularly interesting in normal or typical regulatory development. The child begins to gain control over impulses and actions that are primarily activated situationally, whereby they demonstrate increased capability regarding behavior compliance and delay of gratification. During their preschool experience they begin to engage in more executive or cognitive control of thoughts and actions. It is the emergence of these skills that supports the successful transition to the school and peer environment which demands independent and adaptive behavioral functioning (Rothbart et al, 2000, 2003; Fox & Calkins, 2003; Calkins 2004; Rothbart & Rueda, 2005). Increases in language development, cognitive abilities, and specific self-regulation skills acquired during toddlerhood allow for most children to learn to control early (normal) non-compliant, aggressive, and impulsive tendencies resulting in a decrease in problem behavior (Campbell, 2002).

In conclusion, a child's emotional health is molded by a complex interaction between genetic, constitutional and environmental factors. The environmental factors are double edged offering a compelling influence of risk and protection. These factors are dependent on quality and availability in their command by either protective aspects via buffering and encouraging resilience and typical development or by exacerbating the likelihood of emotional, social and cognitive problems.

CAREGIVER CHARACTERISTICS
- Mental health (emotional/psychological functioning)
- Educational level

3

- Self-efficacy/self-sufficiency
- Resourcefulness and coping
- Health and general well-being

FAMILY FACTORS

- Caregiver–child relationship
- Emotional atmosphere
- Marital quality/task collaboration
- Degree of stress
- Stability
- Sibling issues

COMMUNITY CONNECTEDNESS FACTORS

- Caregiver social support
- Quality of child care
- Child's peer relationships
- Extended family influence
- Cultural/ethnic norms and expectations

ENVIRONMENTAL/NEIGHBORHOOD FACTORS

- Availability and diversity of resources
- Adequacy of housing
- Violence/safety

Attachment

4

At birth, the brain is the most undifferentiated organ. It has a plasticity that enables the creation of neural circuitry throughout life. This means the brain is capable of renewing its structure and function as a result of experiences, in particular, social experiences. Attachment, the emotional bond that is formed between an infant and their primary caregiver, profoundly influences both the structure and the function of the developing infant brain. When that attachment bond is not adequately formed, whether as a result of abuse, neglect, or emotional unavailability on behalf of the caregiver, brain structure and function can be negatively impacted, causing relational or developmental trauma (Diener et al., 2002; Schore, 2001, 2005; van der Kolk, 2005).

The role of attachment in association with emotion regulation during early childhood emphasizes the importance of the context of the parent–child relationship. As the infant develops and directs interest outwards, it is the caregiver who is responsible for helping the infant to regulate the level of arousal. The caregiver accomplishes this by responding to infant cues of distress and providing comfort as well as intense positive arousal experiences. The infant learns from these interactions to trust the caregiver and their help to resolve distressing arousal. This relationship development lays the foundation for establishing an effective attachment relationship, or the dyadic regulation of infant emotion and arousal. As a result, the quality of care provided during this developmental period (dyadic regulation) significantly contributes to the infant's regulatory ability. This relationship has a bidirectional quality for the infant. Not only do they receive from the attuned caregiver, but they directly elicit through their willingness to utilize the caregiver as a secure base, thus allowing them to expand the exploration of their world. As the infant progresses to toddler and then preschooler the role of dyadic regulation and then caregiver-guided self-regulation is replaced with a desire for increased autonomy. The transitional states from dyadic regulation to caregiver-guided regulation to self-regulation are significantly influenced by the quality and consistency of the attachment relationship. Attachment security is associated with effective self-regulation and fewer behavioral problems in preschool. In other words, secure

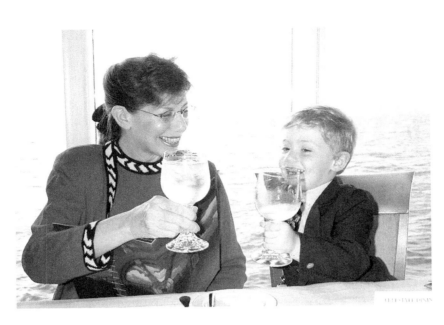

FIGURE 1.1
Family members toast with water glasses.

infant–caregiver attachment is related to lower risk for later peer and behavioral problems. Of course, other features unique to the infant (genetic, temperament, as well as other characteristics) are also a part of this evolving matrix of skill development, or deficiencies in development. Bottom line, competence is associated to healthy developmental trajectories as a protective factor which also increases opportunities for positive interactions and feedback (Mahler et al, 1975; Weinfield et al, 1999; Zeanah, 2000; Schore, 2001) (Figure 1.1).

Schore (2001, 2005; Benson & Haith, 2009) clearly speaks of the relationship between emotion and biology. Multiple regions of the brain and neurohormonal processes are intertwined with emotion and its management. In the nature–nurture scheme, the capacities of emotion regulation unfold along with developmental advances of maturity and the neurobiological influence of attachment. At birth, these systems are active but lack maturity. The HPA (hypothalamic–pituitary–adrenocortical) axis and the subcortical structures such as the amygdala and hypothalamus work together in the activation of the sympathetic nervous system thus arousing the newborn infant. In a manner similar to the activation of sympathetic arousal, the other branch of the autonomic nervous system, the parasympathetic branch, has an inhibitory affect. These immature nervous system responses are the underlying reason for the all or nothing quality of infant response (such as crying). Thus demonstrating that the infant cannot yet regulate manifestations of arousal. An additional feature on the nature side of the equation is the constitution that the infant brings with them, particularly temperament.

Neurological functioning stems from both genetics and environmental influence. Genetics provides innate capacities shaped by experience toward optimal functioning or by limiting capacity. Neurobiology is an integrated network of crucial developmental elements and is the cornerstone of attachment relationships as well as executive functions development. In turn, secure attachments provide the foundation of optimal brain development which facilitates and reinforces skill of executive function such as judgment, planning and management ability of emotional trauma, loss and neglect. Likewise, in the fashion of a negative feedback loop trauma, loss and neglect have the ability to impact negatively neurobiological developmental capacities for attachment, self-regulation and executive function. The demonstration of the neurobiological factors works much like a bidirectional arrow: external (information taken in) ⟷ internal (integrated) ⟷ external (reflected in skill development and risk). A central characteristic of neurobiology is plasticity. Plasticity is a lifelong ability of the brain to reorganize neural pathways based on new experiences (or the ability of the

5

brain to change with learning). Children imitate and internalize influences of their caregiving experiences. Therefore, sensitive responsive care, as well as the opposite, shape brain development (Shore 2001, 2005; Teicher, 2002; Charney, 2004; Lieberman, 2004).

The model of the caregiver–infant attachment relationship (Schore, 2001,2005) facilitates increasing the dimensions of the child's coping capacities. Thus suggesting, "adaptive infant mental health can be fundamentally defined as the earliest expression of flexible strategies for coping with the novelty and stress that is inherent in human interaction". The caregiver role of providing sensory stimulation through physical contact such as bathing, dressing and soothing, and play activity facilitates sensorimotor modulation. The quality of the attachment relationship between an infant and a caregiver is determined by the quality of the caregiver's response to the infant at times when the infant's attachment system is activated (i.e., emotionally distressed, physically hurt, ill, etc.). The integration of the caregiver–infant experiences of touch, movement, auditory stimulation and visual stimulation, which takes place during the first 18 months of life, makes possible the development of self-soothing behaviors (Schore, 2001). Self-soothing behaviors use internal and external resources: visual in the form of looking at sights of interest in their environment; auditory via listening to pleasant or calming sounds; self-touch such as holding on to their own hands or feet, sucking, and holding on to a familiar object such as a blanket or soft toy. Mahler et al (1975) describe face-to-face affective synchrony, symbiotic phase, as beginning at 2–3 months, generating high levels of positive arousal and shared or mutual regulation (attuned) called instances of "optimal mutual cueing". In this pleasurable state of symbiosis (a state in which the infant behaves and functions as if it were one with the caregiver), the infant (Mahler et al, 1975; Polan & Hofer, 1999)

- is in a state of undifferentiation
- is in a state of fusion with the caregiver
- experiences interaction regulation synchronicity
- experiences dual unity within one common boundary
- is within a self-organizing system composed of caregiver and infant as one unit.

This concept of attachment, as a deep and enduring connection established between a child and caregiver, as an interactive regulation of biological synchronicity is possibly best demonstrated by the sharing of facial expressions between caregiver and infant becoming one, or shared-mutual reflection. Attachment refers to the child's thoughts, feelings and behaviors in reflection to significant others, most often the primary caregiver. Early experiences with caregivers shape a child's core beliefs about self, others, and life in general. Experiences of the infant and young child are encoded in the brain. Emotional experiences of nurturance and protection are encoded in the limbic system. Over time, repeated encoded experiences become internal working models or the "lens" through which the child views themselves, others and, overall, their world (Schore, 2001). Healthy social-emotional development for infants and toddlers unfolds in an interpersonal context, namely that of the positive ongoing relationships with familiar, nurturing adults. These expanding capacities help young children to become competent in negotiating increasingly complex interactions. Between the ages of 8 and 18 months, the infant develops the ability to modify responses in relation to events and object characteristics in accordance with intentionality, reciprocal interactions and organized affects. Thus, there is meaning in verbal and contextual cues. This stage is marked by the blossoming of skill development (DeGangi, 2000):

- initiate, maintain, and inhibit physical actions
- the emergence of problem solving
- intentionality
- awareness that actions lead to a goal
- increasing awareness of self as a separate identity (allowing for the differentiation of their own responses from the actions of others).

At about 18 months of age, self-control emerges with the creation of mental images. Mental images have immense utility for homeostasis of the self. They allow the internalization of routines and responding to requests or commands, pretend play and functional language, delaying actions to comply with social expectations (without external cues), and being able to differentiate self from others. Representational thought and recall memory are hallmark features of development at this stage. The role of the caregiver is one of reflective interpretation in pairing affective meaning to situations as well as providing social expectations and values related to particular and specific emotional responses. This caregiver attachment of affective meaning facilitates the infant to label and understand emotion and its context. The instrumental features in achieving emotional regulation are identified as (DeGangi, 2000; Schore, 2002; Thompson et al, 2008):

- *Action schemes*
  - Vocalizations, self-distraction, motoric responses
- *Cognitive organization*
  - Representational thinking and self-monitoring
- *Motivation*
- *Caregiver support.*

Another accepted construct of attachment was set forth by Bowlby (1969). His theory of attachment views the infant's emotional tie to the caregiver as an evolved response that promotes survival. Bowlby's stages of attachment begin as a set of innate signals used by the baby to summon the parent and gradually develops through four stages into an affectionate bond:

1. Pre-attachment (birth to 6 weeks): inborn signaling bringing newborn into close contact with other humans who comfort them
2. Attachment-in-the-making (6 weeks to 6 to 8 months): the baby responds differently to a familiar caregiver than to a stranger and begins to develop a sense of trust
3. Clear-cut attachment (6 to 8 months to 18 to 24 months): the baby displays separation anxiety, becoming upset when the trusted caretaker leaves
4. Formation of reciprocal relationship (18 to 24 months and on): separation protest declines.

Therefore, emotional security is attachment's role in the regulation of emotion. It is a central concept as a regulatory process in normal or typical development and the development of psychopathology. Moreover, failure to acquire mental-age appropriate social-emotional skills may be associated with greater risk for concurrent and later emotional/behavioral problems. For example, secure infant attachment is related to lower risk for later peer and behavior problems. Emotional security serves as a model emphasizing the interplay between social-emotional and biological processes whereby the regulation of emotional well-being and security develop. The experience of this concept is defined from an organizational perspective of the entire person and their unique responses (reactions to events) illustrating a central focus on the impact of marital and parent–child relations on the child's emotional security. There are additional implications for social-emotional development associated with the interaction between attachment and temperament (Cummings & Davies, 1996).

Effortful Control

The study of temperament and the associations to neural circuitry and attentional tasks furthers the examination of development of executive attention and self-regulation. The construct of effortful control tends to increase with age and is associated with several characteristics of children and parents. This construct includes the ability to inhibit dominant responses to act upon subdominant responses, to detect errors, and to engage in planning. Effortful control includes focused attention, perceptual sensitivity, inhibitory

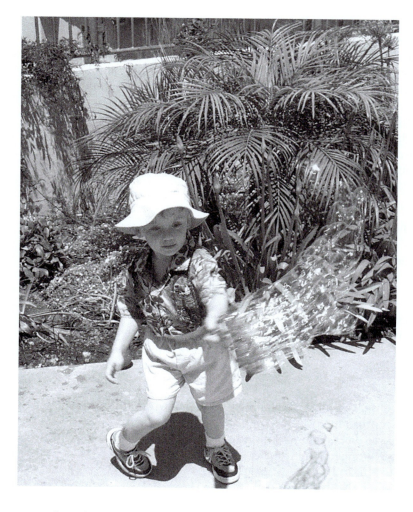

8

FIGURE 1.2
Young boy creates
bubbles.

control, and low intensity pleasure (Figure 1.2). Given the range of abilities in which effortful control plays an important role, it is not unexpected that it is associated to the development of conscience and aggression. It is also a protective factor which promotes following instructions and obedience to caregiver rules.

An infant's ability for focused attention combined with maternal responsiveness and caregiver personality characteristics (such as dependability, effective management and self-control) are also associated with the demonstrated range of effortful control. For example, the influence of affective synchrony in caregiver–infant interaction in the development of effortful control is significant for children demonstrating high negative emotionality in childhood versus the effect of affective synchrony for infants not demonstrating negative emotionality being much smaller. Features defining effortful control include (Rothbart et al, 2000; Carlson & Moses, 2001; Casey et al, 2001; Blair, 2002; Calkins et al, 2002; Fan et al, 2003; Jones et al, 2003; Rueda et al, 2004; Rothbart & Rueda, 2005):

- *Temperament*, or individuality, in constitutional reactivity and self-regulation. Temperament refers to the relatively enduring framework influenced over time by heredity, maturation, and experience. Temperament evolves from genetic provision, however, it influences and is influenced by the individual's experience.
- *Reactivity* refers to the excitability, responsivity, or arousability of the behavioral or physiological systems.
- *Self-regulation* refers to neural and behavioral processes functioning to modulate the underlying reactivity, or the ability to control inner states.

*Competence functions as a protective factor or buffer which supports the understanding of varying developmental trajectories. Competencies also increase opportunities for positive interactions and feedback which serves to diminish problem behavior.

Temperament

Temperament is defined as a constitutionally or biologically based characteristic associated with differences in emotional, motor and attentional reactivity and self-regulation. It is the relatively enduring biological framework influenced over time by heredity, maturation and experience. Infants respond to their environment with reactivity, emotion, and attention with their own unique responsivity from infant to infant. These reactions to the environment, along with the mechanisms that regulate them, make up the child's temperament (Rothbart & Rueda, 2005). Temperament is seen to be relatively consistent across situation and stable over time. It is seen as a key factor in early child characteristics being predictors of later personality development, behavioral patterns, emotional response patterns, adjustment, and the presence as well as severity of clinical symptoms. It is with temperament that the concept of goodness of fit plays a significant role. Goodness of fit refers to the degree of correspondence between child characteristics and parental expectations and demands. Thus, a "good fit" results in a positive adjustment and outcome, whereas, a "poor fit" results in a negative outcome or less than satisfactory adjustment (Wolraich et al, 2008; Benson & Haith, 2009).

With regards to temperament, infants who are easily frustrated use more physical regulation, scanning and caregiver orienting and less distraction. Additionally, they have higher activity levels and demonstrate decreased attention during task exercises. Aside from anger and frustration, other characteristics of temperament include vocal expression/excessive crying, impact of caregiver availability, caregiver attachment quality, and physical stimulation. Constructs of ineffective self-regulation and difficult temperament overlap. Therefore, a child may have a regulatory disorder but not present with a difficult temperament or the opposite can be evident as well (DeGangi, 2000). *Terrikangas et al (1998), in the conclusion of a 15-year longitudinal study, identified infants with difficult temperaments demonstrating an increased risk of developing psychiatric symptoms in adolescence. This risk was diminished for these children when families received mental health interventions.

There exists a direct contribution to social-emotional and personality development by means of temperament and its interactions with caregivers, family, and other environmental factors. For instance, gender differences in temperament of infants/toddlers reveal males to demonstrate higher levels of activity and tendency to approach, while females demonstrate greater hesitation/withdrawal behavior. Furthermore, females show greater fearfulness as well as higher levels of regulation-related skills in early childhood. Individual differences in temperament play a role in children's selection of environment and associated adaptation.

Johnson & Johnson (2011) state that, over the course of the toddler–preschool years, the development of successful regulation of reactive responses is associated with four cognitive skills as the ability to:

- inhibit a preponent motor response
- switch attention
- focus attention
- plan and execute strategies.

The developmental progression of change associated with the growth of these skills is related to parental influence, contextual environmental factors, and underlying neural changes (predominantly maturation of prefrontal cortex areas). Parents offer important input by providing physical comfort, secure attachment, and moderating negative affect or distress. Since the neural structures necessary for successful regulation have not yet developed,

9

parenting behavior allows and supports the child to learn to contain response to arousal, such as distraction and inhibition and is beneficial for regulating negative affect.

Differences in Self-Regulation

Distinguishing, or demonstrating the differences between reactivity and self-regulation is useful for the general conceptualization of development in that early behavior can be seen as reactive to immediate stimulus events and endogenous changes, whereas complex self-regulatory systems develop to modulate reactivity (executive attention system). The development and refining of self-regulatory mechanisms, which transpire over the first two years of life, are associated with physiological maturation, caregiver responsivity, and the infant's adaptation to environmental demands. The self-regulatory systems encompass (Lyons-Ruth & Zeanah, 1993; Rothbart et al, 2000; Rueda et al; 2004):

- affective relationships
- purposeful communication
- use of self and others to control internal states
- an understanding of causal relationships
- development of self-initiated organized behaviors.

The function of emotion regulation is to manage arousal, and assert control over behaviors and reactions, thus defining and adjusting interactions to fulfill appropriately and effectively the needs of the individual as well as social demands. Both intrinsic and extrinsic factors contribute to the development of self-control. Intrinsic factors include the infant's temperament and cognitive processes (attention and inhibitory control). Extrinsic factors involve the caregiving environment, sibling/peer relationships, and cultural expectation of emotional display. The development of emotion regulation evolves from the growth and integration of numerous behavioral and biological processes. Without expounding, the complexity of these systems is a challenge to researchers. Strategies of self-emotion regulation by infants can be observed by their (Rothbart et al, 2000; Thompson et al, 2008):

- passive engagement
- physical regulation/effects of touch
- scanning
- distraction
- self-soothing.

Self-regulation is the infant's first task in learning to modulate themselves and demonstrate an interest in their environment. This ability to control inner states is a critical milestone of development and essential to personality and behavioral adjustment. Associated correlates include competence for engagement and attachment with a demonstrated ability to modulate and process sensory experiences. The caregiver's consistent, sensitive and supportive responding helps to manage emotional arousal within normal limits and these early interactions are important factors in the development of a secure parent–child relationship. An additional aspect of self-regulation is the capacity to coordinate simple motor actions (Figure 1.3). In conjunction, these factors are referred to as "sensorimotor modulation". Touch, vision, hearing, movement, body-awareness, and thought are the building blocks for future learning. Furthermore, the development of this system plays a crucial role in the internalization of moral principles and socialization (Schore, 2001, 2005; Bell & Deater-Deckard, 2007; Benson & Haith, 2009).

As the basic knowledge of brain structure and function are expanded and incorporated into developmental sciences it promotes progress in the complex view of human infancy and increased understanding of the psychoneurobiological mechanisms that are the foundation of infant mental health. Integrated intermodal sensory-motor coordination of the newborn infant's orientation to environmental stimuli and preferential learning of human signals

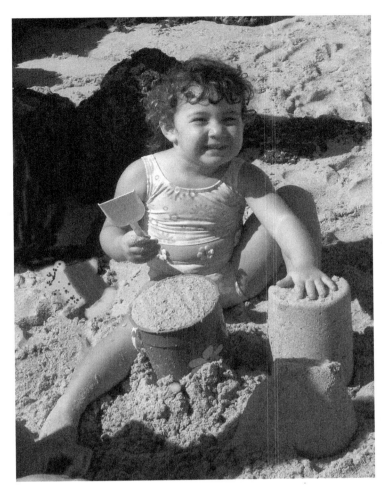

FIGURE 1.3
Young girl makes sand castles at the beach.

demonstrates the capacities for reactive and induced imitation (IMF = intrinsic motive formation developed before birth). In other words, the infant's integrated neural motivating system is viewed as crucial to the development of purposeful consciousness and their ability to cooperate with, and learn from, another person's actions and interests (Trevarthen & Aitken, 2001).

Benson & Haith (2009) offer a diagrammatic depiction of the factors contributing to the development of regulatory processes in young children. The diagram affords a comprehensive view of the complex interaction of factors from biology to developing domains contributing to regulatory processes (Figure 1.4).

Progression of Emotion Regulation

According to Benson & Haith (2009), there are several developmental advancements that demonstrate the progression of emotion regulation throughout infancy and childhood:

- mimic, integration and growth of emotional management by others to increasing self-regulation of emotions
- increasing extensiveness, sophistication, and flexibility in infant/child use of emotion regulation strategies, and their increasing ability to substitute effective for ineffective strategies
- utilizing other developing capacities into emotion regulating efforts, such as emerging language, attentional control, and strategic thinking/planning

Selfhood: Evolving conscious sense of self, agency, and achievements; awareness when help is needed; motivation for mastery; nascent recognition that social relations require balance between self and others' desires.

Biosocial contributions to young children's development.
Species inheritance
Deeply conserved: brain/central nervous system, physiological systems; body structure and functions; basic sensory/perceptual capabilities; social, cognitive, and communicative skills

Family inheritance
Parental gene pool
Sociocultural inheritance
Culturally devised, evolving, flexible patterns of socialization that reflect need for: social cooperation, parental investment including protection of offspring, emotional bonds, specific socialization and learning experiences, and tools for communication

Caregiving practices
Parents, other caregivers: interactive style; protection from harm; type of nurturing; provision of learning, communication, and play experiences; teaching strategies; translation of sociocultural norms for child

Regulatory processes
Physiological, inhibitory, attentional, emotional

Executive functions
Goals, plans, monitoring, evaluation, adaptation

Developing domains: contributions to regulatory processes
Perceptual processes
Cognitions: knowledge of different contexts; production of strategic like behaviors; event memories, etc.
Social/emotional relationships: bonds; social and emotional knowledge
Motor capabilities: expertise in locomotion and grasp
Communication: basic gestural and verbal skills

12

FIGURE 1.4
Comprehensive view of the complex interaction of factors from biology to developing domains contributing to regulatory processes.

- improved sensitivity to context in emotion regulation; social intelligence for emotion management and a finesse in understanding what strategies work best in a variety of situations/social dynamics
- employing emotion specific regulatory strategies, i.e., use of internal dialogue (language connoting "I can do this") and external resources (such as an attuned caretaker) to manage fear
- emerging complexity in both personal and social goals underlying emotion regulation as the toddler/child demonstrates increased ability to regulate their feelings to manage social interactions, support and reinforce self-esteem, and achieve other psychologically sophisticated intentions/purposes
- the emergence and increasing stability of unique individual goals associated with self-regulation, strategies and personal style
- the development of emotion regulation is important because individualized expression of emotion regulation is associated with social competence. Greater skill in emotion regulation is directly proportional to social competence with peers and increased cooperation with caregivers. Additionally, emotion regulation is important to psychological health minimizing risk for affective psychopathology.

It is probable that the most important role of regulatory processes involves assisting executive functions, which are often conscious, self-motivated, supervisory aspects of planning, goal setting, monitoring and evaluation involved in immediate or long-term goals. *Therefore, consider self-regulation processes as underlying mechanisms that facilitate the fulfillment of goals.

Regulation Processes

Benson & Haith (2009; DeGangi, 2000), highlight three regulatory processes.

INHIBITORY CONTROL (IC)

Inhibitory control (IC) reflects the inhibition of acting impulsively, holding one's thoughts, or being vulnerable to inferring stimuli. Inhibitory control is important because it is fundamental to the requirements for effective controlled attention. In other words, a condition for working memory that temporarily maintains the contents of memory "in mind" long enough to focus on and attend to so that the appropriate action can be taken to reach the goal, and for the executive functions associated with planning and evaluating the step-wise progression toward the goal. Problems with IC are identified in young children whose home environments are inadequate for their needs, children with attention deficit hyperactivity disorder (ADHD), prenatal cocaine exposure, severe auditory limitations, and genetic-based disorders (phenylketonuria [PKU], Down's syndrome, etc.). IC appears to have components which, when appropriate, result in the cessation of activity and other times appropriately respond quickly to the task demand (even selecting the most appropriate stimuli to respond to when there are numerous competing stimuli). Inhibitory or effortful control is an antecedent of the internalization of norms of conduct or behavior.

Age Trends Associated With Inhibitory Control

There are age-related trends for response times and error to dissimilar stimuli from ages 3 to adolescence. Age 3 to 5 reveals a more significant improvement rate for error detection than response time. Thus indicating that the actual inhibition of a response may be more difficult for young children than detecting errors of incongruence (for example, the non-corresponding/non-matching of an animal head and body). It has not yet been concretely determined at what age and how a child's participation in the most challenging inhibition circumstances/scenarios begin to create rules that guide behavior. It appears that "rule-like" strategies are more often demonstrated by 5 to 7 year olds than younger children. Additionally, it has been suggested that, by the age of 6 years, children are able to delay without use of strategic behaviors likely relying on internally generated (cognitive rule-based) guidelines. This coincides with other indications of cognitive and social transitions occurring around 7 years of age.

EXECUTIVE ATTENTION (EA)

Executive function skills arise from a combination of genetics and experience. Like all other neurobiological development care, nurturing and support contribute to positive development and growing skills, whereas trauma, neglect and loss contribute to negative consequences with regard to shaping brain development. The term "executive" describes a set of capacities synonymous with being in charge. Executive function is closely related to emotional intelligence.

EA presents with the expected components of function for a regulatory process by being involved with cognitive controls, planning error detection, resolution of conflict, regulation of thoughts and feelings, and prevailing over habitual action. Not unexpectedly, cognitive driven attention influences emotion states demonstrating interconnections between the prefrontal cortex and the amygdala (deep brain structure important to emotion). When investigating the network related to attention, alerting is connected with activation in frontal and parietal areas mostly in the right hemisphere, and oriented to a variety of neuro areas. The study of EA (also focused/controlled attention) specifically with toddlers and young children addresses issues of temperament with executive or effortful attention with aspects of cognitive functioning. Focused attention is fundamental to exploratory, functional and pretend/fantasy play and information obtained from these contexts is beneficial in identifying trends among children.

Age Trends Associated with Executive Attention

In examining age trends related to different types of attention used in play for an entire observation time of 10 minutes broken down into 2 minute segments:

1. Casual; children looking at toys but with limited engagement
2. Settled; pause in casual attention w/steadily looking at a toy and manipulating it
3. Focused; reflecting concentration with an intent facial expression, minimal extraneous body movement, close visual inspection of the toy or talking to themselves (similar to executive attention).

The ages of the children being studied regarding executive attention were 10, 26, and 42 months of age. At 10 months of age, all types of attention demonstrated decline at midpoint of the time frame, possibly due to fatigue. At 26 months of age, there was a crossover time whereby casual and settled attention began to reverse positions, with casual a lower priority activity. At 42 months of age, changes occurred within the blocks of time possibly indicating changing interest in one toy or another and close to the end of the observation time (10 min) overall decreasing interest in the toys. Factors such as diversions/distractions demonstrated a directly proportional trend of increasing settled and focused attention which may bear some relationship to these two qualities of attention being a continuum of controlled attention. This could be an indication that executive attention is not merely a process that is turned on or off, but instead progresses from a less heightened state to an increasing heightened state related to the nature of the demand.

What features influence pattern changes in attention? It could be practice, increased curiosity/interest, selectivity of toys and what can be done with a toy (motivation), and/or improved hand coordination (focus more on manipulation of the toy vs controlling finger dexterity). Regardless, what is most reinforced by this information is the developmental importance of focused attention in the early years.

EMOTION REGULATION (ER)

Through different contexts, ER is seen as an essential, generative regulatory process where children utilize a constellation of means to adapt to their physiological necessities (managing arousal states) to maintain important relationships and meet their own goals (such as learning). Toddlers are set apart from infants by their growing sense of mastery and challenging to caregivers (as they become more mobile, as well as increase their socializing). Negative emotions may increase in association with physical aggression, temper tantrums, and resistance. The toddler's cognitive growth, sense of self and mastery contributes to increased feelings of anger and frustration when their goal directed behaviors are restricted. Five points of the generative process in which ER can occur:

1. making a decision about a situation to attend to or to avoid
2. generating possible ways to avoid a potentially difficult situation
3. modifying one's attentional strategies (i.e., distraction)
4. utilizing cognitive change mechanisms such as reappraisals (cognitive transforming a situation to modify its emotional impact)
5. response focused ER is associated with trying to decrease/suppress emotion expressions that have already been initiated.
   - Younger children attempted to utilize their mothers as a multi-use resource and support system depending on the context. Additionally, the association of language may increase the challenge of ER for younger children.
   - Older children either generated ideas to alter the situation on their own or accepted the directive from an adult while also protecting the self (putting toys away, choosing the sequence).
   - Detached parenting may be particularly detrimental to the developmental process, and may be experienced in the form of especially high levels of explosive behavior and physical aggression.

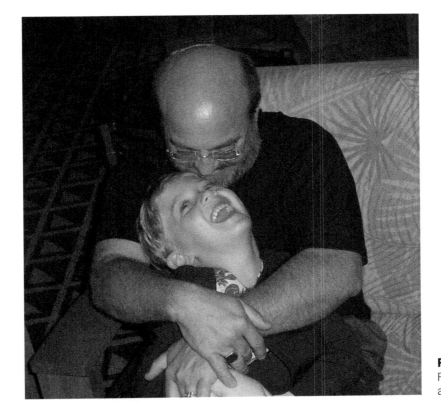

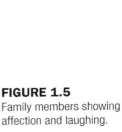

FIGURE 1.5
Family members showing affection and laughing.

Caregiver attunement and self-regulation go hand in hand with attachment. This reciprocal attunement is what children want and need to develop secure attachments (Figure 1.5). A healthy attachment helps children to learn to regulate their emotions. Children who develop capacities for self-regulation will have the capacity to be attuned to others, and therefore, help them self-regulate.

Example: a child chooses to not interact with the caregiver for a brief period of time, turning away. This may be due to feeling over stimulated, tired or a need to self-regulate themselves to a more comfortable state. (+) The attuned sensitive caregiver is respectful of this cue (turning away) and watches the child's stress level go down, thus bringing comfort and relief. (−) The un-attuned caregiver responds intrusively. When the child turns away they continue to try to get the child to acknowledge them instead of respecting the cue to decrease stimulation. *One can see what the impact in these examples of reciprocal attunement and the principle that children learn what they live.

Age Trends Associated With Emotion Regulation

Trends identified in infancy, such as the regulatory mechanism of thumb sucking which is present at birth and offers some protection from the range associated with caregiver attentiveness. During the first year, infants engage in distracting behaviors when mildly distressed. If they experience significantly elevated levels of distress, they are observed to signal cues to caregivers, i.e., visual contact, gesture, crying. Crying and negativism were linked at 21 months. There was a significant decrease in crying at 30 months leaving a remaining high proportion of children across older ages using words or behaviors expressing "no" to any given request. The unrelenting of desires that contributes to the difficult management of the 2 year old is representative of solid growth and development.

Resilience

Another component underlying normal trajectories of development versus maladaptive trajectories of development is resilience (Sapolsky, 2004; Southwick et al, 2005; Charney &

15

Southwick, 2007; Wolraich et al, 2008). In fact, knowledge of internal resources that promote resilience in affected children can enhance preventive efforts by intervening/treating professionals. Key to understanding resilience is the study of individuals who present with a significant degree of risk (adversity such as trauma, social disadvantage, marital transitions, difficult temperament, and significant generational/genetic loading for psychopathology), but defy their at risk potential. It is important to note that resilience does not necessarily mean that a positive outcome will be seen across the board. Instead, it is possible to display resilience in one area and not another. To succeed in life requires resilience. It is the child who develops strengths, acquires the skills to cope, recover from hardship/adversity, and be prepared for future challenges.

Factors that characterize the resilient child are basically the same factors that provide developmental advantage to any child, such as:

- superior intellectual functioning
- positive temperament
- close relationships with caring /protective adults.

Research shows that children have different vulnerabilities and protective systems at different points in development. Resilient children have much in common with other competent children in spite of their differences in life experiences. Adaptive coping mechanisms, related to both physical and psychological well-being, can be generally defined as seeking appropriate social support, problem-focused coping strategies, using rational appraisal to minimize threat, creative flexible narration for long-term problems, a sense of health efficacy, peer-social competence, social and emotional intelligence, attractiveness to others, feelings of self-worth, feeling of hope and meaningfulness, etc. In closing, children are protected not only by the self-righting nature of development, but by their own actions and the action of adults.

The risk factors challenging resilience also reside in every domain. They range from relatively insignificant to severe, such as an irritating experience to the loss of a parent. Overall, the most common detrimental affect is the interplay of relationship to the caregiver(s) whereby the additive impact of minor and major stressors influence the dyadic experience of the child. Therefore, it is not surprising that exposure to psychological and behavioral problems is linked to academic achievement. Table 1.1 shows examples of pediatric risk factors and was adapted from Benson & Haith (2009).

Resiliency and risk, like protective factors and vulnerability, are at every natural developmental stage. When the balance tips in the direction of resilience and protective factors, the potential for a good outcome is improved. Critical transition periods exist for children such as infancy > toddlerhood > preschool > school age > etc. It is during these transitions that resilience and protective factors demonstrate their benefit via increasing skill development and associated self-efficacy (Rolf et al, 1990).

- Resilience
  - Good outcome regardless of presence of risk factors and vulnerabilities
- Risk factors
  - Biological, psychosocial, and environmental factors that increase chance of less than desirable outcome
- Protective factors
  - Modify or improve the child's response to factors that predispose to negative outcome
- Vulnerability
  - Susceptibility to a problem or disorder

Progressive Typical Developmental Stages

Greenspan observed "typical" children to determine their natural developmental stages as they evolve in their sophistication and make sense out of the world around them. These progressive levels demonstrate how risk factors may negatively impact the developing child.

16

TABLE 1.1 Examples of Risk Factors for Children

Domain	Factor
Family processes	Bereavement Family dissolution Maltreatment Harsh parenting Neglect
Parent characteristics	Poor mental health Substance abuse Low education Below average intelligence
Family structure	Single parenthood Numerous stressful life events Household crowding Poverty Transient (moves a lot)
Peers	Peer rejection Delinquent peers
Schools	Always the "new kid" Lower qualified teachers Lack of school resources Negative experiences with teacher Lack of parental support/structure for homework
Community	Violence Poverty Crime Victimization Does not fit in culturally
Societal	Discrimination Racism Prejudice Socio-economic separation Negative social messages (negative placebo)
Environment	War Catastrophic natural events

For example, review each level and then for each factor within a domain ask: "What would be the potential influence(s) of this specific factor?" A summary of the six developmental stages or levels he identified are distilled in the FEAS or Functional Emotional Assessment Scale for Infancy and Early Childhood (Greenspan & DeGangi, 2001; Casenhiser et al, 2007). The typical responses for each level are:

- Level 1: 0 to 3 months Shared attention and self-regulation
  Within 3 months demonstrated mastery of the fundamental building blocks of emotional, cognitive and sensory development. They are able to share interest in their environment such as looking around at what comprises their environment, listening to mommy singing, experience the feeling of being rocked in daddy's arms all while sustaining regulation (being calm, alert and focused).
- Level 2: 2 to 7 months Engagement and relating
  Building upon level 1 skill, the baby uses its ability to engage and relate resulting in the development of relationships with those they share regular contact with – warm and intimate relationships. For example, the baby uses its ability to remain calm and alert to develop relationships by engaging caregivers in social interactions (eye contact, smiling, moving arms/legs in rhythm to a caretaker's voice.

- Level 3: 3 to 10 months Two-way purposeful communication
  Through their smiling and outreach (moving arms and legs in rhythm to a caretaker's voice, etc.) they begin to use their emotion to develop a new ability "two-way purposeful interaction". When a caretaker reaches for them they reach back. When something pleasant or pleasing is said to them they respond by smiling. When they are picked up they explore facial characteristics, hair, beard, jewelry, etc. Their communication is not only in the form of outreach or exploration, but with their emotional answers of making sounds and babbling.

- Level 4: 9 to 18 months Shared social problem solving
  The simple forms of communicating desires experienced earlier becomes more complex as the toddler strings together more body movements such as taking mommy's hand or pointing to the refrigerator for a beverage. Thus, they now have the ability to engage in a continuous flow of complex organized problem solving interactions – using their body to communicate their desires. This also means that they have learned to make relationships by engaging in visual contact, smiling, and moving their arms and legs. This process is a demonstration of using emotions to direct muscles (arms/legs) into more complex and organized movements and behaviors.

- Level 5: 18 to 30 months Creating symbols and ideas
  As the child is approaching 2 years of age they progress from engaging in actions with themselves (such as feeding self) to act upon others. An example of this would be using one doll to feed another doll. Creating symbols and ideas involves creation, elaboration and the sharing of symbols and meanings. At this level, they are using the skills from prior levels (experience the physical sensations of hunger (1), use motion desires communicated through muscle (2), engaging their caretaker visually (3), taking the caretaker's hand and leading them to the refrigerator (4), and now can state "I'm hungry".) This is a demonstration of taking the abstract idea of hunger and separating it from the self to an object (the doll).

- Level 6: 30 to 48 months Building bridges between ideas
  At this level the small child is able to elaborate and, eventually, differentiate the feelings, thoughts and events that come from themselves versus those that come from someone else. This is also an aspect crucial to personality development, distinguishing what is real from what is not, impulse and mood regulation, and a higher order ability to focus attention and to concentrate in order to learn and interact. Emotional thinking allows children to begin to reason right and wrong and think logically.

*Each level builds on the accomplishments of the prior level.

Organizational Model of Sensory and Affective Experiences
A DEVELOPMENTAL–STRUCTURALIST APPROACH

The following information is similar to that printed above by Greenspan and DeGangi but organized differently along a variant of developmental parameters. Greenspan's (Greenspan 2002a; Greenspan et al, 1998; DeGangi, 2000) work over decades emphasizes the relationship between sensory and affective thematic experiences which serve to support the child to organize and regulate emotional processes. This is referred to as the developmental–structuralist approach of psychosocial development. This model is defined by three levels of emotional development:

1. Level of engagement/homeostasis and attachment. As the child forms an attachment to the primary caregiver, social engagement rolls into focus with learning to self-regulate and maintaining homeostasis. The development of complex self-regulatory mechanisms is the result of physiological maturation, parental responsivity, and the infant's ability to adapt to demands from their environment. Early sensory experiences are instrumental in facilitating the infant to distinguish experiences as pleasant (fed or cuddled) or unpleasant (wet or hungry). The reciprocal satisfying experiences between mother and

infant leads to the infant developing special emotional interest in the caregiver. For example, changing sensory processing and modulation (visual, auditory, olfactory, vestibular, proprioceptive), which demonstrate physical and emotional development, would be an infant demonstrating the coordination of simple motor tasks, executing contact or connection, like reaching for a mother's face and cooing at her.

Difficulties

When infants lack the ability to process sensory experiences, seen via maladaptive responses in establishing affective relationships:

○ hypersensitive to touch, sound and movement
○ avoid tactile contact/being held or moved
○ averting visual gaze/avoid face-to-face interactions
○ difficulty with muscle tone or coordination (signaling ability).

The aforementioned difficulties affect a caregiver's ability to respond as a result of misunderstanding signals and the lack of reinforcement found in reciprocal pleasing. The rejection a mother experiences when an infant arches their back and she cannot console or just soothe and hold close results in her feeling like she is an inadequate or bad mother. Likewise, an infant may possess the competence but a depressed mother fails to draw them into a healthy dyadic relationship. Factors that play a role in capacity for infant engagement include physical traits, temperament, ability to self-regulate, sensorimotor abilities, and interactive abilities. *Psychopathology seen in later childhood and even adulthood is rooted difficulties with engagement.

Dr Greenspan describes an "autistic-like" child who presents aloof, distant and isolative, stressed by environmental demands, language problems, participates in play that is not developmentally/socially interactive, unable to adhere to demands, becomes disengaged, etc. Sometimes the child appears mechanical, without reciprocal purpose, emotionally labile or makes demands on the attention of others. Obviously, a child that struggles with stress or demands.

2. Level of intention, interactive, organized behavior and affect. Stage 1 progresses to the second level, age 8 to 18 months, signified by the child developing intentional organized behaviors. Intentional organized behaviors follow with a series of associated milestones such as:

○ flexible reciprocal interactions
○ purposeful communication
○ an understanding of causal relationships
○ development of self-initiated organized behaviors.

Although the child lives in a concrete, here and now with regard to environmental experiences, they begin to attach emotional meaning to a variety of sensory, interactive, play and caregiver experiences, as they engage in interactive cuing using gestures, words and actions. DeGangi utilized the following example to exemplify the factors involved in this stage:

A 9 month old sitting in a high chair with dad at the table, takes his cup and plate – tossing them to the floor expected dad to engage playfully. If dad engages when the child signals with arm waving directing dad to the floor so that he can return them to the high chair tray the stage is set for the scene to be duplicated several times. However, if dad ignores the child's imploring him to participate, initially the child may display anger vocally as well as looking angry or clenching the fist. The infant then begins to organize and communicate its emotions of assertiveness, curiosity, dependency or pleasure. An additional overlay, would be the mother who has been in the background including herself in the infant–dad interaction exclaiming, "did you do that!" resulting in the child feeling encouraged. This is referred to as a distal connection or social referencing, and enables the infant to continue the play routine from across the room (without close proximity to the caregiver). Communication becomes increasingly reciprocal with an ability to receive and give communicated information through gestures, words, sensory, and motor experiences. During this stage, learned messages of love and approval, hate vs rejection, safety vs danger, respect and empathy for self and others vs detachment are discerned.

19

Difficulties

Lack of purposeful interaction seen as disorganization with gestural cues and intentional behaviors. They may be described by stereotypic play, perseverative, unfocused, ignore caregiver cues, ignore/misread receptive communication, temper tantrums or withdrawal from interaction if the child fails to elicit a desired response from their caregiver.

3. Level of representational elaboration and differentiation. The final, and culminating, level takes place from age 18 to 30 months and involves representational capacity, its elaboration and differentiation. In other words, moving from concrete to representational interpretation marked by:
   ○ labeling emotions and feelings
   ○ elaborating on emotions and feelings
   ○ expressing emotions related to such themes as
     - dependency
     - pleasure
     - assertion
     - autonomy
     - anger/control
     - empathy
     - love.

Two way interactive communication now becomes representational in the form of pretend play and the expression of abstract thinking. The young child is able to assign affective meaning to objects, people and events as well as expressing complex emotions such as empathy, and internalization of love for self and others. Later they will be able to experience feelings of loss, sadness and guilt. Pretend play becomes complex drama taken from snapshots of everyday life. A stronger sense of self develops with increased differentiation from others. They are able to go from fantasy play to the reality of the moment (they know what is pretend from what is real). They also begin to understand that their behavior impacts others, saying, "I'm sorry" when they drop something by accident.

Difficulties

Child does not progress from concrete to representational thinking. They get frustrated and either withdraw or become impulsive when confronted with their lack of ability or limitation. Relationship patterns may be fragmented or marked by over-reliance, clinginess, inability to separate from the primary caregiver. The range of affective elaboration is also limited and acting out may be commonplace.

DEFINING REGULATORY DISORDER

To develop an operative conceptualization of regulation requires an understanding of sensory processing. Sensory processing or sensory integration refers to the neurological process of information processing that organizes sensations (experience of senses from their environment: taste, touch, proprioception, gravity, sight, hearing, etc.) which allows for effective use of the body. Through sensory processing/sensory integration many aspects of the nervous system work in concert allowing for effective interaction with the environment and the experience of appropriate satisfaction associated with the rewards of successful management of environmental demands and enrichment (continued learning and skill development). Sensory processing is the manner in which the nervous system receives messages and turns them into motor and behavior responses (Ayers, 2005). Figure 1.6 is a schematic offering the construct of the nervous system as it relates to sensory integration (Taylor & Trott 1991).

Dysfunction can occur at any stage of sensory processing. The stages of sensory processing are defined by the following (Calkins et al, 2002; Rothbart et al, 2005; Bell et al, 2008; Thompson et al, 2008; Benson & Haith, 2009):

• Receiving information from sensory receptors
• Relaying the information from the sensory receptors to appropriate areas of the brain

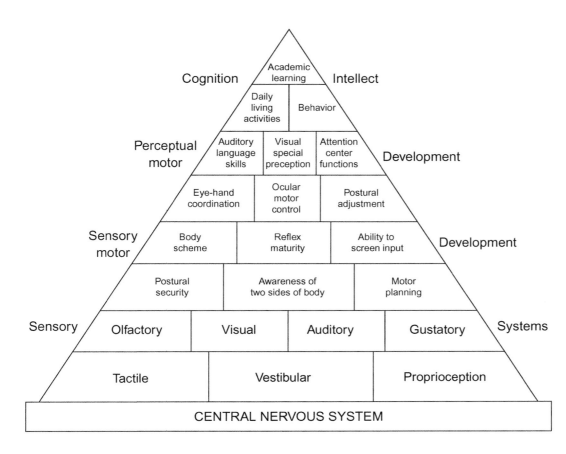

FIGURE 1.6
Schematic offering the construct of the nervous system as it relates to sensory integration *(from Taylor & Trott, 1991).*

- Discriminating (sorting out) what information is important to respond to and blocking non-important information
- Utilizing pre-acquired information to compare/contrast other sensory experiences to develop any necessary plan of action
- Forwarding this synthesized message to the parts of the body needed to carry out the plan of action
- End result: the adaptive response, carrying out all aspects of the planned response.

Abnormal Processes

When an infant/child brain does not process the incoming sensory information normally their ability to self-regulate is diminished and they may not be able to maintain an appropriate level of awareness to meet environmental demands. The types of information shared by distressed parents about difficulties experienced by their children fall into two basic categories:

1. Symptoms of hypersensitivity, defensiveness, or sensory avoiding demonstrating abnormal responding to sensory input
   a. demonstrates limited interests/fatigues easily and appears unmotivated
   b. fear of movement or heights (may get sick in association with movement or heights)
   c. overly cautious and unwilling to try new things or take risks/taking part in unsafe activities (e.g., climbing too high)
   d. withdrawing or responding aggressively when touched
   e. demonstrates a negative response to sounds
   f. selective "picky" eater, overly sensitive to food smells or textures
   g. intolerance to clothing tags, fabric textures, or will only wear certain kinds of clothes

2. Regulatory difficulties

    a. difficulty tolerating or adjusting to changes, even minor changes, in routine

    b. attentional difficulties, easily distracted or becomes fixated on one activity with difficulty changing focus to another activity

    c. impaired ability associated with the interaction with others

    d. disrupted sleep wake cycles

    e. feels uncomfortable in environments with high levels of activity, such as athletic events, shopping malls, celebratory events, etc.

Associated to these regulatory difficulties is the ability to maintain an appropriate level of awareness to meet environmental demands:

- Hides face, isolates from people/activity to avoid interaction and sensory input, may appear to be asleep
- Nervous, anxious, difficulty attending/easily distracted
- Requires cues or direct assistance to remain involved
- May actually go to sleep to avoid sensory input.

As previously stated, the trajectory of normal development for self-regulation exists within a range versus being linear. Clarification of dysfunction is facilitated by a conceptual classification associated with the range of dysfunction to illuminate the progression and degree of impact of regulatory difficulties experienced (Kostuik & Fouts, 2002; Schore, 2002; Bell & Dieter-Deckard, 2007; Woolraich et al, 2008).

- Mild
  - the child is able to adequately maintain while at daycare/preschool, but when they get home or stress escalates they decompensate and "lose it"
  - they feel like they are different from others but are not able to express specifically why, and may experience general unhappiness
  - they maintain strict routines and tend to be compulsive
  - demonstrate a narrow range of interests and activities
- Moderate
  - all areas of life are affected by lack of self-regulation ability (home, school, activities, leisure)
  - avoidant of situations or sensory input which is experienced as aversive
  - negative influence reaches beyond the child to those around them
- Severe
  - requires the assistance of others to participate or complete basic self-care needs
  - obvious discomfort/distress for the majority of the day
  - may engage in stereotypic, aggressive or self-destructive/injurious behavior.

When babies and toddlers are in distress, all of their regulatory resources are devoted to trying to organize and regain equilibrium. For a baby, stress is anything that pulls them out of attunement and into a negative emotional state (fear, anxiety, and sadness create stress). Stress is not exclusively associated to negatively charged events, it could just be the exposure to something new and different. When they are in emotional balance, they are emotionally regulated, and they rely on the relationship with the mother/caregivers to keep them regulated. For example, a mother sets her baby down to answer the phone and the baby begins to cry – signaling the need/requirement for the mother to return and "re-attune" them in order to prevent them from becoming overwhelmed by sadness. If the mother neglects/ignores the cry/plea the crying intensifies and leads to a series of internal reactions at the primary level (survival) focusing the child to direct all resources to basic functioning which unfortunately forfeits the opportunity for potential growth and integration or internalization of self-soothing. As a child continues to grow and develop these needs evolve, but their reliance on the attachment system endures. Healthy attachment resulting from healthy attunement is the key to emotionally healthy babies and toddlers. The child attaches to the regulating mother who facilitates maximal opportunity for positive emotions/security and minimizes negative emotions, thus creating optimal health, security and resilience. A positive note on periods of mis-attunement, as long as they are brief and not chronic it does allow learning self-regulation. Brief periods of mis-attunement followed by re-attunement has the effect of teaching or engendering resilience and may also offer the foundation for developing empathy.

The assumptions underlying developmental psychology, the influence of the dyadic relationship, and the demonstrated impact upon primary areas of function aid in understanding the dynamics of regulation.

Assumptions of Developmental Psychology

A lifespan perspective is beneficial to the understanding of developmental psychopathology with the acknowledgement that the individual participates in their own development and that it is not a linear progression, but instead allows for the interaction between normal developmental milestones, factors associated to context, and psychopathology. Wolraich et al (2008) provide some basic assumptions for developmental psychopathology:

1. Any form of psychopathology is best understood when thoroughly examined via experiences and trajectories influencing and leading up to the identified problems, including the trajectories that follow the problem behavior.
2. The assumption that two children demonstrating the same symptoms at any given time may have a different outcome further in development (multifinality), and that two children with the same outcome may have arrived there by different developmental pathways (equifinality). An additional related common sense assumption is that no single factor will generally be either necessary or sufficient to result in psychopathology.
3. Knowledge is increased when the normative understanding of healthy child development is studied as well as the study of atypical development.
4. Knowledge and understanding of the full range of child and adolescent functioning across numerous areas offers a richness of information not obtained by viewing isolated functioning developmental stages and context.
5. It is important to explore and understand why some children who are at risk or exposed to adversity do not develop psychopathology (understanding the role of resilience and adequate/consistent/caring support).
6. Probability is assumed in association with relations between antecedent events, adaptations, and subsequent psychopathology. One consequence of this is an example provided by early attachment whereby early experiences may have an effect on neurophysiology and ability to regulate emotions, which could result in predictive value to social and individual pathology in some cases.
7. Development takes place through continuous and multiple reorganizations across all domains of child and adolescent functioning (physical, social, cognitive, emotional, neurological).
8. Children play a significant role in their own development and the outcomes of their development. It is a transactional interplay between individual and environment.
9. The multiple transitions during childhood and adolescence provide numerous opportunities for redirection of prior maladaptive trajectories as well as progression toward maladaptive pathways.
10. Factors associated with the onset of a disorder may not be the same factors as those that maintain a disorder.

Regulation capacities increase with age. By age 6 (school age), most children have learned to adjust their behavior and sensory needs. As aforementioned, emotion regulation must be viewed contextually and in association with the infant/child goal for managing feelings.

Therefore, while an infant/child may be perceived as fussy or frustrated, before assigning the interpretation of a problem of emotion regulation seek to understand the context of process and/or their goal (what they are trying to accomplish with their limited skills). Contrary, infants/toddlers with regulatory disorders may continue to have mild to intense difficulties in some areas of sensory, motor, and behavior regulation throughout their childhood. It was the recognition of the persistent characteristics of these difficulties, the presence of sensory reactivity, motor and behavioral patterns across settings and within multiple relationships, that established it as a diagnosis. Regulatory Disorder (Regulatory Disorders of Sensory Modulation/Processing) is a diagnosis from the DC:0-3R (Diagnostic Classification of Mental health and Developmental Disorders of Infancy and Early Childhood, Revised). The diagnosis of regulatory disorder involves a sensory, sensory-motor, processing difficulty and a distinct behavioral pattern indicated by at least one behavioral symptom. The origin of child behavior problems can reside in the child, in the relationship with the caregiver or both. Clearly, clinicians must consider factors beyond the child when diagnosing regulatory problems. Regulatory disordered infants are defined as being behaviorally difficult, displaying sleep disturbance, problems with feeding, difficulties with state-control, deficits in self-calming and mood regulation, as well as indicating poor sensory processing (DeGangi et al, 2006). It has been repetitively demonstrated that excessive crying and feeding problems in infancy exhibit a small but significant adverse effect on cognitive development (Wolke et al, 2009). Likewise, beginning postnatal development with a depressed or abusive caregiver increases the infant challenges for regulating behavior, physiological state, and emotions which are extrapolated from the supposed help of caregivers to the infant taking over these functions themselves with time. There is significant evidence that these early developmental risk factors place children at increased risk for a variety of psychological and social problems, notably emotion dysregulation (Dozier & Peloso, 2006). Emotion dysregulation is defined as the intrinsic and extrinsic processes responsible for identifying, supervising, evaluating, and altering emotional reactions (Thompson, 1994).

"Regulatory Disorder is a diagnostic concept from DC:03, defined by disturbances in the regulation of neurophysiological and emotional-behavioral reactions, which at one end reflect maturity-based and transient deviances in an otherwise normal development and at the other end, more persistent neuro-regulatory disturbances" (Skovgaard, 2010).

This contemporary view of regulatory phenomenon is an integration of biological and behavioral processes (emotion, attention, cognition, action), therefore offering the consideration of risk factors in the environment and within the individual as contributions to the development of psychopathology. This takes place in part through their influences on the capacities and strategies of self-regulation, often involving executive processes, for instance attention control. When the individual modulates internal processes via effective, executive processes the likely result is the child gains knowledge from the experience as well as how to interact in socially appropriate ways. In other words, the child is learning to adjust their internal processes, such as emotion, thought, and respiration in synchrony or coordination with social demands and opportunity. To the contrary, when ineffective executive processes are taking place, the capacity for emotion regulation is negatively impacted and emotions systematize behavior in a problematic manner. Consequently, executive control influences the perception, interpretation, and reinterpretation of situations and experiences that modulate emotion. Thus, disturbances of emotion regulation interfere with striking a balance between protecting the self from negative experiences and encouraging opportunity for positive experiences (Thompson et al, 2008; Cole & Deater-Deckard, 2009).

The Dyadic Relationship

The infant is dependent upon the caregiver(s) for care and emotional management. For it is the caregiver's role to feed, bath, change their diapers, keep warm, rock and protect them. It is

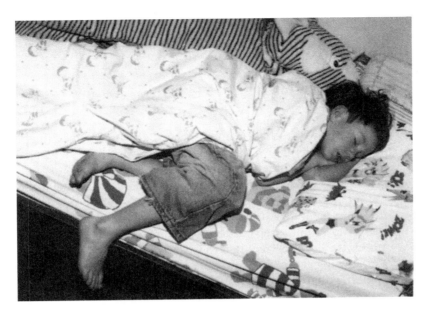

FIGURE 1.7
A child finds comfort sleeping in his own bed with a stuffed tiger and stimulating bed sheets *(from DeGangi, 2002).*

the caregiver(s) who soothe them and alleviate their distress, thus offering the relief provided most specifically in the dyadic relationship, but encompassed by all agents of caregiving in their life. The caregiver manages the infant's stimulation within manageable limits of arousal in frames of social interactions. The attachment relationship is a biologically based process that serves to motivate the infant/child to seek support, comfort, nurturance and protection at times of distress, thus providing psychological security and physical protection. When aspects of this relationship are inadequate, the infant/child experiences difficulties. It is crucial to remember that the dyadic relationship between mother and child is a mutual system. Such systems do not function flawlessly all of the time, everyone is confronted with times of being out of sync or in emotional dysregulation. The primary caregiver alleviates the potential negative outcome by re-attuning the child, thus alleviating or eliminating the distress or dysregulation and thereby teaching self-regulatory skills.

DeGangi (2000) introduces information from the study she participated in which provides a rich clinical presentation of infant challenges of regulation. The study illuminates how difficulties with the most basic task, emotion regulation, exhibit a negative affect on the development of cognition, language, skilled movement, behavioral and emotional control and sensorimotor modulation at 3 years. The earliest emerging disorders of regulation in infancy are associated with basic regulatory functions such as sleeping and feeding (Figure 1.7). These and other primary areas are reviewed in association with regulatory difficulties (DeGangi, 2000; Schore, 2001, 2005; Benson & Haith, 2009).

Primary Areas Associated with Regulatory Difficulties

SLEEP

- Persistent sleep disorders have been linked to biochemical changes in stress hormones, biological rhythms and states of arousal
- Due to difficulty falling asleep and staying asleep the infant becomes overtired and displays fussy/irritable behavior during the day
  - Children identified as exhibiting sleep deficit demonstrate a high state of arousal and lack the ability to inhibit their alert state which would allow sleep
- 15–38% of the infants/toddlers (under age 2) with regulatory disorders wake frequently at night
- 32–47% of subjects 7–18 months of age required extensive help to fall asleep at night (generally over an hour of sleep preparation activity)

- Sleep problems were more common amid mild regulatory disordered infants
- Characteristic problems affecting these infants included
  - Frequent waking in the night
  - Difficulties falling asleep
  - Hypersensitivity to touch
  - Strong craving for movement
  - High separation anxiety
- Different sleep disturbances are associated at different ages, thus supporting the premise that sleep problems are associated to biological and social regulation, and the capacity to form a secure attachment to the caregiver
  - 7 to 9 months: sleep disturbance is commonly related with a high need for vestibular stimulation (caregiver reports of the single was to promote infant sleep was to rock/bounce them for extended periods of time)
  - 10 to 12 months: separation anxiety appeared to compound sleep disturbance. Infants were often reported to be clingy and could only fall asleep when held. Upon awakening at night evidence of distress may have been in conjunction with anxiety finding themselves alone in their crib instead of being held by the caregiver
  - 13 to 18: months many toddlers with sleep problems showed a high need for movement stimulation, which parents reported tended to increase their level of arousal, increasing the challenge to fall asleep. Additionally, distress associated with sounds in the environment was also present at this age, therefore, requiring the use of white noise. Also severe separation anxiety continued at this age, exacerbating sleep disturbance
  - 19 to 24 months: decreased problem associated with falling asleep. However, awakening in the night continued to be problematic. These children commonly craved movement and appeared restless throughout the night.
- Sleep disorders in young children associated with onset of sleep (primary insomnia or sleep refusal) or during sleep such as night wakenings or parasomnias (nightmares/sleep terrors)
- Sleep disturbances may affect both attention and behavior in children. Disturbances of children's sleep may also affect family sleep practices and relationships

*Sleep problems tended to improve with maturity. There were negligible differences between regulatory disordered infants and the normative group after aged 25 months. This maturity factor suggests infants demonstrating a sleep disturbance early in life were likely to exhibit resolution if their regulatory disorder was mild and there were not any other developmental challenges.

FEEDING

(Figure 1.8)

- Difficulty establishing a regular feeding schedule, distress associated with feeding and regurgitation, refusal to eat, and other feeding problems not related to specific allergies or food intolerance
- Resistance to eating a variety of food texture often developed after 9 months. Frequently only eating preferred food (firm, crunchy textures or purees), or spitting out lumpy food textures. This may have been related to tactile hypersensitivity and connected to the preference of certain food textures. *Sometimes growth delay or failure to thrive may be diagnosed in addition to the feeding disturbance
- 13 to 24 months old: 18–46% demonstrated craving for certain foods. Reflux was a problem which was also experienced by toddlers with regulatory disorders
- Feeding disorders can be associated with the context of caregivers who are disengaged from the infant during feeding. Intense conflict between infant and caregiver may also result in feeding disorders

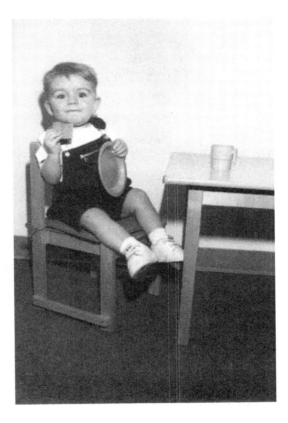

FIGURE 1.8
The toddler develops autonomy by learning to self-feed *(from DeGangi, 2002).*

- It appears that most feeding disorders emerge from a multifactorial origin (for example, sensory processing abnormalities, attachment relationship disturbances, disturbances in state regulation, complicated medical difficulties, etc.)
- Feeding disorders generally result in feelings of inadequacy for caregivers
- Failure to thrive is of the greatest concern due to resulting malnutrition and impaired growth negatively influencing brain development

*Feeding problems included reflux, oral tactile sensitivity in association with refusal to eat certain food textures, as well as the craving for certain foods. Surprisingly, at aged 3 years, the only diagnosis associated to early feeding disturbances was social-emotional disturbances. Follow-up reviews tentatively associated maternal depression and less attachment as being related to both feeding and communication problems. The identification of long-term emotional problems in infants/toddlers who initially presented with feeding disorders indicates the importance of focusing on the parent–child interactive components in treatment once the feeding problem is initially identified.

*In the literature (Armstrong et al, 2000; Hiscock, 2004; Ekvall & Ekvall, 2005) there is also expressed concern for medicalizing normal irritability in infants. In Western countries, an average of 23% to 40% of all babies are identified as having excessive irritability by their primary caregivers leading to incorrect diagnosis of a medical problem and often prescribed medication without any confirmed medical basis. This practice may not only present harm associated with medication, but potentially create lifelong problems (inappropriate labeling of a problem with management) for these infants and their parents.

ATTENTION
(Figures 1.9 & 1.10)

- Research indicated that between 13 and 30 months there is a steady increase in the number of symptoms related to attentional difficulties ranging from being over

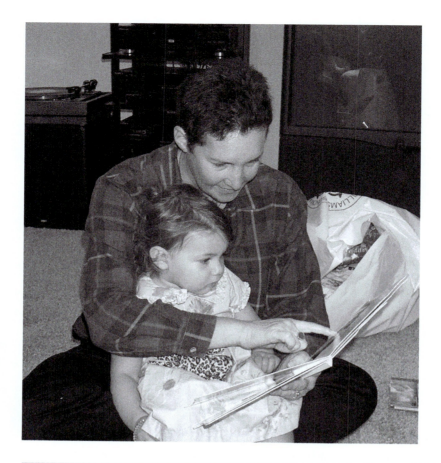

FIGURE 1.9
Woman reads to young child.

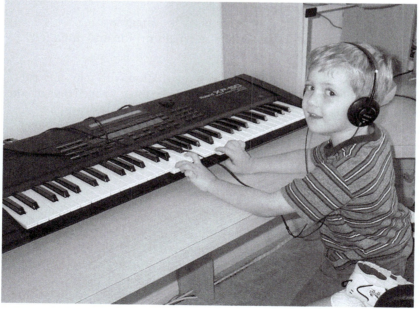

FIGURE 1.10
Young boy plays keyboards.

stimulated by hectic environments to distractibility and problems shifting or engaging attention

○ Infants/toddlers with regulatory problems were described by parents as being intense, wide-eyed, and/or hyper-frequently going from toy to toy, and not playing with any of them long enough to develop a toy preference

- 55 to 64% of subject infants with regulatory disorders displayed problems maintaining attention during novel visual, auditory, tactile, or multisensory activities
- 13 to 31% of aged13 to 30 months were described by caregivers as being extremely distracted by sights and sounds
- 15 to 31% of aged 10 to 30 months demonstrated difficulty with shifting attention to something new
- Maladaptive and developmentally inappropriate level of attention must be carefully assessed to rule out differential diagnoses (anxiety disorders, relationship-based disorders or learning disorders)

*The children who demonstrated distractibility to sights and sounds, excessive arousal in hectic environments and difficulty shifting attention to something new in early life had an increased risk of developing cognitive and motor delays in conjunction with regulatory disorders. Thus signifying the possibility that motor problems recognized at age 3 years were associated to a core deficit in motor planning, which is commonly identified in children experiencing attentional problems.

SENSORY PROCESSING

A child may have the ability to experience all of their senses (sight, hearing, taste, proprioception, etc.), but may have difficulty making sense of the information.

- Infants with regulatory problems fail to demonstrate age appropriate progress in management of distress resulting in the use of negative behavioral responses when confronted with common everyday stimulation (touch/being held by a caregiver, movement/physical play with a caregiver), sights or sounds (stimulating environment such as the marketplace with people/activities)
  - Oversensitivity to loud noises: 53% of subjects 13 to 18 months often become distressed or overwhelmed by loud sounds (siren/horn, public address system, door bell, vacuum, etc.); 31% of normal children demonstrate this at 10 to 12 months
  - Motor planning difficulties: a child with this challenge has a tendency to have difficulty with the process of figuring out, organizing, and carrying out series of actions necessary to complete an unfamiliar activity. This is related to a function known as "praxis" or "dyspraxia". This difficulty is demonstrated by clumsiness learning a new task, avoiding new or unfamiliar physical games or activities
  - Hypersensitivity to light and visual stimulation: 31% of subjects aged 7 to 9 months with regulatory disorders are excessively sensitive to light, while 20 to 44% are excited when in a hectic environments (such as mall, supermarket). Around 30% of subjects aged 10 to 12 months demonstrate the issue of excessive excitation in hectic environments
    - Children with regulatory disorders identified as having visual problems in infancy were commonly sensitive to light which was associated to numerous diagnoses, with the exception of cognitive problems with children in the moderate regulatory disorders group
    - For children diagnosed with pervasive developmental disorder (PDD), visual problems appeared to contribute to the diagnosis of PDD at age 3 years. When the visual problem was coupled with other sensory and regulatory difficulties, it is possible that there may be a general effect on the child's overall processing capabilities
  - Tactile defensiveness or under-activity to touch: tactile hypersensitivities were common among children with regulatory difficulties. Tactile defensiveness tends to vary with age. The tendency to react negatively and emotionally to stimulation from one or more sensory systems that most people have a relatively neutral response to such as taste, touch, smell, sound, movement/gravity, etc., for example, to dislike being held, difficulty tolerating certain textures, refusal to walk on different surfaces such as sand

or grass. For those with auditory sensitivity, they might be seen covering their ears in response to common environmental sound such as the vacuum or telephone, and demonstrate an irrational fear of heights, body movement or swinging

- Tactile hypersensitivities may be demonstrated in a number of ways for young children with regulatory difficulties
- 7 to 12 months: tactile problems were demonstrated by a dislike for being held/ having their face washed/resistance to being dressed/placed in certain body positions, and these difficulties continue into year 2 along with other symptoms of tactile defensiveness
- 13 to 24 months: those with regulatory difficulties demonstrated a dislike for wearing clothes/hated the car seat/avoided touching textures/getting hands messy
- Tactile problems were found to be common in children with both regulatory disorders and PDD, as well as being related to a range of clinical diagnoses
- 18% aged 13 to 18 months may dislike wearing clothes
- 14 to 41% aged 10 to 30 months resist cuddling
- 38 to 59% aged 7 to 18 months hate having their faces washed
- 41 to 100% aged 7 to 18 month disliked being stroked on the body
- A smaller number of children with regulatory disorders present as being undersensitive to touch and do not experience the pain of receiving a shot or falling down

*Data indicate that primary process deficits in any one or more of the senses (tactile, vestibular-proprioceptive) can have a significant impact on later developmental outcomes.

○ Gravitational insecurity or underreactivity to movement. The child diagnosed with regulatory disorders may display an overactivity to postual changes and a fear of body movement
- 55 to 95% of the study sample exhibited hypersensitivity to movement
- 20 to 25% aged 30 months displayed fear of movement
- 43 to 46% aged 7 to 9 and 13 to 24 months demonstrated underactivity to movement
- Regulatory disordered responses to movement stimulation ranged from fear of movement to craving of movement with many children demonstrating a combination to both (often craving linear movement such as swinging/rocking/ bouncing and preferred upright body postures). However, they showed fear when moved in planes that involved neck and trunk rotation or quick unexpected movement
- Some children displayed an underactivity to movement such as craving of movement activity/need to be in motion
- 18 to 24 months of age were reported to demonstrate clumsiness and poor balance
- Problems with vestibular sense appeared to be related to later problems with self-regulation, motor and language delays, and social emotional problems

○ Motor planning problems
- 50% of the sample subjects displayed difficulty sequencing and organizing purposeful movement
- 38% aged 19 to 24 months exhibited clumsiness and poor balance as reported by caregivers

ATTACHMENT/EMOTIONAL FUNCTIONING

- Infants with regulatory problems demonstrated poor social interaction as evidenced by poor eye contact, dull affect, difficulties initiating and sustaining reciprocal interactions, aggressive behavior, difficulty responding to limits and boundaries, a need to be the focus of attention, fearfulness of new people and situations, difficulty adapting to the demands of others, severe separation anxiety

- 7 to 9 months of age: the caregivers reported experiencing difficulty reading the infant's cues which may be related to the child having difficulty organizing clear gestural cues
- 19 to 24 months of age: toddlers demonstrated difficulty organizing reciprocal interactions
- 7 to 30 months of age: infants with regulatory disorders displayed increased non-contingent responses, more aggression, less tactile exploration, and flat affect only when engaged in tactile play situations (no difference was found in infant behavior during symbolic or vestibular play). *One explanation is that children with regulatory disorders experience increased distress in everyday sensory experiences, thus affecting their ability to organize appropriately and effectively social interchanges.
- Moderate regulatory disorders appears to be underlying the wide range of behavioral and emotional diagnoses

*The only diagnosis that was not related with early behavioral and emotional difficulties for children with moderate regulatory disorders was sensory integration dysfunction. It seems likely that dysfunctions of sensory integration are usually developed over time. However, it may endure if it was present at birth.

Some of the risk to infants/children are related to genetic and biological issues. But the risk factors related to poor parenting, marital discord, domestic violence, socioeconomic disadvantaged and the increased loading associated with a mentally ill parent or just an emotionally distant parent have the potential for significant consequences. The stress diathesis theory describes the child's vulnerability due to genetics and early childhood environmental stressors which can precipitate risk or actual onset of illness. The predominant risk is likely associated with poor parenting. An outline of the psychiatric and non-psychiatric factors that can increase parenting risk have been adapted from Benson & Haithl (2009) and is shown in Table 1.2.

Another view of parents at high risk for substance abuse, serious mental health issues, and environmental strife such as domestic violence and low self-esteems might demonstrate the following types of "danger signs" (Knitzer, 2000):

- An inability to make and keep professional appointments, lack of follow through on other important responsibilities (paperwork for welfare benefits, not paying bills, etc.)
- Repeated job loss after brief intervals of work, inability to accept supervision or authority in general, difficulty getting along with employers (chip on shoulder, non-responsive, ignores, etc.)
- Deficient in basic literacy skills, even when opportunities have clearly been available
- Chronic oppositional behavioral problems (adolescent type of responses), requiring to be asked to leave the premises of school or other environments
- Unstable housing patterns, evictions, bumming off of friends and family, etc.
- Severe personality disorders, addicted to crises/substances, chronic victim, unable to form stable relationships (even with guidance and emotional support)
- Chronic impulsive behavior, problems with time sequencing and planning, attention deficit (adult ADHD), magical thinking
- Evidence of fetal alcohol syndrome (FAS).

According to Kostuik and Fouts (2002), if an infant is unable to master the important task of emotional regulation "deleterious emotional arousal and the misleading identification and misdirection of emotion" can cause the potential outcome of socially inappropriate behaviors along with a limited or diminished ability to adapt to spontaneous experiences. The clinical significance of ineffective regulation of arousal is exhibited by an elevated incident of children with sleep disturbances who have behavioral disturbances, ADHD, and depression. When infant problems are associated with regulatory sensorimotor systems, hypersensitivity to stimulation, there is an identified association in school-aged children

TABLE 1.2 An Outline of the Psychiatric and Non-Psychiatric Factors that can Increase Parenting Risk

Psychiatric factors that can increase parenting risk

Dual diagnosis
A comorbid substance abuse problem
Active psychotic symptoms
Aggressive or violent behavior
Poor insight into the mental illness
Including a child in delusions
Parent has command hallucinations
Lack of response to treatment
Non-compliance with treatment
Low level of adaptive functioning
Below average intellectual functioning

Non-psychiatric factors that can increase parenting risk

Neglect of the baby's basic needs
Apathy or hostility toward the baby
A projection of feelings onto the baby (e.g., "he hates me")
A refusal to hold and engage the baby
Parent has an intrusive or hostile interactive style
Parent has expectations that the child should provide the parent with comfort and support
Parent lacks basic knowledge about the child or holds unrealistic expectations about child
Parent has difficulties in meeting their own basic needs
Parent utilizes extreme disciplinary measures
Parent has a small or unviable support network
Parent has difficulties in establishing and maintaining supportive relationships
Parent denies he or she has problems
Domestic violence
Marital disharmony and conflict
Birth is consequence of sexual assault
Parent has too many children along with a lack of intrinsic and extrinsic resources

regarding the development of emotional difficulties (DeGangi, 2000). Developmental research on emotion regulation is increasingly refining a system perspective that integrates behavioral and biological factors of emotional self-control (Thompson et al, 2008). These biological correlates combined with an infant history of regulatory problems appear to increase the risk of later problems (Becker et al, 2010).

Regulatory Disorders of Sensory Processing

The regulation disorders of sensory processing in infants and young children is a diagnostic classification which identifies recurring patterns in children with regulatory disorders based upon different behavioral and sensorimotor profiles or summaries. These patterns of behavior are generally diagnosed in infancy and early childhood. These diagnostic classifications are not in the Diagnostic and Statistical Manual of Mental Disorders, but rather a diagnostic category in the DC: 0-3R. Not surprisingly, there is conflict and controversy over these diagnostic classifications. Infants and children with regulation disorders are identified as having a pattern of behaviors and responses observed over time and in different settings that act to interfere with normal growth and development. The observed problems are seen in three areas – sensory, motor, and behavioral responses. Physiological problems associated with this diagnostic classification involve sleep, eating, elimination, and language (expressive and receptive). Cognitive function is not a part of this diagnostic criterion, but may be present in children with a regulatory disordered diagnosis. The Regulation Disorders of Sensory Processing categories and subtypes are as follows (Sensory Processing when coupled with parent/child interaction) (DeGangi, 2000; Reebye et al, 2007):

AXIS I

400. Regulation Disorders of Sensory Processing
- Difficulties in regulating emotions/behaviors in response to sensory stimulation, leading to impairment in development and functioning
- Behavior patterns exhibited across settings and within multiple relationships
- Requires presence of the following
  - sensory processing difficulties
  - motor difficulties
  - specific behavioral patterns.

410 Hypersensitive Subtype

These infants and children exhibit hypersensitivity to various stimuli, resulting in them either being fearful and cautious or negative and defiant. These children
- are overreactive to touch, sound, visual stimuli, and sensory input associated with taste or smell
- may demonstrate problems with motor planning and gross motor play as well as rejecting movement
- tend to demonstrate extreme responses that interfere with self-care, play and learning activities
- in making transition from one activity to another may result in anxiety or negative reactions.

*411 Type A: Fearful/Cautious

Sensitivity/shyness introverted. They have a dislike for routines, are fearful of new people and situations, and demonstrate severe separation anxiety. This child is easily upset and irritable as well as experiencing difficulty in self-calming. The sensory characteristic which may occur with these characteristics is an overactivity to touch, movement, loud noises, and bright lights. There may also be a difficulty displayed by motor planning problems.

*412 Type B: Negative/Defiant

This child demonstrates difficulty tolerating change, is extremely irritable, and is very controlling of the environment. They may exhibit being overreactive to touch and sound as well as motor planning problems.

420 Hyposensitive/Underresponsive Subtype

ADD (inattentive type; sensitivity/shyness/social withdrawal). These infants and children
- appear self-absorbed, withdrawn and are challenging to engage
- are underreactive to stimuli such as sound, taste, smell, touch, visual stimuli, and proprioception
- may appear sad
- once in preschool, the child may exhibit a reduced or restricted range of fantasy and seek repetitive sensory patterns (which are often determined by sensory idiosyncracies). Such responses in conjunction with their unresponsiveness to the environment, peers and adults must be diagnostically distinct to differentiate regulatory disordered from developmental delay or pervasive developmental disorder.

430 Sensory Stimulation-Seeking/Impulsive Subtype

ADD (specifiers; with hyperactivity, overactivity, unspecified). These infants and children
- actively seek high intensity, frequent input to satisfy sensory needs and to be engaged. Crave high intensity stimulation
- are often the clinic referred population
- exhibit impulsive and disorganized behavior in associated with motor responses
- tend to be accident prone (likely poor motor planning skills)
- may demonstrate aggression toward peers before their peers can be aggressive to them
- attention seeking/impulsive stimulus seeking behavior mimic children with ADHD.

*Conversely, caregivers of children with regulatory disorders describe that their children exhibit these behaviors from early infancy, while the parents of the child with ADHD report that these behaviors only appeared once the child was mobile.

- Sensory Reactivity Patterns: under-reactivity to touch, smell, sound, taste, movement, proprioception
- Motor Patterns: high need for motor discharge, diffuse impulsivity, accident proneness without clumsiness
- Behavioral Patterns: high activity levels, high risk behaviors, seeks constant contact with people/objects, seeks stimulation through deep pressure, recklessness; disorganized behavior as a consequence of sensory stimulation.

Symptoms of Neurological Deficits of Sensory Processing

Ayers (2005; May-Benson et al, 2006), a neurological disorders specialist (and a pioneer on the topic of sensory processing), developed the sensory integration theory to explain the dynamic relationship between behavior and brain/neural functioning. Sensory integration dysfunction is one example, but a significant one, of what can go wrong with neural processes. The brain mediates how we process environmental and internal information resulting in a significant impact on feelings, thoughts, and actions. Some of the symptoms or manifestations of the neurological deficits of sensory integration dysfunction are:

Sensory defensiveness: The highly aroused nervous system which remains on alert (fight or flight survival oriented) erroneously applied to basic behaviors. For example, the stress that is experienced with an activity as simple as crossing the street with their mother being experienced as if the body is preparing for survival. Such a problem negatively impacts daily routines.

Attention and regulatory problems: Refers to a problem in responding to sensory input without the benefit of screening ability. This can produce distractibility hyperactive or unihibited output. They may lack the ability to self-calm or self-sooth, thus being predisposed to overreact or be non-responsive. Attention and regulatory problems in the modulation, inhibition, habituation or facilitation brain processes.

Activity levels: A child may appear disorganized, lacking purpose or goal directedness in their activity. They don't engage in exploring their environment or play in a variety of activities. Following physical activity they may experience difficulty calming down or seek excessive amounts of sensory input. These characteristics are associated with improper functioning in any of the sensory systems (or a combination of them).

Behaviors: Negative behaviors (lack of flexibility, explosiveness, difficulty with transitions) demonstrated by a child may have an underlying cause. They may be irritable or crying for no apparent reason. The underlying reason for such responses could be due to being fearful to certain sounds or visual stimuli or intolerant to something as simple as wrinkles in their shirt. These behaviors are an obvious contribution to a lack of emotional stability and social skills. Given the reciprocal interaction between people their interactions bear an influence on how others respond to them. While these seem to be behaviors that would be unavoidable to acknowledge they could be subtle. Regardless, they could result in the child being treated in an insensitive or unfair manner.

Sensory Modulation: Refers to an inability to regulate sensory input properly, and inability to maintain appropriately. These children have senses that respond randomly with variable effectiveness.

Sensory integration is the organization of sensations for use: Sensations are constantly, at a rapid rate, coming to the brain. These sensations need to be acted upon, organized, and coordinated (with caregiver support) to learn efficiency. When well managed, the brain takes these sensations to form perceptions, then concepts and derive meaning, allowing for learning. With sensory integration problems the child experiences ineffective learning ability. Here, the sensations flowing to the brain do not consistently activate the normal potentials, thus the knowledge is not correctly interpreted meaning that the knowledge is not effectively used to direct the body and mind.

Efficiency of modulation: When sensory modulation is at a level of adequate efficiency there is less sensory overload. Communication is a pervasive/all encompassing activity, however, these factors overlap with the concept of sensory integration, thus illuminating the degree of struggle with these problems can exhibit.

The ear: The vestibular system of the inner ear which affects balance, gravity response, and muscle tone is an aspect of sensory process important to learning disorders and is associated with concentration and emotional well-being. Auditory sensory integration will influence developmental problems, speech and language disabilities.

In order to conceptualize the specific types of symptoms of sensory integration that might be seen as associated to sensory input:

Auditory
○ Responds negatively when exposed to unexpected or loud noises
○ Holds hands over ears demonstrating a lack of tolerance
○ Cannot walk without background noise
○ Appears oblivious/detached within an active environment

Visual
○ Prefers to be in the dark/avoids bright lights
○ Is reluctant to go up/down stairs
○ Stares intensely at people or objects
○ Avoids eye contact

Taste/Smell
○ Avoids certain tastes/smells that are common to their diet
○ Commonly smells non-food objects
○ Seeks out/drawn to certain tastes/smells – does not want to try anything new
○ Does not seem to smell strong odors

Body Position
○ Continually seeks out all kinds of movement activities
○ Hangs on other people, furniture, objects, even in familiar situations
○ Seems to have weak muscles, tires easily, demonstrates poor endurance
○ Walks on toes

Movement
○ Becomes anxious or distressed when their feet leave the ground/clinging and appearing fearful
○ Avoids climbing or jumping
○ Avoids playground equipment
○ Seeks a variety of movement to the degree that it interferes with daily life
○ Takes excessive risks while playing – lacks awareness for safety

Touch
○ Can't stand to be messy, avoids getting messy in glue, finger paint, tape, dirt, etc.
○ Is sensitive to certain fabrics (clothing, bedding, clothing tags)
○ Touches people and objects at an irritating level
○ Avoids going barefoot, especially disliking grass or sand on feet
○ Has decreased awareness for pain or temperature

Attention/Behavior, and Social
○ Distractibility, jumping from one activity to another frequently and interferes in the play of others
○ Has difficulty paying attention/easily distracted
○ Is overly affectionate with others
○ Appears anxious
○ Is accident prone
○ Has difficulty making friends/does not express emotions

Compare and Contrast Sensory Integration Dysfunction vs Attention Deficit Disorder

Kranowitz (2003) takes to task a comparison of two diagnoses, sensory integration and attention deficit disorder, that offer a similar presentation of symptoms. She describes sensory integration dysfunction as the inefficient neurological processing of information. This information is received via all senses and results in learning, development, and behavioral problems. She defines ADD as a constellation of symptoms characterized by serious and persistent symptoms that, likewise, negatively impact aspects of development, learning and behavior. Notably, both can be manifested by inattention, impulsivity, fidgety movement, etc. Therefore, these diagnoses may look alike because of the symptom overlap. A careful assessment is required to determine diagnostic clarification before an accurate treatment plan is developed and initiated. Additionally, medication (as an aspect of the treatment profile) does not fix sensory integration dysfunction. Thus demonstrating a need for a conservative approach initially to insure the appropriate interventions.

With regards to sensory integration disorder, according to Kranowitz (2003), it is important to acknowledge and consider the following:

- The child with sensory integration dysfunction need not demonstrate every symptom or feature of the diagnosis
- There are times when a child will not exhibit symptoms in a similar manner everyday. Inconsistency is a common characteristic of most neurological dysfunctions
- A child may demonstrate features/symptoms of a specific dysfunction but not have that dysfunction (withdraw from being touched but not have a tactile problem but an emotional problem instead)
- A child may exhibit symptoms of hyposensitivity and hypersensitivity (very sensitive to a light touch on the shoulder, but be indifferent to getting a shot at the doctor's office)
- No one is regulated all the time, therefore, everyone experiences some sensory integration difficulty from time to time.

Impact of Dyadic and Family Influence

Benson & Haith (2009; Mahler et al, 1975; Zeanah, 2000; Shore, 2001; Greenspan 2002b) assert the importance of understanding the dynamics of the caregiver–child relationship because of the crucial role of this primary relationship (parent–child) in both normal development and the emergence of psychopathology (Figure 1.11). Therefore, it is necessary to evaluate, diagnose, and treat disorders associated with the dyadic relationship, parental psychopathology, and/or developmental disorders of the child. Keren et al (2010) reported, that infants referred to a clinic whereby relational factors were assessed found that family functioning and mother–infant relational patterns demonstrated deficits in all domains of emotional and instrumental communication regardless of diagnosis. On the dyadic level, the mothers were more intrusive and the infants more withdrawn. Additionally, the diagnostic impressions of the mothers indicated higher levels of depression and phobia. Thus highlighting the importance of clinicians addressing both family level and dyadic level of functioning. While it is not possible to predict at age 3 exactly what a child's functioning will be in grade school or high school, early assessment creates the opportunity to help children and their families to avoid or reduce difficulties seen in older children.

Another factor to consider is the impact of the child's daily care environment. Greenspan (2003) reviewed two studies on day care suggesting that young children appear to demonstrate increased aggressive behavior proportional to the time spent in day care. This increase in aggressiveness was related to increased levels of cortisol. It was noted that factors likely to increase risk included sensory processing and modulation challenges, family stress, a lack of sensitive/nurturing interactions (associated with lower quality day care). He further set forth, 85 to 90% of current day care is not considered high quality and, therefore, families

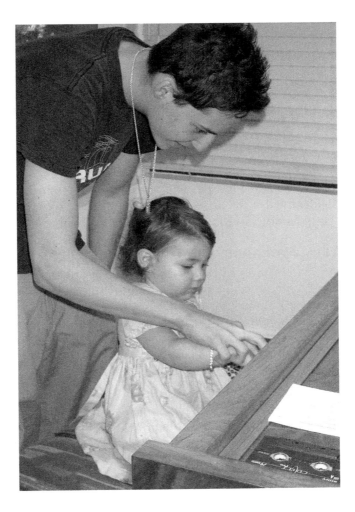

FIGURE 1.11
Little girl at keyboard with adult helping her.

need to be encouraged to consider carefully and explore child-care options, especially providing direct care to their children at least half of the day.

In an epidemiological study (a study of patterns of disease in human populations) on mental health problems and psychopathology in infancy and early childhood (Skovgaard, 2010), literature from 1967 to 2007 was reviewed to investigate aspects of psychopathology in children 0 to 3 years (under 4 years). The study found:

1. Infants and toddlers suffer from mental illness like older children do. Standardized measures and clinical assessments revealed mental health disorders (ICD-10 and DC:03R) can be detected in the general population of children as young as 1½ years of age. Notably, the distribution and frequency of diagnostic categories are consistent along several features to what has been identified in older children. General developmental disorders and eating disorders exhibited the highest frequency. Pervasive developmental disorders were diagnosed with more frequency the older the age, whereas eating disorders and attachment disorders demonstrated increased frequency in younger children. Additionally, regarding gender distribution, neurodevelopmental disorders were diagnosed more frequently in males, while eating disorders were diagnosed more frequently in females.

2. Disorders of neurodevelopment: mental retardation, pervasive developmental disorders (PDD), and ADHD are demonstrated in the first year of life. Disorders of neurodevelopment were recognized in 7% of general population children age 1½ years. Among these, 2.8% were diagnosed ADHD, and no children were diagnosed with

autism-spectrum disorders at this age. For children who had been referred between the ages of 0 and 3 years, there was a 0.03% incidence of ADHD. Additionally, the frequency of PDD was 0.1%, with frequency increasing with age. Significant early risk biological factors associated with neurodevelopmental disorders (birth to 10 months) were similar to what has been found in older children. Amid the referred children, the identified increased risk of neurodevelopmental disorders in males (known in older males) was recognized at child ages 0 to 3 years.

3. Evidence of risk factors and predictors of child mental illness can be detected in the first year of life. Cross-sectional data obtained from parents at the time of child assessment (age 18 months) and predictors were studied on information collected by health nurses from infants aged 0 to 10 months. The early influences of recognized risk factors can be identified in the first 6 months of age. There is concordance with reviewed results from epidemiological studies of older children with regards to pathways of risk.

Early Symptoms and Their Relationship To Later Diagnostic Outcomes

When an infant is regulatory disordered they lack the capacity to modulate mood, self-calm, delay gratification and tolerate transitions in activity. Unlike most babies, they are not able to engage in simple self-calming behaviors such as sucking on their fist, putting their hands together, holding their feet, rocking, looking at/listening to soothing visual or auditory stimuli. Once upset the effort required by the caretaker to calm and sooth the distressed infant could be 2 to 4 hours/day. Older infants may display severe temper tantrums (DeGangi, 2000):

- Most Pervasive Infant Trait: Fussiness. Between 23 and 54% of the regulatory disordered infants displayed problems with fussiness/irritability. They were described by their caregivers as escalating from a pleasant mood to intense crying (27 to 57%) and to exhibit difficulty self-calming (20 to 46%).
- Maternal Perception of Difficultness: Caregiver reports need to be confirmed by the use of temperament scales (for example, Bate's Infant Characterisitcs Questionnaire, fussy/difficult subscales) (Bates, 1984). When caretakers do not interpret the infant's behavior as difficult regardless of clinical evidence of mood regulation, further investigation is necessary to rule out the source of the identified problems as caregiver inexperience, denial, maternal depression or other problem. Generally, the fussiness/irritability results in family distress.
- Symptomology of Infants/Toddlers with Regulatory Disorders: A high percentage of the subjects in the study exhibited irritability, inconsolability, demandingness, and poor self-calming ability in the first year. Infants/toddlers between 10 and 24 months experienced an increased number of symptoms when a regulatory disorder was present under 30 months of age. Problems with irritability, crying, and self-calming were still present at 24 months. As these challenges in behaviors were ameliorated at 25 to 30 months, there was an emergence of problems tolerating change. As the subject matured to 25 to 30 months of age, there was a decrease in regulatory problems which may be related to cognitive development increasing their ability to modulate distress and tolerate change. Regulatory Disordered Sample versus Normal Sample and Emotion Regulation Profile as provided by DeGangi, 2000.

Review of Epidemiological Research

According to Skovgaard (2010), risk factors identified in the general population aged 0 to 3 years appear to be similar to findings in literature reviews of older children. Additionally, there appear to be specific psychopathological pathways of biological and psychosocial risks. Moreover, epidemiological study results suggest the parent–child relationship disturbances play a major role in early childhood as a mediator of psychosocial difficulties. Data gleaned from life experience with the outcome being a mental disorder at 1½ years indicate developmental predictors of neuropsychiatric disorders being concordant. Ultimately, this information adds to the understanding of developmental pathology early in life with a focus on factors associated with the parent–child relationship, identification of early risk factors, assessing biological risks and extrapolating the potential outcome to older children. Epidemiological research has shown the significance of childhood psychopathology demonstrating an overall prevalence in psychiatric disorders in school-aged children and adolescence (16 to 18%) along with a high risk of continuity in mental health problems from school aged > adolescence > adult (Costello et al, 2005a,b). All of which reinforces earlier literature review findings by DeGangi (2000), that children with early characteristics of regulatory disorders are at an increased risk for developing long-term emotional and developmental problems, and the group that demonstrates the greatest risk for later developmental problems were the infants/toddlers who had moderate to severe regulatory disorders.

Taking into consideration emotion regulation is multifaceted biologically as well as behaviorally serves as a foundation that the generation and regulation of emotion interact with each other via a feedback process. Therefore, self-regulation develops in an organized manner through the interaction of multiple factors versus the exclusive maturation of higher order control mechanisms (Thompson et al, 2008). DeGangi (2000) cautions that although some normal infants display regulatory disorder symptoms, it is the number and intensity of symptoms that signify one child from another in developing a regulatory disorder.

The key findings in Skovgaard's (2010) review of epidemiological research demonstrate significance of childhood psychopathology in the determination of mental health later in life. The distribution of varying problems during the age period of 0 to 2 months, 2 to 6 months, and 6 to 10 month was presented. The major findings across the first 10 months of life as recorded by health nurse visits were:

1. 30% demonstrated feeding/eating problems
2. 13% exhibited some problem with overall development
3. 11.7% exhibited abnormal development of verbal and non-verbal communication
4. 10% demonstrated problems in the interaction between mother and child. *Predictors of neurodevelopmental disorders and parent–child relationship disturbances can be identified in the first 10 months of life from the general population.

When psychopathology was reviewed for children aged 1½ years, the most frequent DC:0-3 diagnoses were those of regulatory disorders. Comorbidity of axis I primary child diagnoses and axis II parent–child relationship disturbances revealed:

1. 19.1% hyperactivity/attention deficit disorder (ICD-10 F90)
2. 14.5% disorders of conduct and emotion (ICD-10 F92-93)
3. 6.3% regulatory disorders (DC:0-3 400)
4. 2.2% developmental disorders (ICD-10 F88-89)
5. 1.3% disorders of eating and sleeping (ICD-10 F51; F98.2).

There was significant comorbidity evidenced between the parent–child relationship disorder and child mental health disorders, in particular ADHD, disorders of conduct and emotion, and regulatory disorders. In accordance with Skovgaard's review, it appears that many of the presented problems reside within the child as well as potentially residing in their environment. For instance, the interaction of family variables with child characteristics:

- Excessive tantrums, oppositional behavior, aggression, family trauma, accident proneness, and toilet training problems
- Parenting skills, physical abuse, poor attachment, sexual abuse, separation anxiety, custody issues, and fearfulness
- Hyperactivity, parental depression/anxiety, feeding problems, chronic illness, and excessive shyness.

Regarding the associations of biological and psychosocial risks with mental health disorders and relationship disturbances for age 1½ years, biological risk was associated with an increased risk of mental health disorder (only neurodevelopment diagnoses), and psychosocial risk was significantly associated with a mental health disorder in the child and with a parent–child relationship disorder (Figures 1.12 and 1.13). The most robust associations were among relationship disorders and child mental health disorders in the area of emotional, behavioral, eating and sleeping disorders. *The most frequent mental health problem was relationship disorders, found in 8.5% of parent–child pairs. Studies of children, aged 5 years and older in the general population, found a 16% prevalence of mental disorder. Skovgaard (2010) further states in her review, "studies of older children have shown an overall distribution of diagnostic categories which are comparable to the results from the present study, with emotional, behavioral, and adjustment disorders being the most common, and neurodevelopmental disorders, including attention deficit hyperactivity disorders, affecting a minor proportion of disordered children".

The demonstrated significant associations between relationship disorders, child mental health disorders and psychosocial adversity in the present study (Skovgaard, 2010) of general population children are aligned with empirical statistics from clinical populations of infants of parents who are psychosocially disadvantaged (i.e. mental illness, alcohol/drug abuse, low education, etc.). This information is fundamental to the understanding of interactive factors associated with infant/child mental health problems and psychopathology which further result in later diagnostic outcome. Early relationships are critical to the developing infant, and positive consistent relationships are key to healthy growth, development and learning. Responsive caregiving supports infants in their initiation of regulating their emotions and contributes to the development of a sense of predictability, responsiveness, and safety in

40

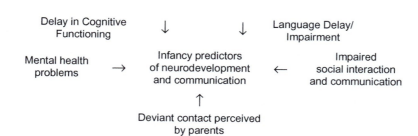

FIGURE 1.12
Associations of neuropsychiatric disorders at age 1½ years. *(Adapted from Skovgaard, 2010.)*

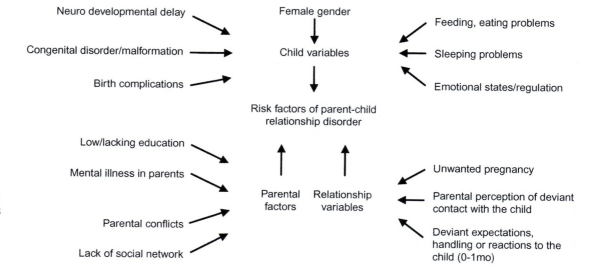

FIGURE 1.13
Associations of child–family variables recorded 0–10 months and a relationship disorder diagnosed at age 18 months. *(Adapted from Skovgaard, 2010.)*

their environments and social exchanges. For example, high quality relationships increase the likelihood of positive outcomes as infants and children learn about social relationships and emotions through exploration and predictable interactions.

"Infants are dependent on caregivers for help with regulating behavior, physiological state, and emotions. With development, children increasingly take over these functions themselves. When a caregiver is unresponsive (as often happens with a depressed caregiver) or frightening (as often happens with a maltreating caregiver), children may not receive the help they need in taking over these regulatory functions. There has been strong evidence that these and other early environmental risk factors place children at increased risk for a host of psychological and social problems"

(Dozier and Peloso, 2006).

When neurodevelopment disorders were investigated, impaired social interaction, delays in cognitive functioning and language impairment predicted all of the neurodevelopment disorders except ADHD. The factor which did predict ADHD was the parent perception of deviant contact with the child (recorded 0 to 10 months of life). Additionally, these predictors of neuropsychiatric disorders have also been exhibited in longitudinal studies of adolescents and adults, therefore, confirming risk of pathogenesis of neurodevelopment disorders and indicating global predictors for neuropsychiatric disorders/disturbances in the first year of life.

Reviewing Early Risk Pathways

INFANTS AND CHILDREN SUFFER FROM MENTAL ILLNESS JUST LIKE OLDER CHILDREN DO

The reluctance to diagnose mental illness in children has played a role in the discrepancies between disorders in the primary health service setting versus general population. Infants and toddlers suffer from mental illness just as older children do. When standardized measures and clinical assessments are used, mental health categories in ICD-10 and DC:0-3 are detected in the general population as early as aged 1½ years. Additionally, the distribution and frequency of the constellation of symptoms required to meet diagnostic criteria correspond with several features found in studies of older children (Costello et al, 2005a,b; Suniga et al, 2006; Rutter et al, 2006; Skovgaard, 2010).

For children diagnosed in a hospital setting the following patterns were identified:

- *Younger children* demonstrated increased frequency of eating disorders and attachment disorders
- *Older children* demonstrated increased frequency of pervasive developmental disorders
- *ADHD* severity in preschoolers is predictive of oppositional defiant disorder (ODD), and the combination of ADHD and ODD predicts the persistence of both in middle childhood.

ROLE OF GENDER

The gender distribution identified from studies on older children was already evident in children aged 0 to 3 years. Boys more frequently met the diagnostic criteria for neurodevelopmental disorders, and girls more frequently met the diagnostic criteria for eating disorders (Rutter et al, 2003). Epidemiological studies on young children compared to older children find that older children demonstrate different pathways of risk (i.e., biological risks associated with neurodevelopment disorders and psychosocial risk associated with emotional, behavioral, eating, sleeping and adjustment disorders) exhibited by predictors which could be identified in the first 6 months of life (Chatoor & Ganiban, 2004; Rutter 2005; Costello et al, 2006; Skovgaard, 2010):

- ADHD occurs 2 to 4 times more commonly in boys than girls
- Male to female ratio 4:1 for the predominantly hyperactive type
- Male to female ratio 2:1 for the predominantly inattentive type

- ADHD is one of the most common disorders of childhood. (In the USA approximately 8 to 10% of children satisfy diagnostic criteria for ADHD).

Parent observations suggest that males act out more aggressively than females, have more behavioral and attentional problems, may demonstrate motor skills deficits, and have more expressive language problems (mumbling and stammering), whereas females often demonstrate increased impulsivity that may result in danger to themselves, and they have more difficulty shifting mental set (vacillating between new information or mentally going back and forth between information content). *Approximately 40 to 50% of ADHD-hyperactive children will have (typically non-hyperactive) symptoms persist into adulthood.

According to Wolke et al (2009) both in males and females, shortened gestational age, neonatal neurological complications, and poor parent–infant relationship were factors predictive of regulatory problems at 5 months and lower cognition at 56 months.

Disorders of neurodevelopment in children aged 1½ years in the general population (mental retardation, PDD, ADD):

- Identified in 7% of children aged 1½ years
- ADHD found 2.8% of children aged 1½ years, but no children were diagnosed at this age with an autism-spectrum disorder
- Referred children aged 0 to 3 showed an ADHD incidence of 0.03% and an overall incidence of PDD of 0.1%, and incidence increased with age
- Associated with biological risk factors similar to what has been identified in studies focused on older children
  - significant early predictors of deviant neurodevelopment were identified 0 to 10 months
  - documented studies of older male children demonstrated an identified risk for neurodevelopmental disorders by 0 to 3 years of age.

*These results are indicative of the validity of neurodevelopmental disorders in early age.

ROLE OF RELATIONSHIP DISTURBANCE

Relationship problems between parent and child identified in infants aged 0 to 10 months were associated with twice the risk of a child disorder at aged 18 months, and a ten times increased risk of a comorbid mental disorder (Skovgaard, 2010; Zeanah, 2000):

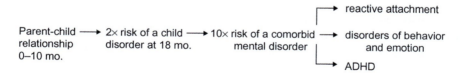

*These findings suggest age-specific differences along with gender demonstration and identification of psychopathology seen in studies of older children are evident in very early childhood (Rutter et al, 2003). In a longitudinal study aiming to examine regulatory problems in infancy as a predictor of hyperkinetic symptoms in childhood and pre-adolescence (hyperkinetic behavior problems assessed at the ages of 2, 4, 5, 8, and 11 by standardized parent interview), the impact of early family adversity factors explicitly outweighed that of infant psychopathology on later behavior disorder. Infant regulatory difficulties at 3 months of age (determined by multiple sources of information including an observational procedure used to assess the quality of mother–infant interaction) found the following (Becker et al, 2004):

- At the age of 3 months, 17% of infants suffered from multiple regulatory problems
- Compared to a control group, these children presented more hyperkinetic symptoms throughout childhood

- Negativity in the mother–infant interaction and early family adversity each contributed to later hyperkinetic symptoms.

*When controlling for family adversity, the association between infant multiple regulatory problems and later hyperkinetic problems was statistically insignificant.

The parent–child relationship is a focal point in development. It is the impact of the infant's experience of environmental risk factors and intrinsic factors in association with the parent–child relationship that manifests in regulatory disorders (examples of environmental risk are poverty, domestic violence, caregiver depression; examples of intrinsic factors are biological difficulties, complications of prematurity, caregiver exposure to substances, etc). All of these interactions, at different levels, act as the moderator with problematic outcomes associated with a less supportive caretaker relationship and a more positive outcome when the caregiver relationship is adequately supportive (Benson & Haith, 2009).

ROLE OF EARLY FEEDING AND EATING PROBLEMS

Almost one-third of all general population children aged 0–10 months were reported to exhibit a feeding problem (CCC, 2000; Chatoor & Ganiban, 2004; Olsen et al, 2007; Wolke et al, 2009).

- General population children aged 1½ years demonstrated a 2.8% incidence of eating disorders (the most common infant problem of feeding and eating) diagnosed at hospitals. *Children referred to treatment of an eating disorder at a hospital (possibly weight instability/failure to thrive) aged 0 to 12 months suggest an early manifestation of severe eating/feeding problems
- Feeding problems recorded by a health nurse at age 8 to 10 months were the only significant infant predictor of an eating disorder at age 18 months. The mechanism could be: (1) unstable weight/failure to thrive within the first 2 months of life (early signs of neurodevelopmental impairment such as oral–motor conditioned feeding problems) or pre/perinatal adversities; (2) compromised parent–child interactions (developing over time in an otherwise healthy child)
- Excessive crying and feeding problems in infancy have a small but significant adverse effect on cognitive development.

Skovgaard's (2010) conclusion following the extensive literature review was that risk factors of relationship disorders at aged 1½ years can be identified before the birth of the child and, additionally, the predictors can be identified by health nurses from age 0 to 10 months. Therefore, demonstrating in the general population that children as early as 18 months may suffer from mental illness as seen in older children. In other words, it is possible to identify risk factors and predictors of mental illness in infants 0 to 10 months, and the associations of risk found in older children appear to operate or function from birth. Skovgaard et al (2010) state that predictors of neurodevelopmental disorders and parent–child relationship disturbances can be identified in the general population at 0 to 10 months of age. Further, unwanted pregnancy along with parental negative expectations of the child recorded in the first month of life were identified as significant predictors of relationship disturbances at 18 months. Additionally, Flaherty et al (2006) offer that a number of studies demonstrate an association between early adversity and problematic child health outcomes. Wolke et al (2009) also weigh in on this topic, "both in boys and girls, shortened gestational age, neonatal neurological complications, and poor parent–infant relationship were predictive of regulatory problems at 5 months and lower cognition at 56 months".

Information from the field of molecular biology continues to progress and reinforce not only the biological aspects of psychopathology, but the interplay with mitigating environmental risk factors. For example, research by Becker et al (2010) revealed the following in their study of 300 children examining the potential moderating effect on ADHD measures: "in children with the DRD4-7r allele, a history of regulatory problems in infancy was unrelated to later

ADHD. But in children with regulatory problems in infancy, the additional presence of the DRD4-7r allele increased the risk of ADHD in childhood". Such information bears special significance in association with early detection and intervention for the child and their family proactively to prevent predictive problems and enhance a positive outcome from an educational and quality of life perspective.

Long before a clinical diagnosis is made, parents of a regulatory disordered child have observed their child does not react like their siblings at the same age or other children of a similar age. Some examples of parental descriptions of these children at discrete stages of age and development suggest a spectrum of symptoms that are excessive in comparison to appropriate responses of children approximately the same age (DeGangi, 2000; Calkins et al, 2002; Cesari et al, 2003; Rutter et al, 2003; Chatoor & Ganiban, 2004; Skovgaard, 2010). For clinicians working with the pediatric population the following case will serve as an example of the type of case that may be referred to them.

Eric

Eric was referred at 22 months by his daycare for biting other children. Eric's teacher told his mother that she needed to remedy the problem or he would not be allowed to attend their daycare. The biting appeared to be associated with Eric experiencing difficulty when other children wanted something that he had or another child was playing or sitting too close in proximity to him.

When Eric's parents were being interviewed he was out of control. Eric was running all over the office, pulling books off of the shelf, hanging off of chairs, etc. The parents barely acknowledged his behavior making almost no effort to contain his behavior. During the floortime play with the clinician there was a dramatic change in his behavior. At the close of the meeting, the clinician offered the parents information about emotionally connecting and bonding with their son with an opportunity to practice it before the meeting terminated. Neither parent had any success of accomplishing what was instructed during this time.

Eric's history revealed that as an infant he utilized primitive mouthing strategies to explore his environment. He continued this behavior into his second year and exhibited difficulty functioning when his mother would leave the room. Eric had difficulty going to bed and staying asleep, as well as an inability to use expressive language to communicate what he wanted and needed. Eric's mother had utilized breast feeding him to calm him. However, during such an episode, when he was about 1 year old, he bit her. To her recollection this is when the "biting problem" originated.

Eric's mother appeared appropriately invested in his best interest and providing him with the best environment possible. However, she experienced difficulty with emotional closeness to him. Eric's mother offered more negative descriptions about him than his father. Additionally, self-reports indicated that she was under stress and had a history of depression. When she described her time with Eric she appeared angry that she couldn't get a break from him whether this was breast feeding, she never had any time for herself or he interrupted her sleep (this was complicated by the fact that he at times slept with his parents). She struggled with setting limits and boundaries for him and herself. Her frustration with him had appeared to result in her emotional distancing (rejection) of Eric. The father expressed feeling helpless and ineffective to impact any positive change when his son was distressed.

Eric's parent's gave a release so that the daycare teacher could be contacted for further information. Apparently, when Eric got stressed at daycare he was unable to regulate emotion and anxiety in his interactions with other children. The regulation difficulty, biting behavior, had now been identified with his mother, other children, and other care providers (beyond the parent–child relationship).

Diagnosis:

Axis I Affect Disorder of Mixed emotional Expressiveness ....R/O Regulatory disorder Type II (hyperactive, defiant, negative)

Axis II Relationship Disorder, Mixed Relationship Type

Parental Descriptions of Child Behavior

INFANCY

Active, fussy/rigid, excessive crying, sleep problems (needing complete darkness, being driven around in a car/movement vibration to fall asleep, white noise to calm them), eating problems, touch sensitivity, colic-like symptoms, irritability, inconsolable, demanding, sensory hypersensitivity to touch or light, a high need for movement, fear of novelty, deficits in giving clear gestural and vocal signs, severe separation anxiety. They may also have difficulty regulating their eating and elimination and difficulty self-calming. Therefore, difficulties with basic characteristics of homeostasis.

TODDLER AND PRESCHOOL

Demonstrate a lack of awareness for personal space, safety and judging distances, tactile sensitivity, noise sensitivity, fine motor problems, food allergies, dislike for new food textures, excessive movement in sleep, night terrors, dislike for restraint (car seats, being dressed), distress with loud noises, fear of movement, lack of reciprocal interaction (interaction problems), difficulty with clear gestural signs, difficulty with limit setting, advanced in cognitive areas but poor social skills, seek out and play with younger or older children, an almost desperate drive to seek control of their environment, may be engaging and charming but can rapidly switch to violent outbursts/reactions, noticeably aggressive and/or negative, conversational ability may be high but their goal directed activity is slow. Therefore, persistent problems with homeostasis in conjunction with difficulties in gestural communication, affective expression, attentional capacities, reciprocal play and negotiating autonomy and control.

OLDER PRESCHOOL

Difficulty tolerating the feeling of certain clothes, difficulty with temperature control/ perspire a lot, want to only eat certain foods, fearful of flushing the toilet, hate to have their teeth brushed, refuse/complain excessively about having their hair brushed or cut, become perseverative or get stuck in a play routine (repeating the same play routine over and over), play with only certain toys, fear the unknown (like the confusing distortions of the human form such as a clown or Santa Claus), crave the feeling of gravity for long periods of time (swinging, amusement rides).

PRIMARY SCHOOL YEARS

Difficulty with making transitions, reactive to noise, reactive to touch, demonstrate fine and gross motor skill problems (in comparison to peers), impulsive responses (often interpreted as aggressive behavior), exhibit poor social skills, can attend to play for short periods of time, but interrupted by shifting to their need for personal attention, cannot stand to be wrong or lose face, find something wrong with everything, excessive behaviors with an over focus or preoccupation with a particular method/routine or behavior, verbally adept and intelligent. Because of their aggression and impulsivity it is difficult to include them in shopping or other outside events. Their perspective does not allow for a smooth social flow and their bossy or aggressive behavior results in few sustained friendships.

Due to the dynamic aspect of presentation (changing from day to day), and the complex and individual nature of their sensory and behavioral responses, these children are difficult to describe precisely by parents. However, the parental descriptions offered in combination with their own level of associated distress offers the necessary point of early intervention, notably the earlier the better with regard to improvement/amelioration and prevention.

DeGangi (2000) asserts, in a basic manner which binds the aforementioned information, in studies on regulatory disordered infants, "that children with regulatory disorders have underlying deficits in self-regulation, attention and arousal, sensory processing, and emotion regulation". Further adding that different symptoms can be identified at different ages and developmental levels of the child. *Therefore, highlighting the importance of understanding how such symptoms maintain a certain continuity but change over time.

Children with Regulatory Disorders and Underlying Deficits
REGULATION DISORDERS AND ADHD

The child diagnosed with both of these disorders offers more clinical complexity than with either single diagnosis. Not all children with Regulatory Disorders of Sensory Processing (RDSP) will have a diagnosis of ADHD or the converse. The common presentation of ADHD involves problems with attention, impulsivity and hyperactivity. The child with RDSP and ADHD may demonstrate more problems as a result of the factors of dysregulation, temperamental difficulties, sensory, motor and spatial problems that interact and complicate the problems created by ADHD.

REGULATION DISORDERS AND AUTISM SPECTRUM DISORDERS (ASD)

Unfortunately, sometimes children with RDSP are misdiagnosed with an ASD. This may happen because a child is slow to respond to sensory input and presents as being withdrawn, listless, and appears to lack interest in the environment (only self-interested). Children with an under-responsive pattern, slow motor pattern of limited exploration or limited play repertoire also exhibit responses similar to children with ASD. An additional diagnostic dilemma is associated with children diagnosed with Multisystem Developmental Disorders (MSDD) because of the similar presentation to RDSP and ASD. *Many of the social-cognitive deficits manifested by ASD are embedded in the incapacity to organize and directly grasp the intrinsic goal related organization of motor behavior (Diamond, 2009).

Examples of Other Factors Influence Regulation
Numerous factors can wield an influence on regulation, for example:

IMPACT OF PRENATAL ALCOHOL/SUBSTANCE EXPOSURE UPON REGULATION

1. As evidenced by finding a "blunted" response to a heel lance (viewed as an acutely painful event) suggests prenatal alcohol exposure may alter the brain's pain regulatory system
2. In the study of acute pain reactivity and stress regulation in newborns of depressed mothers taking an SSRI (such as Prozac) during their pregnancy. SSRIs and alcohol alter the serotonin thereby blunting pain pathways
3. Prenatal alcohol exposure may be destructive to neurotropins (peptides) that influence the growth, development, and functional plasticity of the fetal brain
4. Prenatal methamphetamine exposure results in children demonstrating brain abnormality that may be more severe than alcohol exposure
5. Heavy prenatal alcohol exposure may lead to fetal alcohol syndrome (FAS). Sometimes it can lead to cognitive and behavioral deficits in absence of craniofacial characteristics
6. Fetal exposure to alcohol may result in memory and information processing deficits in children as well as negative influences in visual perception and control of attention

7. Prenatal drug exposure is associated with sleep problems in children (Science Daily, 2010).

INFANTS/CHILDREN OF DEPRESSED MOTHERS

1. More often than infants of well mothers these infants and children present as having difficult temperaments, dysregulated emotions, less secure attachments
2. Exhibit a higher rate of atypical frontal lobe activity, lower motor and mental development
3. React more negatively to stress and have less effective self-regulation skills
4. Show fewer interpersonal skills in interactions with peers
5. Demonstrate a lack of social competence (aggressive, withdrawn, and inappropriate behavior with peers)
6. Females may be more vulnerable to the effects of maternal depression because of gender role modeling
7. More likely to develop patterns of undercontrol (aggressive, oppositional, disruptive, and impulsive) and overcontrol (withdrawal, regulation or suppression of negative emotion). They are also seen to reflect compliance or other forms of effortful control of their social environments such as being well behaved, caring, and considerate of others. This may be associated with overinvestment in the well-being of others (peacemakers or a pseudo-parent role reversal before they are developmentally prepared to perform these roles)
8. Prosocial development whereby caring behavior for the caregiver, empathic overinvolvement, becoming more frequent over the second year begins to include cognitive and affective aspects. A result may be child development of anxiety, helplessness and misplaced sense of responsibility (Cummings et al, 2000; Zahn-Waxler, 2000).

Other Factors That Impact Development

LOW BIRTH WEIGHT (WOLRAICH ET AL, 2008)

Very low birth weight (VLBW < 1500 g). With the increasing rate of survival of premature and low birth weight infants there are associated numerous consequences. These consequences take the form of:

- significant neurodevelopmental difficulties
- during school-age years, the appearance of social, academic and behavioral difficulties not previously identified.

GENETICS (WOLRAICH ET AL, 2008)

Genetic studies are highly complex. As researchers strive to identify and understand the relationship between abnormal genetic mechanisms and disorders of development and behavior, two examples are:

- allelic differences associated with reading disorders, ASD, ADHD
- multigene disorders which are associated with reading, ASD, ADHD.

As noted earlier, with advances in medical knowledge and treatment, there is improvement in life expectancy and quality of life. Wolraich et al (2008) provided a summary of aspects of genetically based phenotypes. A few examples from their summary:

- circumscribed behavior
    - self-injury in Lesch–Nyhan syndrome
    - spasmodic "self-hug" in Smith–Magenis syndrome
    - hand-wringing in Rett syndrome
- cognitive/neuropsychological
    - phonological/verbal memory impairment in Down's syndrome
    - spatial memory and visual-motor impairments in Williams syndrome
    - non-verbal learning disability profile in Turner syndrome

- developmental/behavioral
  - emergence of hyperphagia and resolution of severe hypotonia in preschool-aged children with Prader–Willi syndrome
- temperament and personality
  - sociability in Williams syndrome
- biobehavioral
  - sleep disorders and melatonin dysregulation in Smith–Magenis syndrome
  - pharmocogenic effects (differences in hepatic metabolism).

INFECTIOUS DISEASE AND ASSOCIATED DEVELOPMENTAL AND BEHAVIORAL OUTCOMES (WOLRAICH ET AL, 2008)

Infectious diseases can adversely impact the growth and development of children. Of particular interest are those of the central nervous system that are associated with long-term consequences (resulting from the infectious disease) that impacts cognition, learning, and behavior. The consequences of infection are associated with the complex interplay of illness, family, health, and quality of social system.

As has been established many infants demonstrate difficulty with self-regulation, whether seen in the lack of ability to regulate their emotional state or how to organize effectively a response to a variety of environmental demands. While many of these problems are resolved as the infant matures, for many, these difficulties persist beyond 6 months of age and into early childhood where they are considered maladaptive and may be indicative of a regulatory disorder. Infants and young children with regulatory disorders are challenged by behaviors such as persistent irritability and impulsivity which impedes adaptive functioning. The result is an increased risk for a number of problems such as developmental delays. Therapists and other professionals who intervene with families presenting with infants and small children demonstrating disorders of affect and behavior are challenged by the task of identifying regulatory disorders, diagnosis, and treatment planning.

DEFINING EMOTION

This discussion on emotion was purposefully saved as a reinforcing element to be an integrated aspect of preparing the intervening professional to investigate with care an interest not only what the child is experiencing functionally but their emotional experience of it. Emotion is the color palette of life experience. Emotions (DeGangi, 2000; Greenspan, 2002b) influence how a child experiences the world within and the world around them. Emotions provide motivation, meaning and regulatory function as they guide thoughts and behaviors. The expression of emotion reveals coping mechanisms, self-concept and self-regulation. The manner in which a person of any age experiences and expresses emotion and interacts with others is unique to the individual. Disposition may be predominantly happy or sad, content or angry, curious or withdrawn, flexible or destructive, compulsive or disorganized. However, what is most common is that different emotions and behavior will be associated with the situational experience combined with the prevailing mood at the time. Overall, emotions mediate the individual's ability to adapt and adjust or respond to a multitude of experiences. DeGangi (2000) describes five major areas related to emotional regulation.

1. Cognitive Appraisal (CA)

CA takes place when an individual is confronted with a situation/stimulus. It is the reading of social cues. The CA determines the intensity and quality of the emotional reaction. CA and associated analytical skills continue to develop and is refined over time based upon knowledge obtained over time in the form of similar situations, memory file of past experiences, and perceptual skills of environmental cues. This means that, over time, appraisal is demonstrated by numerous different emotional responses as an individual thinks about past and current experiences. An example:

A child experiences a new situation that results in an emotional experience of fear/dread/ misgiving/angst. If the child had experienced something similar in the past they may (a) remember that they were able to deal with and felt successful in managing their distress, or (b) that they were frustrated, unable to cope, and felt unable to manage their distress. In the aforementioned response they initially feel distressed but deal with it, in the second depiction they likely seek to avoid a replay of the negative emotions.

How would this be translated to a child preparing to attend school with time to prime a foundation of support and change, thus increasing their preparedness for school?

Ethan, a four year old, already has a history of difficulty coping with stress. He has experienced difficulties with peers at preschool and does not want to go to school because it has been a distressing and negative experience. Ethan was disorganized and unable to progress through the preschool activity program with his peers, experienced difficulty sharing and, when upset, would act out such as sometimes biting one of his peers.

SOLUTION

A full time aid was assigned to Ethan to help him make adjustments and take the time to guide him in modulating his emotional reactivity. Upon reintroduction to school, the challenge was to alter his self-concept. This was accomplished by utilizing a stepwise progression into the school environment. At first, he only attended pre-kindergarten for 2 hours/day to program an increased possibility of success. Initially, 2 hours/day was manageable in addition to utilizing positive reinforcement from his aid to accomplish programmed tasks like his peers. Breaks were built into his schedule to provide time for him to reorganize and calm himself. A school and home program was developed for consistency and reinforcement. The program reinforced positive behavioral responses (not acting out or biting peers), making transitions (picking up toys and putting them away in a timely manner to have a snack with his peers), and self-soothing when upset/agitated (choices like time alone in a decision chair to think about things and be reinforced in his decision making by the assigned aid). It did not take long for Ethan's compliance to increase dramatically at school and at home, thus, altering his self-concept into a positive self-statement about a little boy who was excited about going to school.

With this scenario what changed? His experience and, thus, his interpretation or perception of his experience has been changed. Fundamental aspects of these changes include Perceptual Understanding of Facial Expressions. This is a fascinating developmental learning progression allowing the child to discriminate emotion which is defined by:

a. Perceptual understanding: at 4 to 7 weeks of age an infant can discern the facial hair outline. At around 5 months, the infant has developed the notion of "faceness" whereby they are putting together the features of the face and are particularly interested in the mouth. By 7 months of age, the facial feature progression includes the detection of variations in facial poses (angles)

b. Recognition of affective expressions: understanding the difference between a smile and a frown. This ability is more complicated than it appears. It is the integration of auditory and visual perception skills in the context of time and space. Because facial changes are discrete (facial changes demonstrate a beginning and an end), the infant is able to develop a catalog composite of sorts that includes association to quality of voice to an increasing number of distinguishing faces and associated interpretations

c. Simultaneous perception of vocal expressions, speech content, gestures, and postural changes: a common experience following the birth of an infant is the ability of the infant to recognize their mother's voice. This distinguishing ability expands to the detection of synchrony of a moving face and its voice and the matching of facial and vocal expressions, thus utilizing visual and auditory cues

d. Understanding the meaning of facial expression during interpersonal interactions: the ability to discriminate quality or meaning increases. For example, the difference between an authentic smile versus an ingenuous one. This skill draws and builds from the face time with caregivers. Particularly during interaction with the mother, the baby mimics the movements of the mouth and tongue instinctually. This increasing discrimination of meaning in facial expressions is matched by the baby's responsiveness to various facial expressions. This early interaction or mirroring with the primary caregiver significantly influences the child's own facial expressions. The happy mother who has positive energy, smiles and talks to her baby elicits a similar response from her baby. Whereas, the depressed mother who has negative energy, and looks sad will result in a baby having more sadness or anger and not remain fixed eye to eye (avert gaze). *Difficulty in the perception of facial expression is experienced in some children with mood-regulation problems. The disconnect in being able to understand facial and emotional expression results in feeling overwhelmed, leading to avoidance of eye contact and other behavioral cues associated with non-verbal cues. Parents may report this as their child does not listen to them, ignoring their efforts to set boundaries, and may react with inappropriate emotional responses as well. A child may also not recognize what should be identified as a familiar face or misread other social cues. Unfortunately, this lack of accurate perceptual ability results in a lack of being able to progress in emotional intelligence which bridges expressive emotion to more subtle emotional cues and from predictable events to the non-predictable, thus resulting in feeling overwhelmed. The reading of social cues can be remedied by pertinent fantasy play allowing repetitive opportunity for practice and reinforcement

e. Neural mechanisms underlying perception of facial expressions: as previously stated, the multifaceted composite pattern recognition and synchronization of visual and auditory input is required for accurate processing of emotional expression. The right and left hemispheres of the brain possess different dominant or central properties. The right brain plays a principal role in recognition of visual-spatial and auditory patterns and integrating perceptual properties, whereas the left hemisphere holds a significant role in the cognitive appraisal of emotion. This is an important consideration when preparing a treatment plan and using it as an opportunity to acknowledge and understand the impact of compromised neural mechanisms.

2. Physiological Aspects of Emotions (PAE)

PAEs are the autonomic nervous system (ANS) responses corresponding to emotion. For example, heart rate, blushing, gastric responses to emotional distress. This is all indicative of the neural pathways between the brain and associated emotion:

a. Mediation of emotions through autonomic responses: while there may not be consensus regarding what takes place first emotion or the autonomic response, the autonomic responses are valuable to the person in identifying feelings and labeling them

b. Specificity of emotions: there is a close association between autonomic activity and facial expression (neural mechanisms controlling facial muscles and the ANS). In other words, when emotion is experienced, specific facial expressions and associated unique configuration of autonomic activity are elicited based on the emotional state. Purposefully engaging in certain facial expressions, for some, may result in changing ANS changes. This could explain why some people feel better when choosing to smile, thus changing their physiological response by experiencing an elevation in mood

c. Polyvagal theory of emotion: the connection between the ANS activity and social communication is in the polyvagal theory of emotion. The vagal system plays a role in digestion and decreasing cardiac output in novel or threatening situations. This theory describes three stages of neural development (i) exemplified by immobilization responses, (ii) mobilization represented by the fight or flight response when confronted with a threatening object, (iii) neurological foundation of early life mother–infant interactions and the development of multifaceted social behaviors. The resulting contributions include emotional expression, vocal communication, and dependent social behaviors

d. Neural mechanisms underlying physiological changes: neural mechanisms (afferent feedback) from facial and postural muscles play an important function in modulation of emotion and the mechanism is central to the self-monitoring of emotional expression and in organizing purposeful exploration. Increased maturity should be demonstrated by greater regulation, decreased variability in autonomic responding, commensurate with learning to adapt to a range of novel or stressful situations.

3. Expression of Emotion (EE)

The affective demonstration of emotion (outward display of emotion) includes factors such as facial expression (primarily), gestures, posture, movement and vocal responses. All of these components work together clearly to convey the message. Affective expression is associated with the internal emotional experience. The facial expression is interpreted as a reflection of the internal experience. An example of clear emotional expression decreases confusion by a toddler:

A parent clarifying a limit, "furrowed brow, unhappy facial expression, body posture explicitly directed toward the toddler, the shaking of a finger and the resounding statement "no!"

Facial expressions that are universal to all cultures include surprise, fear, distress, anger, disgust, and happiness. Developmental differences in affective expression: (a) neonates express an array of emotions such as distress and pleasure, (b) different types of crying exhibited by babies are expressions of sorrow, fear, anger, pain. Differences in emotional expression are associated with individual learning experiences anchoring different meanings to events.

4. Socialization of Emotions (SE)

The interactions between an infant and a parent is the fertile ground for socialization adaptations. The optimal time for instrumental conditioning is less than half a second. Mothers smiling and talking to their infants are reinforcing positive affect (emotional expression). Infants elicit the attention of their parents by facial expressions as an expression of need, requiring the caregiver to be sensitive to reading these cues and appropriately engaging. Mothers must be prepared to compensate for an infant who is less capable of initiating these emotional expression cues (such as a Down's syndrome baby). The real challenge is when the mother has an irritable baby. In this circumstance, mothers were found to do the exact opposite of what the baby was trying to elicit from them. Additionally, there was a tendency to overstimulate the baby with too much talking versus active play. When a mother has difficulty reading her baby's cues seeking a certain response, the mother's capacity to support their child's competence to self-regulate or organize planned actions to decrease distress is diminished. The unfortunate result is a lack of synchrony between a mother and a child.

a. Inhibition of affective expression: it is very difficult to totally prevent or inhibit the expression of emotion. Often it is the tone of voice which is the give away when all other affective expression is suppressed. It is more difficult to inhibit facial expression that other body signs (like posture)

b. Neural mechanisms mediating affective expression: affective expression is a building integration of cognitive, perceptual and motor skills resulting from the expanding connections of regions in the brain. Both hemispheres of the brain contribute in different ways to both the experience and expression of emotion. Posture also contributes to the regulation of affect. For example, slumping, caved inward, sad body posture versus a happy posture, holding the body high and open. These postures impact proprioceptive discharge or feeling. The therapy technique of muscle relaxation works to unblock negative emotion by purposefully using posture. Muscle tone and motor planning are particularly important in children identified as having sensory integration dysfunction. They exhibit difficulty in modulating affective expression as a result of ineffective feedback associated with posture(s) that do not match facial expression of emotion. Case example:

Suzie is a 5-year-old kindergarten student. She is described as bright, accident prone with severe motor planning difficulty and slow to learn tasks. Recently, she began to dress herself, but couldn't tie her shoes and button a shirt, also age appropriate delayed skills. She exhibited a high degree of anxiety, behaviorally oppositional, and learned helplessness when confronted with any task requiring motor planning. She would become overwhelmed and afraid whenever she had to climb stairs, even expressing that she was going to be sick (vomit). She would cling to her parents and cry to go home. She felt nauseous while traveling in a car and when she had been swinging. Her behavior seemed extreme with demands, screaming and aggressiveness or passive and submissive. The focus of treatment was to enhance awareness to feedback from her own body and physical functioning while at the same time working on appropriate means to manage her environment and relationship interactions.

5. Modulation of Emotion and Mood States (MEMS)

The modulation of emotion is closely linked with the process of self-directed regulation (internalized regulation). It must be kept in mind, if a person has not been exposed to information or a skill they lack knowledge and must rely on others for the accurate cue to communicate emotional meaning. Encouragement from a caretaker for persistence in trying to accomplish a task until there is success is a deterrent to frustration, tantrums and other negative behaviors. Interestingly, the infant that has already learned how to self-soothe via thumb sucking or decreasing stimuli by looking away may have the frustration tolerance to persist in task completion (reaching for an object) without caregiver encouragement.

a. Regulation of negative affect: the development of self-regulation is a complex interaction involving vocalizing, self-distraction, manipulating an object, or removing oneself from a situation. All of these actions work together to decrease the level of arousal associated with potential distress. As the child learns adaptive functioning and coping they are able to organize and monitor their own actions/responses and regulate negative emotions. This is an example of social learning. When skills are utilized to deal successfully with a situation, thus decreasing feelings of frustration and reinforcing feelings of self-efficacy, they are likely to utilize the technique or strategy when presented with the same or similar stimuli. An example would be a child to hold their own hands when given a set limit of not touching an identified object, thus demonstrating an adaptive response

b. Emotion regulation and adaptation: successful experience. Emotions experienced while engaged in a particular action reinforce adaptive regulation or ability to respond to a specific situation. As skill increases behavioral responses are generalized. Internal goals motivate activity to obtain that goal. Such goals may be at the foundation level of safety, security and homeostasis or for mastery and accomplishment of skill. When learning a new skill one can experience frustration or anger when acquisition of the skill feels elusive versus the experience of a positive emotional state (joy/interest) which serves to motivate the child to engage in the activity to be repeatedly practiced. When the infant feels overwhelmed by the bar being too high to accomplish, the result is feelings of sadness and defeat, even withdrawal from the activity

c. The role of arousal in the socialization of emotion: the infant's first goal is to learn affective tolerance (AT), whereby they take an interest in their environment and regulate their level of arousal and feeding and sleep cycle. AT refers to learning to tolerate the intensity of arousal and being able to regulate their internal state allowing them to maintain the interaction and derive pleasure from it instead of feeling overwhelmed. Initially, the parent helps the infant to maintain maximum internal arousal while continuing engagement in the interaction, thus facilitating their secure attachment. If the primary caregiver provides excessive or minimal stimulation, the infant's response is to withdraw from the stimulation. The optimal infant threshold for arousal, tolerance for stimulation and ability to self-regulate varies individually, thus requiring an attuned primary caregiver who effectively reads their infant's cues signaling the need for more or less arousal or engagement

d. Mood regulation: first define the difference between emotions, feelings and moods. Emotions last only a few seconds, and the associated ANS responses last a bit longer. There is a direct proportional relationship between the length of emotion and the feeling of the emotion. In other words, the longer an emotion is experienced the more intense the feeling. Additionally, feelings occur when emotion is being expressed. When a feeling lasts for a long period of time (an hour or more) it becomes a mood. Duration is an operational issue in emotional disorders where the emotion is intense and interferes with level of functioning. Memories associated with events may bring forth associated feelings. Also, sights, sounds (words/phrases/or other sounds), and smells may provoke a reaction resulting from the elicited feelings.

It is hoped that saving the discussion on emotions as a closing topic reinforces the importance of consolidating immensely complex information for a working model of assessment and intervention. To create an opportunity for a small child and their family system to be assessed in order to understand what is working and what is not could be a turning point which alters their quality of life. For an assessment and ensuing interventions to provide an optimal and enduring change requires depth of understanding of the child's internal and external experience.

Bibliography

Armstrong, K. L., Previtera, N., & McCallum, R. N. (2000). Medicalizing normalcy? Management of irritable babies. *Journal of Paediatrics and Child Health, 36*, 301–305.

Ayers, A. J. (2005). *Sensory integration and the child: Understanding hidden sensory challenges.* Los Angeles: WPS.

Bates, J. E. (1984). *Infant characteristics questionnaire, revised.* Bloomington: Indiana University Press.

Becker, K., Blomeyer, D., El-Faddagh, M., Esser, G., Schmidt, M. H., Banaschewewski, T., et al. (2010). From regulatory problems in infancy to attention-deficit/hyperactivity disorder in childhood: a moderating role in the dopamine D4 receptor gene? *Journal of Pediatrics, 156*(5), 798–803. e2

Becker, K., Holtmann, M., Laucht, M., & Schmidt, M. H. (2004). Are regulatory problems in infancy precursors of later hyperkinetic problems? *Acta Paediatrica, 93*(11), 1463–1469.

Bell, M. A., & Deater-Deckard, K. (2007). Biological systems and the development of self-regulation: integrating behavior, genetics, and psychophysiology. *Journal of Developmental and Behavioral Pediatrics, 28*(5), 409–420.

Benson, J. B., & Haith, M. M. (2009). *Social and emotional development in infancy and early childhood.* San Diego: Academic Press.

Blair, C. (2002). School readiness: Integrating cognition and emotion in a neurobiological conceptualization of children's functioning at school entry. *American Psychologist, 57*, 111–127.

Bowlby, J. (1969). *Attachment and loss: Volume 1: Attachment.* The Hogarth Press and the Institute of Psychoanalysis.

Calkins, S. D. (2004). Early attachment process and the development of emotional self regulation. In R. F. Baumeister & K. D. Vohs (Eds.), *The handbook of self-regulation.* Hillsdale NJ: Lawrence Erlbaum.

Calkins, S. D., Dedmon, S. E., Gill, K. L., Lomax, S. E., & Johnson, L. M. (2002). Frustration in infancy: implications for emotion regulation, physiological processes, and temperament. *Infancy, 3*(2), 175–197.

Campbell, S. B. (2002). *Behavior problems in preschool children: clinical and developmental issues.* (2nd ed.). New York: Guilford.

Carlson, S. T., & Moses, L. J. (2001). Individual differences in inhibitory control in children's theory of mind. *Child Development, 72,* 1032–1053.

Casenhiser, D., Breinbauer, C., & Greenspan, S.I. (2007). Evaluating Greenspan's social emotional Growth Scale/chart as a screening for autism. Presented at the ICDL 11th Annual International conference: Critical Factors for Optimal Outcomes for Children with Autism and Special Needs. Tyson Corner, VA: November 2007.

Casey, B. J., Durston, S., & Fossella, J. A. (2001). Evidence for a mechanistic model of cognitive control. *Clinical Neuroscience Research, 1,* 267–282.

CCC. (2000). The Copenhapen Child Cohort 2000 (former CCCC 2000) Longitudinal study of 6090 children. CCC 2000 Study Team – E.M. Olsen, T. Houmann, E. Christiansen, S.L. Landorph, K. Heering, S. Kaas-Nielsen, V. Samberg, A. Lichtenberg, T. Jorgensen, & A.M. Skovgaard. Correspondence to: Anne Mette Skovgaard, Child and Adolescent Psychiatric Centre, University Hospital of Copenhagen, Glostrup, DK: 2600; Tel: +4543233747/3759; +4543233973; email: ames@glo.regionHdk.

Cesari, A., Maestro, S., Cavallero, C., Chilosi, A., Pecini, C., & Pfanner, L. (2003). Diagnostic boundaries between regulatory and multisystem developmental disorders: a clinical study. *Infant Mental Health Journal, 24*(4), 365–377.

Charney, D. (2004). Psychobiological mechanism of resilience and vulnerability: implications for successful adaptation to extreme stress. *American Journal of Psychiatry, 161,* 195–216.

Charney, D., & Southwick, S. (2007). Social support and resilience to stress: from Neurobiology to clinical practice. *Psychiatry, 4*(5), 35–40.

Chatoor, I., & Ganiban, J. (2004). The diagnostic assessment and classification of feeding disorders. In R. Carmen-Wiggins, & A. Carter (Eds.), *Handbook of infant, toddler, and preschool mental health assessment.* Oxford University Press.

Cole, P. M., & Deater-Deckard, K. (2009). Emotion regulation, risk, and psychopathology. *Journal of Child Psychology and Psychiatry, 50*(11), 1327–1330.

Costello, E. J., Egger, H. L., & Angold, A. (2005). The developmental epidemiology of anxiety disorders: phenomenology, prevalence, and comorbidity. *Child and adolescent psychiatric clinics of North America, 14,* 631–648.

Costello, E. J., Egger, H., & Angold, A. (2005). 10-year research update review: the epidemiology of child and adolescent psychiatric disorders: I. Methods and public health burden. *Journal of the American Academy of Child & Adolescent Psychiatry, 44*(10), 972–986.

Costello, E. J., Foley, D., & Angold, A. (2006). 10-year research update review: the epidemiology of child and adolescent psychiatric disorders: II. Developmental epidemiology. *Journal of the American Academy of Child & Adolescent Psychiatry, 45*(1), 8–25.

Cummings, E. M., Davies, P. T., & Campbell, S. B. (2000). *Developmental psychopathology and family process: theory, research and clinical implications.* New York: Guilford Press.

Cummings, E. M., & Davies, P. (1996). Emotional security as a regulatory process in normal development and the development of psychopathology. *Developmental psychopathology, 8,* 123–139.

DC: 0-3R. (2007). Department of Community Health-Mental Health Services to Children and Families. December 18, 2007. http://www.mi-aimh.org/documents/crosswalkaccess_elegibilitywithdch_title_121807

DeGangi, G. A. (2000). *Pediatric disorders of regulatiion in affect and behavior.* San Diego: Academic Press.

DeGangi, G. A., & Kendall, A. (2006). *Effective parenting for the hard to manage child.* New York: Routledge Press.

DeGangi, G. A., Porges, S. W., Sickel, R. Z., & Greenspan, S. I. (1993). Four year follow-up of a sample of regulatory disordered infants. *Infant Mental Health Journal, 14*(4), 330–343.

Diagnostic Classification of Mental Health and Developmental Disorders of Infancy and Early Childhood. Revised 0-3 DC:0-3R. (2005). National Center for Infants, Toddlers, and Families. Washington DC: 20005–1013.

Diamond, A. (2009). The interplay of biology and the environment broadly defined. *Developmental Psychology, 45*(1), 1–8.

Diener, M. L., Mangelsdorf, S. C., McHale, J. L., & Frosch, C. A. (2002). Infants' behavioral strategies for emotion regulation with fathers and mothers: associations with emotional expressions and attachment quality. *Infancy, 3*(2), 153–177.

Dozier, M., & Peloso, E. (2006). The role of early stressors in child health and mental health outcomes. *Archives of Pediatrics & Adolescent Medicine, 160*(12), 1300–1301.

Ekvall, S., & Ekvall, V. (2005). *Pediatric nutrition in chronic diseases and developmental disorders.* Oxford University Press.

Fan, J., Fossella, J. A., Summer, T., & Posner, M. I. (2003). Mapping the genetic variation of executive attention onto brain activity. *Proceedings of the National Academy of Sciences of the United States of America, 100,* 7406–7411.

Fenichel, E., & Eggbeer, (1990). *Preparing practitioners to work with infants, toddlers, and their families: issues and recommendations for educators and trainers.* Washington DC: ZERO TO THREE/National Center for Infants, Toddlers and their Families. author initial.

Flaherty, E. G., Thompson, R., Litrownik, A. J., Theodore, A., English, D. J., Black, M. M., et al. (2006). Effects of early childhood adversity on child health. *Archives of Pediatrics & Adolescent Medicine, 160*(12), 1232–1238.

Fox, N. A., & Calkins, S. D. (2003). The development of self-control of emotion: intrinsic and extrinsic influences. *MotivatEm otions, 27*(1), 7–26.

Greenspan S.I. (2002a). Meeting learning challenges: working with the child of alcoholic parents. Scholast Early Child Today, Jan/Feb.

Greenspan, S. I. (2002). The affect diathesis hypothesis: the role of emotions in core deficit in autism and the development of intelligence and social skills. *Journal of Developmental and Learning Disorders, 5*, 1.

Greenspan, S. I. (2003). Child care research: a clinical perspective. *Child Development, 74*(4), 1064–1068.

Greenspan, S. I., & DeGangi, G. A. (2001). Research on FEAS: test development reliability and validity studies. In S. Greenspan, G. DeGangi, & S. Wieder (Eds.), *The Functional Emotional Assessment Scale (FEAS) for infancy and early childhood. Clinical and research applications* (pp. 167–247). Bethesda: Interdisciplinary Council on Development and Learning Disorders (ICDL).

Greenspan, S. I., Wieder, S., & Simon, R. (1998). *The child with special needs.* Reading, MA: Merloyd Laurence.

Hiscock, H. (2004). Problem crying in infancy. *Medical Journal of Australia, 181*(9), 507–512.

Johnson & Johnson Pediatric round Table Series <www.JJPI.com> ph 1-877-565-5465 accessed 8/17/11.

Jones, L., Rothbart, M. K., & Posner, M. I. (2003). Development of executive attention in preschool children. *Developmental Science, 6*, 498–504.

Keren, M., Dolberg, D., Koster, T., Danino, K., & Feldman, K. (2010). *Journal of Family Psychology, 24*(5), 597–604. article title

Knitzer J. (2000). *Children and Welfare Reform, Issue Brief No. 8. Promoting resilience: helping young children and parents affected by substance abuse, domestic violence, and depression in the context of welfare reform.* NCCP: National Center for Children of Poverty. Columbia University: Mailman School of Public Health.

Kostuik, L.M., & Fouts, G.T. (2002). Understanding of emotion regulation in adolescent females with conduct problems: a qualitative analysis. The Qualitative Report 7(1). <www.niva.edu/ssss/QR/QR7-1/kostiuk.html>

Kranowitz, C. (2003). *The out of sync child has fun.* New York: Penguin Group.

Lieberman, A. F. (2004). Traumatic stress and quality of attachment: reality and internalization in disorder and infant mental health. *Infant Mental Health Journal, 25*(4), 336–351.

Lyons-Ruth, K., & Zeanah, C. H. (1993). The family context of mental health, I: affective development in the primary caregiver relationship. In C. H. Zeanah (Ed.), *Handbook of infant mental health* (pp. 14–37). New York: Guilford.

Mahler, M., Pine, F., & Bergman, A. (1975). *The psychological birth of the human infant.* New York: Basic Books.

May-Benson, T., Koomar, J., & Teasdale, A. (2006). *Prevalence of pre-/post-natal and developmental factors in 1000 children with SPD.* Watertown MA: The Spiral Foundation.

Olsen, E. M., Petersen, J., Skovgaard, A. M., & Jorgensen, T. (2007). Failure to thrive: the prevalence and concurrence of anthropometric criteria in the general population. *Archives of Disease in Childhood, 92*(2), 109–114.

Polan, H. J., & Hofer, M. A. (1999). Psychobiological origins of infant attachment and separation responses. In J. Cassidy, & P. R. Shaver (Eds.), *Handbook of attachment: theory, research, and clinical applications* (pp. 162–180). New York: Guilford.

Reebye, P., & Stalker, A. (2007). *Understanding regulation risorders of sensory processing in children.* London: Jessical Kingsley Publishing.

Rolf, J., Masten, A. S., Cicchett, D., Neuchterlein, K. H., & Weintraub, S. (1990). *Development and Psychopathology* (vol 2). Cambridge University Press. (copywrited by the American medical Association).

Rothbart, M. K., Derryberry, D., & Hershey, K. (2000). Stability of temperament in childhood: laboratory infant assessment to parent report at seven years. In V. J. Molfese & D. L. Molfese (Eds.), *Temperament and personality development across the lifespan* (pp. 85–119). Hillsdale, NJ: Erlbaum.

Rothbart, M. K., Ellis, L. K., Rueda, R., & Posner, M. I. (2003). Developing mechanisms of temperamental effortful control. *Journal of Personality, 71*(6), 1113–1144.

Rothbart, M. K., & Rueda, M. R. (2005). The development of effortful control. In U. Mayr, E. Awh, & S. Keele (Eds.), *Developing individuality in the human brain: a tribute to Michael I. Posner* (pp. 167–188). Washington DC: American Psychological Association.

Rueda, M. R., Fan, J., McCandliss, B., Halparin, J. D., Gruber, D. B., Pappert, L., et al. (2004). Development of attentional networks in childhood. *Neuropsychologia, 42*, 1029–1040.

Rutter, M. (2003). Commentary: Causal process leading to antisocial behavior. *Developmental Psychology, 39*, 372–378.

Rutter, M. (2005). Categories, dimensions, and the mental health of children and adolescents. *Annals of the New York Academy of Sciences, 1008*, 11–21. doi:10.1196/annals.1301.002. Published online Jan 2006.

Rutter, M., Kim-Kohen, J., & Maughan, B. (2006). Continuities and discontinuities in psychopathology between childhood and adult life. *Journal of Child Psychology and Psychiatry, 47*(3-4), 276–295.

Rutter, M., Avshalom, C., & Moffitt, T. (2003). Using sex differences in psychopathology to study causal mechanisms: identifying issues and research strategies. *Journal of Child Psychology and Psychiatry, 44*(8), 1092–1115.

Sapolsky, R. (2004). *Why zebras don't get ulcers*. New York: MacMillan.

Schore, A. N. (2001). Effects of secure attachment relationship on right brain development, affect regulation, and infant mental health. *Infant Mental Health Journal, 22*(1-2), 7–66.

Schore, A. N. (2002). Dysregulation of the right brain: a fundamental mechanism of traumatic attachment and the pathogenesis of posttraumatic stress disorder. *Australian and New Zealand Journal of Psychiatry, 36*(1), 9–30.

Schore, A. N. (2005). Attachment, affect regulation, and the developing right brain: linking developmental neuroscience to pediatrics. *Pediatrics in Review, 26*, 204–217.

Science Daily. (2010). Prenatal alcohol exposure can alter the brain's developing pain regulatory system. January 28, 2010. <http://www.sciencedaily.com/releases/2010/01/100127164017.htm>

Skovgaard, A. M. (2010). Mental health problems and psychopathology in infancy and early childhood. *Danish Medical Bulletin, 57* B4193. <anne.mette.skovgaard@regionh.dk>

Sonuga-Barke, E., Thomson, M., Abikoff, H., Klein, R., & Miller-Brotman, L. (2006). Nonpharmacological interventions for preschoolers with ADHD: The case for specialized parent training. *Infants and Young Children, 19*(2), 142–153.

Southwick , S. M., Vythilingam, M., & Charney, D. S. (2005). The psychobiology of depression and resilience to stress: Implications for prevention and treatment. *Annual Review of Clinical Psychology, 1*, 255–291.

Taylor, K. & Trott, M. (1991). (Pyramid) Maryann Trott at 1621 Richmond Drive SE, Albuquerque, NM 87106 USA.

Teichner, M. H. (2002). Scars that won't heal: the neurobiology of child abuse: maltreatment at an early age can have enduring effects on a child's brain. *Scientific American, 286*, 68–76.

Terrikangas, O. M., Aronen, E. T., Martin, R. P., & Huttunen, M. (1998). Effects of infant temperament and early interventions on the psychiatric symptoms of adolescents. *Journal of the American Academy of Child & Adolescent Psychiatry, 37*(10), 1070–1076.

Thompson, R. A. (1994). Emotion regulation: a theme in search of definition. *JSTOR Monographs of the Society for Research in Child Development, 59*(2/3), 25–52.

Thompson, R. A., Lewis, M. D., & Calkins, S. D. (2008). Reassessing emotion regulation. *Child Devel Perspect, 2*(3), 124–131.

Trevarthen, C., & Aitken, K. J. (2001). Infant intersubjectivity: research, theory, and clinical applications. *Journal of Child Psychology and Psychiatry and Allied Discipline, 42*(1), 3–48.

van der Kolk, B. A. (2005). Developmental trauma disorder. *Psychiatric Annals, 35*, 401–408.

Weinfield, N. S., Sroufe, L. A., Egeland, B., & Carlson, E. A. (1999). The nature of individual differences in infant-caregiver attachment. In J. Cassidy, & P. R. Shaver (Eds.), *Handbook of attachment: theory, research, and clinical applications*. New York: Guilford Press.

Wolke, D., Schmid, G., Schreier, A., & Meyer, D. (2009). Crying and feeding problems in infancy and cognitive outcome in preschool children born at risk: a prospective population study. *Journal of Developmental & Behavioral Pediatrics, 30*(3), 226–238. doi:10.1097/DBP.obo13e3181a85973.

Wolraich, M. L., Drotar, D. D., Dworkin, P. H., & Perrin, E. C. (2008). *Developmental-behavioral pediatrics: evidence and practice*. Philadelphia: Mosby, Inc.

Zahn-Waxler, C. (2000). The development of empathy, guilt, and internalization of distress: implication for gender differences in internalizing and externalizing problems. In R. J. Davidson (Ed.), *Anxiety, depression, and emotion*. Oxford: Oxford University Press.

Zeanah, C. H. (2000). Psychopathology. In C. H. Zeanah (Ed.), *Handbook of infant mental health* (2nd ed.). New York: Guilford Press.

Further Reading

Cohen, J., Ngozi, O., Clothier, S., & Poppe, J. (2005). Helping young children succeed: strategies to promote early childhood social and emotional development. National Conference of State Legislatures. A project of NCLS and ZERO TO THREE.

National Institute on Early Childhood Development and Education. Office of Education Research and Improvement. U.S. Department of Education. 555 New Jersey Ave., N.W., Washington, D.C. 20208. <www.ed.gov/office/OERI/ECI>

CHAPTER 2

Assessment and Diagnosis

With contributions from Sara Katz, M.A. and Jamie Mize, M.A, CCC-SLP

The healthy infant is able to regulate physiological homeostatic functions. As they mature their regulatory abilities expand in complexity to include emotion regulation, self-soothing, sensorimotor integration, motor planning, regulation of sleep/wake cycles, and hunger/satiety cycles. All of these dynamic changes in competence are necessary for challenging multifaceted social, behavioral, and emotional interactions (DeGangi, 2000; Benson & Haith, 2009). Infants with regulatory disorders left untreated face the possibility for later developmental, sensorimotor, and/or emotional and behavioral problems in the area of cognitive abilities, attention span, activity level, emotional maturity, motor maturity, and tactile sensitivity. Therefore, the early identification of social and emotional problems in infants, toddlers and young children is crucial to facilitating the appropriate interventions and level of support necessary for building their social and emotional competence and decrease the likelihood of placement in special education programs.

The task at hand is an immensely important undertaking, and one that has the potential to alter the quality of life. If the assessment scope was narrowed to include only the capability of sustained attention many children would not find themselves placed within the category of special education. It is a challenge to identify early life cognitive functioning which would distinguish them as being at risk for later cognitive delays. DeGangi (2000) asserts these infants and toddlers often score well within the normal range on assessment instruments measuring motor and cognitive development, however, if left untreated they are at risk to develop attentional, behavioral, and developmental deficits before they reach school age. Therefore, if infants or toddlers present with regulatory difficulties or have been exposed *in utero* to substances, they are candidates for, and should receive, a neurobehavioral assessment to evaluate the type and degree of their atypical behavior (Greenspan, 2003).

Individual differences are not strong determinants because the circumstances and context in which infants/young children are observed can have a significant impact upon their ability to manage their feelings. For example, whether or not their environment is familiar or unfamiliar, a caregiver is present or absent, as well as the type and degree of the stimuli all bear potential influence. Therefore, behavior manifestations of emotion regulation should be interpreted with caution, especially when attempting to measure across situations because they may demonstrate better management of feelings in some situations and offer a relatively poor performance in others (Reebye & Stalker, 2007; Benson & Haith, 2009; Gleason & Zeanah, 2005; Gross et al., 1993). The following scenario offers clarification of a situation where a regulatory disorder is of concern and emphasizes the aforementioned contextual experience:

> Rebecca, a fearful, anxious infant is brought to the clinic/office to be assessed. She startles every time she is touched by someone she doesn't recognize or when she hears an unexpected loud noise. However, when the trained clinician who has

Therapist's Guide to Pediatric Affect and Behavior Regulation. DOI: http://dx.doi.org/10.1016/B978-0-12-386884-8.00002-1

taken time to establish a bond/build rapport within the context of a comfortable and trusting relationship examines her, she does not demonstrate any defining evidence of sensory hyperactivity or processing difficulties. Thus, the suspected regulatory problems are determined to be secondary to anxiety and/or fears. In conclusion, Anxiety Disorder of Infancy would be regarded as the first diagnostic option.

When working with children, parental/caregiver observations and their levels of functioning are an important component of the clinical picture. Caregivers can be of tremendous benefit regarding the identification and intervention of children with regulatory disorders. Unfortunately, many mentally ill adults are parenting children, either alone or with the support of others. As mentioned in Chapter 1, substance abuse and depression have been identified as contributing factors in creating an environment which lacks consistency and enrichment, negatively impacting the parent–child relationship, and increases the risk of child neglect and abuse. Therefore, highlighting the importance of assessing the interactions of parental/caretaker functioning, environment, and who composes the family system.

The need for comprehensive assessment has led to an appropriate focus on screening and assessment tools to assure the identification of problems which can be treated in a preventative manner, as well as accurately assessing regulatory disorders comprised of self-regulation, sensory processing, attention, and emotion regulation. The US Education Department (2007) reinforces this concept by asserting the importance of a thorough evaluative process. The goal is to promote school readiness. School readiness includes cognitive readiness and knowledge, as well as social and emotional development as important antecedents of a child's emotional intelligence.

Assessment of development and behavior is generally a multistage process structured to acquire sufficient information and understanding of a child so that appropriate and effective decisions can be made. Different methods of information collecting result in a different constellation of information. Therefore, it is of utmost importance to utilize methods and procedures which are "best suited" to a child's developmental stage and referral question(s). DeGangi (2000) outlines a comprehensive assessment model which serves to:

1. Evaluate performance in sensorimotor, regulatory, and attentional processes impacting functional learning and behaviors
2. Incorporate behavioral observation of parents regarding how the child behaviors affect the manner in which he/she functions in the family system and in the home environment.
3. Examine parental characteristics (stress, and how they interact with the child) in addition to their ability to participate in the assessment and treatment process.

ASSESSMENT STRATEGIES FOR THE REGULATORY DISORDERED INFANT/CHILD

The assessment and intervention of infants and young children are oriented toward prevention. It is a time marked by rapid developmental change and lays the foundation for future development. Therefore, the clinician's primary focus is aimed at facilitating change(s) toward healthy, optimal development and strengthening caregiver and environmental support systems. Since caretakers are central to the treatment team and a conduit of change they are always considered in the assessment and intervention of infants and toddlers. Caregivers of infants and toddlers often feel anxious or guilty because they believe that problems exist because of inadequate parenting skills. The development of a respectful relationship with the caregiver(s) is invaluable. The respect is built upon their knowledge of the child, being a central influence in the child's life, their desire for a better life and opportunities for their child, along with having unique values, preferences, and cultural beliefs.

With regard to the child, it is imperative to assess the nature, severity, and developmental impact of the child's behavioral difficulties, functional impairment, and subjective distress on the child and on the family. Therefore, there is a need to identify the risk and protective factors that, during the process of development, contribute to or ameliorate the current concerns. Ultimately, the value and integrity of the assessment will be revealed in the accuracy of the diagnosis and the associated interventions.

Due to the complexity of infancy/early childhood, assessments should be reflective of all potential contributing factors and take into consideration that, in infants and young children, developmental changes take place quickly, developmental appropriateness of behaviors change over time, and the environmental context influences developmental progress. Preferably assessment data are obtained from multiple perspectives and integrated into relevant clinical decisions. Assessment and diagnosis must be guided by the awareness that all infants and toddlers are participants in relationships, usually within families, and that these families are part of a larger community and culture. Therefore, all infants and children exhibit their own developmental progression which demonstrates individual differences in their motor, sensory, language, cognitive, affective and interactive patterns.

Those performing pediatric assessments seek to identify the following in association with the presenting problem(s) (DeGangi, 2000; Frankel & Harmon, 2006):

- child's performance in sensorimotor, regulatory, and attentional processes that affect functional learning and behaviors
- speech, hearing, auditory processing
- medical history
- pregnancy (prenatal through labor and delivery)
- multiple areas of development (psychological and developmental status)
- temperament
- progression toward developmental milestones
- socioemotional milestones
- medical problems/neuropsychological deficits
- resiliency/strengths/talents
- individual differences
  - temperament, constitution
  - behavioral goals, skills associated with getting needs met age appropriately
  - language issues
- regulatory patterns
  - sleep/wake cycles
  - feeding/satiety cycles
- quality of infant-caregiver(s) relationship
  - affective tone
  - rhythms/expectancies/contingencies
  - comfort seeking
  - secure base, exploration
  - social referencing
  - relating to others
- infant's contextual experiences
  - parent(s) level of psychological functioning
    parent characteristics (parental stress/interactional style)
    parent history of mental illness
    parent history of substance abuse
    parental response to child across situations
    parent conception and birth experience (and its impact on the infant–caregiver relationship)
    parental expectation of child
  - family as a caregiving support system

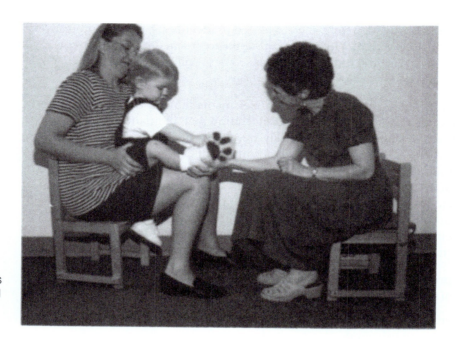

FIGURE 2.1
Infant demonstrating organized motor and tactile response on items from adaptive-motor and visual-tactile integration subtests.

      ○ behavioral observations of the child and how their behaviors affect the way in which they function within the family and home environment
      ○ cultural, community, and ethnic influences.

*With a non-verbal child, it is necessary to gather from the caregiver data about the caregiving environment including information about the caregiver's mental health status.

The assessment process is initiated by the referral question and begins with a comprehensive interview of the caregivers, includes behavioral observation of the infant/child and the use of various assessment tools depending on the referral question (Figure 2.1). Potentially, a skilled multidisciplinary treatment team may be involved in the assessment. This team of skilled professionals could include: clinical/school psychologist, neuropsychologist, developmental specialist, occupational therapist, education specialist, speech pathologist, and an infant/child mental health specialist. Assessment is generally a multistage process in which information from clinical sources and tools from numerous perspectives are integrated into clinical decisions. The systematic assessment process includes the following types of information sources (DeGangi, 1991, 2000; Wolraich et al., 2008; Meschan & Perrin, 2010):

- The intake interview (infant/child)
- The home visit
- Clinical assessment of the child
- Self-regulation and sensory processing and reactivity
  - Parent report measures
  - Instruments for direct clinical observation of the child
- Child temperament
  - parent report measures
- Sustained attention
  - Parent report measures
  - Instruments for direct clinical observation of the child
- Parent–child interactions
- Medical examination (medical problems and vision, hearing, speech processes)
- Neurological examination

- Executive function
- Speech pathology
- Special education
- Occupational therapy.

The Intake Interview

Caregiver-report instruments and interviews offer a critical source of information about the young child's social-emotional and behavioral development. Caregivers have the greatest range of historical and cross-contextual views of the child's experience. This allows them to provide information about (low) base-rate behaviors not likely to be observed in a formal or professional setting. Additionally, the meanings and interpretations that caregivers attribute to behavior play a central role in how they respond when the child is engaging in that behavior. Thus enriching the clinical perspective and information to be considered diagnostically.

The goal of a thorough assessment and accurate diagnosis is the development of a comprehensive treatment/case plan. This requires clinicians to identify internal and external risks and adversities as well as strengths, competencies and resilience processes in multiple realms or settings. The result is a treatment/case plan that fully utilizes resources to manage risk and adversities in order to promote and reinforce optimal functioning and development. The interview plays an important role in the course of assessment. However, caregiver-report instruments should never be used as the only source in determining if a child is evidencing difficulty. At the very least, a second source of information should be obtained. Nevertheless, caregiver-reports can provide starting points for early detection and should be included as part of the clinical evaluation.

The interview method could be accomplished by a formal structured or semi-structured instrument. However, when numerous family system issues are evident it will likely be more beneficial to take the time to develop trust and positive regard demonstrated by the observer's genuine concern and interest. This will allow for a more cooperative clinical environment in which to explore the more intimate details of their daily lives, family background and other pertinent history. DeGangi (2000) offers an example outline of an assessment interview with considerations which should play a role in all clinical contacts with the perspective of meeting the client where they are which means being sensitive to wording, the type of information being sought, and the emotional cues being reflected during the interview. In other words, use common sense in this semi-structured interview to adapt questions to the circumstance and response. DeGangi's intake interview can be found in the business forms section.

Family assessments are based on a combination of observations, interviews, self-report measures and social history. Assessing the family is essential to determine the range of services that are needed for the family system, determining potential level of compliance (need for monitoring and support), to explore options and to make suggestions/recommendations. In some cases, a family assessment suggests that family factors are at the source of the problem, acutely precipitated the problem, and have maintained the problem. Such findings indicate the need for an intervention to alter patterns of family interaction. Therefore, to make sure there is an outcome of adequate information from the parents/caregivers acquired during the intake interview, the person conducting the interview needs to be able to answer the following questions when the interview is concluded:

- Are there safety and protection issues that must be addressed?
- What are the relative strengths and weaknesses of the family?
- What are the family's needs?
- Can the family meet the needs of the child?
- What are the resources available to the family (extended family, church, community, etc.)?

- Does this family have a functional hierarchical structure?
- Is the family enmeshed or disengaged?
- Are major mental health problems present in the family?
- Are there any substance abuse problems present in the family?
- Is there any evidence of personality disorder(s) present in the parents/caregivers?
- Is the family competent to provide for basic needs?
- Do the parents/caregivers have the ability to manage problem behaviors in age-appropriate ways without any safety risks?
- Is there any evidence of multigenerational patterns of abuse or neglect, substance abuse, etc.?
- Parental/caregiver ability to empathize
- Parental/caregiver ability to nurture
- What resources have been helpful to this family system in the past?
- How does this family system cope with stress and crises?

The Greenspan Floortime Approach

The Greenspan Floortime Approach course (www.stanleygrenspan.com; Wieder & Greenspan, 2001) is a comprehensive developmental approach to assessment and diagnosis for infants and children which tailors or individualizes interaction. It acknowledges that it is essential for all interactions and learning to understand a child's sensory profile as well as emotion playing a central role in the development of intelligence, language, motor and sensory processing. The Floortime Approach by Greenspan (www.stanleygreenspan.com) and DeGangi (2000) concur regarding the importance of developing a thorough clinical understanding of infant/child sensory regulation and response to stimuli and how it influences behavior, attention, impulse control, postural control, motor control, motor planning and sequencing, and functional skills, as well as an emphasis on auditory processing, visual-spatial, and executive functioning. Additionally, the assessment of an infant/child must include the attachment relationship. All of this information is necessary for accurate assessing and diagnosing so that an effective plan of treatment and intervention can be planned.

The DIR Floortime Approach includes a method for clinical assessment and outlines the basic frame of the diagnostic profile:

The DIR Model

- D = Functional Developmental Stages
- I = Individual differences in the areas of auditory processing, motor planning, and sensory modulation
- R = Relationships, dynamic, evolving/ever changing learning interactions and family patterns

Clinical Assessment Approaches

- Evaluating adaptive development (motor, affective, sensory, language, cognitive, and sense of self)
- Observing infant/child behavior, affects, and developmental patterns
- Comprehending infant/child-caregiver interactions and family patterns
- Discovering constitutional and maturational differences
- Taking the initial interview and extracting the developmental history
- Assessing clinical challenges (for example, the differences between developmental variations and what constitutes disorders)
- Utilization of the Functional Emotional Assessment Scale (FEAS) and the Social-Emotional Growth Chart

Diagnostic Profile

- Determining functional developmental levels (in comparison to age-appropriate or age-expected levels)
- Determining the range, flexibility, and stability of adaptive and coping strategies

- Assessing the contribution of family patterns and all other environmental patterns, stresses, conflicts, constitutional patterns and maturational patterns
- Evaluating emotional and developmental delays as well as disorders

Motivational Interviewing

This approach to interviewing has long been used in medical settings and associated substance abuse treatment and harm reduction. It is a client-centered method of interviewing which is brief and directive. It is designed to improve and increase intrinsic motivation for behavior change by exploring the positives and negatives associated with change and decreasing ambivalence to change. This client-centered approach is accomplished by eliciting information in an empathic, accepting, and non-judgmental manner as a collaborative plan for change. While motivational interviewing would not be a process used in engaging children, it would be useful in interviewing parents and increasing their investment in the change process (Miller & Rollnik, 1991; Johnson, 2005, Wolraich et al., 2008).

The Home Visit

Development of a clear picture of the home environment and to assure an adequate provision of services requires a home visit. A home visit should be conducted by someone trained to observe and assess the home environment. This is an important assessment because whatever resources are provided to the family and home environment must meet the goal(s) to assist in the management of the child's behaviors or to benefit and improve the parent–child interaction with the overall goal of optimal functioning and development of the child. Caldwell & Bradley (1978, 1984, refer to HOME) developed the *Home Observation for Measurement of the Environment* (HOME) which is a useful scale for this very purpose. There is an infant/toddler (IT HOME) version, the early childhood (EC HOME) version, the middle child (MC HOME) version, and the early adolescent (EA HOME) version. Information is obtained during a 45–90-minute home visit at a time when the target child and the child's primary caregiver are present and awake. The procedure is a semi-structured observation and interview designed to be minimally intrusive, thus allowing family members to proceed as they normally would. Observations of parent–child interaction and discussion with the parent about objects, events, and transactions that occur are explored and interpreted from the child's point of view. The intent is to understand the child's experiences and opportunities. Additionally, this home interview tool offers interview techniques to clarify parental concerns. Therefore, parents often speak freely about their concerns and difficulties, feeling they are not alone and the presenting problems will be ameliorated and/or resolved (DeGangi, 2000).

Recognizing the importance of parental observations, their evaluation and observations are enhanced by the intermittent use of evidenced-based screening tools along with parent questionnaires. These informational resources are extremely valuable to the intervening professional in combination with professionally administered screening tools and assessment tools. Family self-reports and a history are insufficient without observing the family in action. The assessment needs to be dynamic and fluid, and demonstrate the family energy, style, behavior communication style, skill level, etc. Additionally, screening tools can be administered intermittently to supplement data, in a targeted manner to explore in depth parental concerns, or to assure early detection.

Clinical Assessment

SCREENING AND ASSESSMENT

The Early Intervention Program (EI) has existed since 1994 (for all states and the District of Columbia) to provide screening, evaluation, and intervention to infants and toddlers with disabilities (0–36 months) (Figure 2.2). While the program has expanded, data show that only 2.5% of age eligible children receive EI services. It is estimated that 13% of

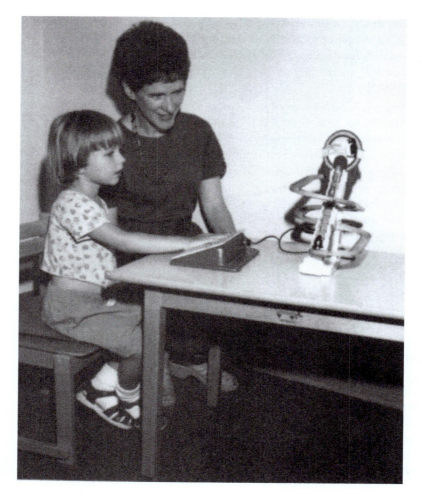

64 FIGURE 2.2
Child attending to visual attention task on the Test of Attention in Infants.

young children aged 9–24 months have developmental delays identifying them as eligible for EI services and that one child in ten with delays received necessary intervention by age 24 months. One study cited young children referred to developmental specialists by their pediatricians and found a 15.5 month delay between parental concern and the child receiving a developmental evaluation (Shavell et al., 2001; US Education Department, 2007; Rosenberg et al., 2008). Therefore, early identification of social and emotional problems in infants, toddlers and young children is fundamental if they are to be assisted in building social and emotional competence. The need for prevention or early elimination of social or emotional problems in young children is an international concern, addressed in the USA by the Individuals with Disabilities Education Act (IDEA) Amendment of 1997 (PL 105-17). In the 1980s, the developmental evaluation of infants and children found increased interest with the 1986 Education of Handicapped Act Amendments (Public Law 99-457) and continues with the Individuals with Disabilities Education Improvement Act of 2004 (Public Law 108-446), a revision of IDEA. To determine if a child qualifies for services from 0–5 years five major areas of development are assessed: cognitive, communication, physical, social-emotional, and adaptive. Thus making developmental evaluation critical. *State and/ or federal law regulates determination of services eligibility for support program under the No Child Left Behind (such as Title I, Migrant and Bilingual, and American Indian Services, as well as early intervention and special education services).

Screening tools are informal instruments that are utilized to define better the types of behaviors or characteristics that may indicate sensory processing difficulties. Screening involves procedures to identify infants/children who are at risk for a particular problem with associated targeted interventions. It is recommended that sensory issues always be considered in young children because it is early identification and intervention that offer the opportunity to promote optimal development versus developmental dysfunction. Even when dysfunction cannot be prevented the measured outcome of effective intervention demonstrates benefit to the child as well as improved family functioning. Additionally, children identified with environmental risk also benefit from early intervention (Wolraich et al., 2008). Therefore, observations and screenings offer the opportunity to attend to caregiver opinions and concerns (a source of valued information as well as a resource to facilitate/shape necessary changes), provide the prospect to detect developmental problems, and thereby, lead to promotion and guidance of the most favorable results being achieved and reinforced. As noted by Wolraich et al (2008), the concerns and opinions of parents are to be considered within the context of cultural influences, along with the understanding that their appraisals and descriptions are influenced by expectations of normal development. In other words, they may demonstrate differences not only from the individual perspective, but from a cultural and ethnic perspective as well.

According to Achenbach (2000) and DeGangi et al (2000), to make informed decisions regarding preventive and intervention referrals for services requires the identification of the three following groups of young children:

- Children who are exhibiting social-emotional and or behavior problems
- Children whose parents interpret their typically developing behaviors as evidence of social-emotional and/or behavioral problems
- Children who do not exhibit social-emotional or behavioral disturbance, but who are failing to acquire age-appropriate social-emotional competencies.

*Remember, identification of problems in young children does not imply that the source of the problem necessarily resides in the child. Additionally, a caregiver's negative appraisal of a child (the caregiver's internal working model of the child) is likely to influence not only parenting practices but subsequent child behavior as well. Another *very important* factor associated with caregivers is the notion of bias. Clinicians are quite aware that caregivers are at times motivated to accentuate and potentiate or deny the degree of difficulty a child has. When seeking services, caregivers may support more severe symptoms than are actually experienced. To the contrary, when caregivers are concerned about the stigma of having a child with serious enough problems to warrant special programming/interventions, they may fail to acknowledge such problems. There could be other reasons for the minimizing of difficulties:

- Cross-cultural contexts which may be due to a lack of familiarity (culturally may not view the problem behavior as a problem)
- Caregiver sensitivity to low base rate of delay or deviance
- Caregiver lack of familiarity typical developmental norms.

In order to advocate adequately for young children and their families requires questionnaire-based assessments to initiate a more formalized assessment process. This begins with questionnaire-based assessments for the early detection of children who may be evidencing, or be at risk for, social, emotional and behavioral disturbances. There are numerous comprehensive lists and descriptions of screening and assessment instruments available at the National Early Childhood Technical Assistance Center (NECTAC), from the Compendium of Screening Tools for Early Childhood Emotional Development at http://www.first5caspecialneeds.org/documents/IPFMHI-CompendiumofScreeningTools. pdf, the Children's Health Fund (Sosna & Mastergeorge, 2005; Glascoe, 2006; Wolraich et al., 2008, etc.). For example, Ringwalt (2008) compiled a summary of developmental screening and assessment instruments for NECTAC with an emphasis on social and emotional development for young children ages to be completed by parents/caregivers, and professionals, which is shown in Table 2.1.

TABLE 2.1 Summary of Developmental Screening and Assessment Instruments

I. Multidomain screening instruments that may be completed by families or other caregivers

Name of instrument	Description	Age range	Time frame	Scoring	Psychometric information	May be administered by
Ages and Stages Questionnaire (ASQ) – 2nd Ed.	The Ages and Stages Questionnaire (ASQ) system is designed to be implemented in a range of settings & can easily be tailored to fit the needs of many families. Clear drawings & simple directions help parents indicate children's skills in language, personal-social, fine & gross motor, & problem solving. The ASQ involves separate copyable forms of 30 items for each age range (tied to well-child visit schedule). The measure can be used in mass mail-outs for child-find programs as a first-level screening tool to determine which children need further evaluation to determine their eligibility for early intervention or preschool services. The questionnaire can also be used to monitor the development of children at risk for disabilities or delays. Published in English, Spanish, French & Korean, other translations are in development. A video is available that demonstrates completion of the questionnaire for two children. Their family is introduced & guided through questionnaire completion by a home visitor. Viewers discover how to explain the ASQ screening process, redefine items to reflect a family's values & culture, create opportunities for child learning & development, & promote positive parent-child interaction	Birth to 60 months	≈15–20 minutes, less if parents complete independently (each questionnaire takes 10–20 minutes to complete, with 2–3 minutes to score)	A 2 SD below the mean cut-off score is used for questionnaires at 4, 8, 12, 16, 24, 30, & 36 months. A 75 developmental quotient is the cut-off for questionnaires at 6, 10, 14, 18, 22, 27 & 33 months. Scores provide guidance on which children to refer for diagnostic testing, which to provide with skill-building activities & recommend to re-screen, & which children simply to provide activities for	The normative sample consisted of educationally, economically, and ethnically diverse families (Caucasian, African American, Hispanic, and Native American), but the sample was not nationally representative. Test–retest reliability, inter-rater reliability, and internal consistency: acceptably high to strong results. Internal consistency and predictive validity: moderate results. Under-referral rates ranged from 1% to 13% across the age intervals; over-referral rate ranged from 7% to 16%. Sensitivity ranged from 38% to 90% across the intervals, while specificity ranged from 81% to 90%. Concerns: the normative sample was not nationally representative — parents from Asian backgrounds appear underrepresented. Product information: http://www.brookespublishing.com/store/books/bricker-asq/index.htm	Parents; home visitors; other providers; requires a 6th grade reading level. Professionals score the questionnaires
Child Development Inventories (CDI)	Three separate instruments [the Infant Development Inventory (IDI), Early Child Development Inventory (ECDI), & the Preschool Development Inventory (PDI)] each with 60 yes–no descriptions. Inventories measure a child's development in five domains: gross motor, fine motor, language, comprehension, and person-social. Items tap the better predictors of developmental status only. A 300-item assessment-level version may be useful in follow-up studies or subspecialty clinics & produces age equivalent & cutoff scores in each domain	3–72 months; IDI for 3–18 months; ECDI for 18–36 months; PDI for 36–60 months	≈10 minutes, less if parents complete independently	The ECDI & the PDI produce a single cut-off tied to 1.5 standard deviations. T-scores may be calculated from this information. The IDI provides cut-offs for each of five developmental domains & illustrates both significantly advanced & delayed development	The normative sample reported in 1995 consisted of 1322 children; it was three times larger than the original MCDI sample for the same ages (1–4 years), and represented a broader range of demographics. A February 2006 article in the *Journal of Clinical Psychology* reports that a review of 132 cases utilizing parental report on the CDI found these data to be highly correlated (r = 0.92) with mental ages obtained during formal psychometric evaluation. Product information: http://ags.pearsonassessments.com/group.asp?nGroupInfoID=a9670	The CDIs can be mailed to families, completed in waiting rooms, administered by interview or by direct elicitation

Measure	Description	Age Range	Time	What It Provides	Psychometrics/Standardization	Settings/Notes
Kent Inventory of Developmental Skills – 3rd Ed. (KIDS)	Completed by the child's caregiver, and based on repeated observations of behavior across a wide range of conditions. The 252 items on the KIDS questionnaire assess the following domains: motor, self-help, cognitive, communication, and social skills. Linguistically adapted and standardized versions are available for the Netherlands, Spain, Russia, and Hungary	Infancy through 15 months (or up to age 6 when a severe developmental delay is present)	45 minutes	Developmental age scores and standard scores which highlight a child's strengths and needs. Provides information about whether a child has developmental delays, is at risk for delays, or is not delayed	Standardized on 706 infants in the USA and in Europe. The reliability of the domains is particularly high for infants between 2 and 12 months; for those older than 12 months the analysis of the Motor and Self-Help domain is less reliable. Internal consistency = 0.95 for full development scale & between 0.93 and 0.99 for the 5 domains. Test-retest reliability between 0.86 and 0.98. Scale validity: 0.95 for the full scale and somewhat lower values for the 5 domains (between 0.80 and 0.88). Product information: http://portal.wpspublish.com/portal/page?_pageid=53,1050083&_dad=portal&_schema=PORTAL	Parent or other caregiver who spends significant amounts of time with the child. Can be completed at home or elsewhere and returned for scoring
The Ounce Scale	The Ounce Scale is an observational, functional assessment that can be used effectively with children living in poverty, children at risk or with disabilities, and children growing and developing typically. The Ounce Scale is organized around eight age levels and six areas of development: Personal Connections – How children show trust; Feelings about Self – How children express who they are; Relationships with Other Children – How children act around other children; Understanding and Communicating – How children understand and communicate; Exploration and Problem Solving – How children explore and figure things out; and Movement and Coordination – How children move their bodies and use their hands. English and Spanish versions available	Birth through 42 months – divided into 8 intervals	The Ounce Scale involves ongoing observation that is periodically summarized	The Ounce Scale has a twofold purpose: (1) to provide guidelines and standards for observing and interpreting young children's growth and behavior; and (2) to provide information that parents and caregivers can use in everyday interactions with their children. It is not scored, but provides rating on individual indicators	Pilot and field testing of the Scale occurred over two years across 5 states in early childhood sites. Validation and reliability studies underway. Product information: http://pelcatalog.pearson.com/program_multiple.cfm?site_id=1021&discipline_id=802&subarea_id=0&program_id=942	Early interventionists, Early Head Start programs, child-care centers, Even Start programs, home visiting programs, and family child care homes
Parents' Evaluations of Developmental Status (PEDS)	This screening & surveillance tool provides decision support & both detects & addresses a wide range of developmental issues include behavioral & mental health problems. It promotes parent-provider collaboration & family-centered practice by relying on 10 carefully constructed questions eliciting parents' concerns. Domains screened include: global/cognitive, expressive language and articulation, receptive language, fine motor, gross motor, behavior, social-emotional, self-help, and school. In English, Spanish & Vietnamese with additional translations in development	Birth to 8 years	2–10 minutes, less if parents complete independently	Yields high, moderate, & low risk for developmental & behavioral/mental health problems. A longitudinal score & interpretation form organized by the AAP's well-visit schedule remains in the medical record. Identifies when to refer, screen a second time, advise or support families, postpone referral, and/or monitor development,	Normative sample: not nationally representative. Inter-rater reliability, internal consistency, and predictive validity: acceptably high to strong results; concurrent validity: moderate results. Concerns: diversity of normative sample. Product information: http://www.pedstest.com/	Written at the 4th to 5th grade level, parents can complete the measure while they wait for appointments

(Continued)

TABLE 2.1 (Continued)

Name of instrument	Description	Age range	Time frame	Scoring	Psychometric information	May be administered by
	behavior, & academic progress. Resources on the PEDS can be downloaded from: http://www.pedstest.com/content.php?content=download_resources.html					
Pediatric Symptom Checklist	This tool, which consists of a 35-item checklist for emotional and behavioral problems, screens for social-emotional delays or disorders in order to identify need for additional assessment. English, Spanish, and Japanese versions available	4–16 years	10–15 minutes	Items are rated on a 3-point scale of "never," "sometimes," or "often"	Test–retest reliability and internal consistency: acceptably high to strong results; predictive validity: moderate results. Product information: http://psc.partners.org/	Parent or caregiver, with interpretation by a practitioner with advanced training and experience in psychology
II. Multidomain screening instruments to be completed by professionals						
Battelle Developmental Inventory Screening Test (BDIST)	The 96 items use a combination of direct assessment, observation, & parental interview. The BDIST taps a range of discrete domains including receptive & expressive language, fine & gross motor, adaptive, personal-social, & cognitive/academic. It is intended to identify children at risk for delay and in need of full evaluation with the full-scale Battelle Developmental Inventory (BDI)	12–96 months	≈20 minutes	Yields cut-off scores and age equivalents. Cut-offs at 1.0, 105, & 2.0 SD below the mean, with 1.5 providing optimal sensitivity & specificity. Test also produces age equivalents	Normative sample of 800 children is nationally representative, and based on the BDI. Test–retest reliability and concurrent validity: acceptably high to strong results. The receptive language subtest appears accurate as a brief prescreen. Concerns: the age equivalent scores appear deflated & thus are best used only when cut-offs fall at or below 1.5. In addition, while the normative sample is considered nationally representative, the sub-sample of children at any particular age may be quite small. Furthermore, Asian or Native American families were not included in the sample. Product information: http://www.assess.nelson.com/test-ind/bdi.html	Members of multidisciplinary evaluation teams; can be administered by paraprofessionals who have had supervised practice
Bayley Infant Neurodevelopmental Screener (BINS)	The BINS is designed to identify infants who are developmentally delayed or who have neurological impairments. It emphasizes a process approach by considering how an ability is expressed, rather than simply whether the ability is exhibited. Each of the six item sets that comprise the BINS is appropriate for different developmental ages; each covers a 3–6 month age range. The sets contain 11 to 13 items. The four conceptual areas of ability assessed by the BINS are basic neurological functions/intactness; receptive functions; expressive	3–24 months	≈10 minutes/set	Cut scores of low, moderate or high risk for each of the domains. Items are scored as optimal/non-optimal. Those performed optimally by the infant are summed, & the total score is located in relation to the cut scores to determine the infant's risk classification	Normative sample is nationally representative. Test–retest reliability, inter-rater reliability, internal consistency: acceptably high to strong results. Concurrent validity: moderate results. Product information: http://harcourtassessment.com/haiweb/cultures/en-us/productdetail.htm?pid=015-8028-708	A professional with training & credentials & meeting the requirements specified by the particular test instrument or test company

Instrument	Description	Age range	Time	Scoring	Standardization	Administration
	functions; & cognitive process. A single form covers all age ranges & a carrying case of needed materials is provided. A videotape is also available to facilitate learning to administer the measure. The BINS is published in English only					
Birth to Three Assessment and Intervention System, 2nd E. (BTAIS-2), Screening Test of Developmental Abilities	The Screening Test of Developmental Disabilities consists of 85 items for identifying problems in the following areas: language comprehension; language expression; non-verbal thinking; social/personal development; and motor development	Birth to 3 years	15 minutes	Instrument is norm-referenced and yields standard scores. It can be scored by observation or parental report, with the score for each subtest plotted on a graph to show child's performance level in months	Normative sample of 357 typically developing children from 4½ to 36 months from 3 states. Children were evenly divided between rural and urban, male and female, with children from various ethnic backgrounds and socioeconomic status. Concerns: limited evidence for both validity and reliability. Because no children younger than 4 months were included in the normative sample, then the screening may not be appropriate for very young infants. Product information: http://psycan.com/Default.aspx	A professional with training & credentials & meeting the requirements specified by the particular test instrument or test company
Brignance Screens	Nine separate forms, ≈ one for each 12-month age range, the Brignance Screens tap speech-language, motor, readiness & general knowledge, & for the youngest age group, social-emotional skills. All Screens use direct elicitation & observation except the Infant & Toddler Screen, which can be administered by parent report. All Screens are available in English & Spanish	Birth to ≈90 months	≈10 minutes/screen	Cut-off, age equivalents, percentiles, & quotients in motor, language, & readiness at all age levels except Infant & Toddler, which provides scores for non-verbal & communication. Cut-off scores should identify at least 75% of the children who need further evaluation and 82% of those who do not. Overall scores generated at all age levels. The screens also provide criterion-referenced and norm-references scores and growth indicator scores to measure a child's progress	The 1995 standardization sample (for children two and older) included 408 children and families, representing the geographic regions of the USA and the demographic characteristics of the US population as a whole. The parents of children in the normative sample reflect the current US demographics (educational attainment, ethnicity, etc.). In 2001, the Infant/Toddler Screens were standardized on children from 29 sites across the country. Testing results reflect the average performance of children according to ethnicity, gender, age, socioeconomic differences, etc. Product information: http://www.curriculumassociates.com/products/detail.asp?title=Brig ScreenInfant&Type=SCH&Cust Id=9875991229081714082 93	Widely used in educational settings & often administered by paraprofessionals (a video is available to facilitate learning the test). I/T screen can be done by parent report

(Continued)

TABLE 2.1 (Continued)

Name of instrument	Description	Age range	Time frame	Scoring	Psychometric information	May be administered by
Denver Developmental Screening Test II (DDST-II)	The purpose of the DDST-II is to screen children or possible developmental problems, to confirm suspected problems with an objective measure, to monitor children at risk for developmental problems. 125 Performance-based and parent report items are used to screen children's development in four areas of functioning: fine motor-adaptive; gross motor; personal-social; and language skills. There is also a testing behavior observation filled out by the test administrator. English and Spanish versions available	1 month to 6 years of age	10–20 minutes	Child's exact age is calculated and marked on the score sheet; for premature infants, scorer should subtract the number of months premature from the infant's chronological age. Scorer administers selected items based on where the age line intersects each functional area. The scorer can then determine if child's responses fall into or outside of the normal expected range of success on that item for the child's age. The number of items upon which the child scores below the expected age range determines whether the child is classified as within normal range, suspect, or delayed. Those with suspect scores are monitored by more frequent screening, while those with delayed scores are referred for further assessment	Normative sample: Originally, 1036 English-speaking children from Colorado, approximating the occupational and ethnic distribution of that state. 1990 re-standardization included 2096 children, also from Colorado. Test–retest reliability and inter-rater reliability: acceptably high to strong results. Concerns: normative sample not nationally representative – re-standardization sample overrepresented Hispanic infants, underrepresented African American infants, and had a disproportionate number of infants from Caucasian mothers with more than 12 years of education. In addition, the screening is reported to miss children with developmental delays. Product information: http://www.denverii.com/DenverII/html	Trained paraprofessionals and professionals administer the test
Developmental Indicators for the Assessment of Learning – 3rd Ed. (DIAL-3) and Speed DIAL	Screens all five early childhood areas: motor, language, concepts, plus self-help and social development. The test also includes a 9-item rating scale of the child's social-emotional behavior and a rating of the child's intelligibility. The Speed DIAL, included with the DIAL-3, is a brief screen. English and Spanish versions available	3.0 through 6.11	20–30 minutes; Speed DIAL: 15–20 minutes	The DIAL-3, like DIAL-R, provides scores for *Motor, Concepts, Language*, plus an overall composite, and behavioral observation cut-offs. The DIAL-3 also provides standardized scores for *Self-Help* and *Social Development*, assessed by a Parent Questionnaire. Percentile ranks and standard scores are also provided. Speed DIAL yields one total score	Normative sample: 1560 English-speaking and 605 Spanish-speaking children throughout the USA, based on 1994 Census Data. The Speed DIAL total score is reported to be reliable and highly correlated with the DIAL-3. Internal consistency for the scales ranges from 0.66 to 0.87. Content and concurrent validity are reported to be good. Product information: http://ags.pearsonassessments.com/group.asp?nGroupInfoID=a13700	Useful for early childhood specialists, preschool and kindergarten teachers, Head Start programs, and child development centers. Speed DIAL is appropriate for quick screening in smaller settings such as departments of public health, pediatric offices, health fairs, homes, and classrooms.

Instrument	Description	Age Range	Administration Time	Scores	Standardization / Product Information	User Qualifications
						The supervisor of those who use these screening instruments should have completed graduate training in measurement, guidance, individual psychological assessment, or special appraisal methods
Developmental Profile 3 (DP-3)	Adaptive behavior scales, in 5 domains: physical, self help skills, social, academic and communication	Birth to 12 years	20–40 minutes	The DP-3 yields norm-based standard scores (including a General Development Score) that can be used to determine eligibility for services; percentiles, stanines, age equivalents, and descriptive ranges	Standardized on a nationally representative (in terms of ethnicity, geography, and socioeconomic status) sample of 2216 children who were typically developing. Product information: http://portal.wpspublish.com/portal/page?_pageid=53,1866018&_dad=portal&_schema=PORTAL	Interview or parent/caregiver checklist (to be used when an interview is not possible). User should have training in child development and experience interviewing families
Early Childhood Inventory-4 (ECI-4)	Modeled closely on the *Child Symptom Inventory-4* (CSI-4), the Early Childhood Inventory-4 (ECI-4) screens for emotional and behavioral disorders in children from 3 to 5 years of age. A Teacher Checklist and a Parent Checklist, based on DSM-IV criteria, cover symptoms for the same disorders as the CSI-4, except that they do not cover schizophrenia but add reactive attachment disorder, selective mutism, and eating, sleeping, and elimination problems. In addition, a brief developmental section gives a global impression of the child's speech and language abilities, fine and gross motor coordination, and social skills	3 to 5 years	10–15 minutes for each checklist	The ECI-4 offers a Screening Cut-off Score and a Symptom Severity Score; together these provide a picture of the child's symptoms and groundwork for a DSM-IV diagnosis	The ECI-4 Manual addresses appropriate concerns and cautions about applying DSM-IV diagnostic criteria to preschool children. Product information: http://portal.wpspublish.com/portal/page?_pageid=53,694698&_dad=portal&_schema=PORTAL	By a professional, using checklists completed by parents and teachers
Early Screening Inventory – Revised (ESI-R)	ESI-R is designed to be a brief developmental screening tool that accurately identifies children who may need special education services in order to perform successfully in school. The test consists of performance-based items that test the child's capabilities in the areas of visual motor/adaptive, language, and cognitive development. It enables programs to address quickly any possible learning blocks, such as developmental delays, learning problems, or lack of school preparedness. Parents are present for the test administration and fill out a Parent	3–6 years	15–20 minutes	Norm-referenced rating scale. This instrument has two versions, each normed for a different age range: ESI-P is for children ages 3 to 4 ½ ESI-K is for children ages 4 ½ to 6	Normative sample: 5034 children enrolled in 60 sites from 10 states. Classrooms were drawn from Head Start (N = 20), public schools (N = 26) and other child-care and early childhood programs. This sample included approximately equal numbers of girls and boys. Seventy percent of the children were white (non-Hispanic), 16% were African American, 32% were enrolled in Head Start programs, and 20% had mothers who had less than a high	Individuals who have some background in early childhood behavior and development can administer the scale, such as teachers, students of child development, school psychologists, or allied health professionals.

(Continued)

TABLE 2.1 (Continued)

Name of instrument	Description	Age range	Time frame	Scoring	Psychometric information	May be administered by
	Questionnaire, which is used for supplementary information. English and Spanish versions available				school education. Reliability data indicate that the inventory is a highly stable and consistent screening device. The test accurately identified 9 out of 10 students who were "at risk" of school problems and also correctly excluded most students who were not at risk from further assessments. Reliability: inter-rater = 0.97–0.99; Test-retest = 0.87–0.98. Validity: predictive = 0.73. Sensitivity: 92–93%. Specificity: 80%. Product information: http://www.pearsonearlylearning.com/	Experienced paraprofessionals have also been successfully trained to administer the scale
ESP: Early Screening Profiles	A comprehensive, yet brief, multidimensional screening instrument for children. The ESP is a tool that uses multiple domains, settings, and sources to measure cognitive, language, motor, self-help, and social development. It also surveys the child's articulation, home environment, health history, and test behavior. The three basic components, called Profiles, are supplemented by 4 Surveys. You can administer all of the profiles and surveys, or just the ones you need. The Profiles are: Cognitive/Language, Motor, and Self-Help/Social. The 4 Surveys are: Articulation, Home, Health History, and Behavior. Only available in English	2.0 through 6.11	For most children, administration of the Profiles takes 15–30 minutes. The Surveys require an additional 15–20 minutes	Two levels to choose from: Level I – Screening indexes of one to six corresponding to standard deviation units on the normal curve; Level II – Standard scores with confidence intervals, percentile ranks, and age equivalents	Normative sample of 1149 children, stratified by gender, geographic region, parental education level, and race/ethnic group, ages 2 years 0 months through 6 years 11 months. Reliability: internal consistency = 0.60–0.90; Test-retest = 0.55–0.93; Inter-observer = 0.80–0.99; Validity: studies are extensive and correlations vary. Sensitivity: 53–92%. Specificity: 65–88%. Product information: http://ags.pearsonsassessments.com/group.asp?nGroupInfoID=a3500	Useful for early childhood specialists, preschool and kindergarten teachers, Head Start programs, hospitals, clinics, and family health centers. Supervisor should have completed graduate training in measurement, guidance, individual psychological assessment, or special appraisal methods
Infant – Toddler and Family Instrument (ITFI)	ITFI allows family service providers to gather information and impressions about a child and family and their home environment that help providers decide whether further referrals and services are needed. The areas screened include gross and fine motor, social and emotional, language, coping, and self-help. Components include a Caregiver Interview (covering home and family life, child health and safety, and family issues and concerns), a Developmental Map, a post-visit Checklist for	6–36 months	Two 45- to 60-minute sessions to conduct the Caregiver Interview and the Developmental Map; one 45- to 60-minute session to	Scoring for the ITFI is completed using a three-part Checklist for Evaluating Concern, after the provider leaves the family's home. The checklist summarizes the provider's impressions of family and child strengths and concerns based on information from the	Not normed; field test involved 55 Connecticut families with 59 children ages 6 to 36 months. Product information: http://www.brookespublishing.com/store/books/apfel-4935/index.htm	Family service providers. Can be used in home visiting or center-based programs by family service providers from different fields, with varying levels of education and experience

Instrument	Description	Age range	Scoring	Duration	Psychometrics	Administration
	Evaluating Concern to alert providers to areas that are or may become problems and should be monitored, and a Plan for the Child and Family		share findings and develop a plan		Caregiver Interview, the Developmental Map, and observations of the caregiver–child interaction and the home environment. For each item in the checklist, the provider indicates whether the condition is present, is of concern, or if the provider is unsure of its presence	Normative sample: not nationally representative. Inter-rater reliability and internal consistency: acceptably high to strong results; concurrent validity: moderate results. Concerns diversity of normative population. Product information: http://www.riverpub.com/products/ida/index.html
Infant–Toddler Developmental Assessment	Screens developmental functioning in several domains: gross motor, fine motor, relationship to inanimate objects (cognitive), language/communication, self-help, relationship to persons, emotions and feeling states, and coping. Identifies the need for additional assessment and intervention. Two or more professionals perform six phases of screening: referral and pre-interview data gathering; initial parent interview; health review; developmental observation and assessment; integration and synthesis; and sharing findings, completion, and reporting. Available in English and Spanish versions (parent report)	Birth–42 months	Varies		Child's behavior rated as "present and observed", "not present and not observed", "reported present and not observed", "emerging", or "refused"	Administered, scored, and interpreted by highly trained individuals, using parent report and observations

III. Social-emotional screening instruments that may be completed by families and other caregivers

Instrument	Description	Age range	Duration	Scoring	Psychometrics	Administration
Ages and Stages Questionnaires: Social-Emotional (ASQ-SE)	Parent completed questionnaires designed to identify children in need of additional assessment. Personal-social areas assessed include self-regulation, communication, autonomy, coping, and relationships. Varies from 21 to 32 items, depending on age interval. English and Spanish versions available	3–66 months	10–15 minutes	Scores on the ASQ: SE can be compared with empirically derived cut-off scores that indicate whether a child needs additional evaluation	National normative sample of 3014 children from diverse backgrounds. Validity and reliability established in supporting studies. Sensitivity = 0.75–0.89; specificity = 0.82–0.96; alpha = 0.67–0.91; test-retest reliability = 0.94. Inter-observer reliability under study. Internal consistency, concurrent validity, and predictive validity: acceptably high to strong results. Concerns: normative sample not nationally representative. Product information: http://www.brookespublishing.com/store/books/squires-asqse/index.htm	Parent, caregiver; requires a 5th–6th grade reading level

(Continued)

TABLE 2.1 (Continued)

Name of instrument	Description	Age range	Time frame	Scoring	Psychometric information	May be administered by
Behavioral Assessment of Baby's Emotional and Social Style (BABES)	Behavioral screening instrument, consisting of three scales – temperament, ability to self-soothe, and regulatory processes. This instrument is intended for use in pediatric practices, clinics, and early intervention programs. Available in both English and Spanish	0–36 months	10 minutes	The maximum possible score for this instrument is 48, with higher scores indicating more problematic behaviors	Standardized on 128 caregivers (primarily mothers) in California. Concerns: psychometric data are limited; additional standardization has been reported to be underway. Product information: California School of Professional Psychology – Los Angeles (818) 284-2777, extension 3030	Parent or other caregiver
Brief Infant/Toddler Social Emotional Assessment (BITSEA)	This screening assessment, designed to assess quickly emerging social-emotional development, encompasses 60 items. It is intended to identify children who may need further, more comprehensive evaluation. The Parent Form includes 42 items and can be completed in the home or clinic. The Child Care Provider form allows screening across multiple settings. The available online items are from the Infant/Toddler Social Emotional Assessment – Revised (ITSEA-R), a comprehensive measure. Areas assessed are problem and competence, including activity, anxiety, and emotionality. Available in English, Spanish, French, Hebrew, and Dutch	12–36 months	7–15 minutes	Yields both problem and competence total scores	Clinical groups in the normative sample included young children who had delayed language, were premature, and those who had other diagnosed disorders. Adequate validity and reliability. Internal consistency for Problem = 0.83–0.89; for Competence = 0.66–0.75. Test-retest reliability, inter-rater reliability, internal consistency: acceptably high to strong results. Concurrent validity: moderate results. Concerns: normative sample of 600 children (1280 in the ITSEA normative sample) was not geographically representative. Product information: http://harcourtassessment.com/ haiweb/cultures/en-us/productdetail. htm?pid=015-8007-352	Parent, caregiver, child-care provider; requires 4th to 6th grade reading level
Carey Temperament Scales	These scales consist of questionnaires for five age groupings: *The Early Infancy Temperament Questionnaire* (EITQ) for infants 1–4 months; the *Revised Infant Temperament Questionnaire* (RITQ) for infants 4–11 months; the *Toddler Temperament Scale* (TTS) for children 1–3; the *Behavioral Style Questionnaire* (BSQ) for children 3–7; and the *Middle Childhood Questionnaire* (MCTQ) for children 8–12. Each questionnaire comprises 75–100 behavioral descriptions that are rated on a 6-point frequency of occurrence scale. Available in English	1 month–12 years	20 minutes	Provides norms for nine categories of behavioral style as defined in the classic *New York Longitudinal Study* (NYLS). May be scored by hand or by computer. Items are tabulated to yield a category score for each of the nine areas. The Caregiver Report includes the temperament profile and an interpretive report of scores written for the caregiver. The authors emphasize the importance of supplementing the results from the CTS with	Normative sample: not nationally representative. Reliability: internal consistency (Cronbach's alphas): EITQ: scale ranged from 0.43 to 0.76 (median = 0.62); RITQ: scale ranged from 0.49 to 0.71 (median = 0.57); TTS: scale ranged from 0.53 to 0.86 (median = 0.70); BSQ: scale ranged from 0.47 to 0.80 (median = 0.70); MCTQ: scale ranged from 0.71 to 0.83 (median = 0.82). Test-retest reliability: EITQ (20-day test interval): scale ranged from 0.64 to 0.79 (median = 0.68); RITQ (25 day interval): scale ranged from 0.66 to 0.81 (median = 0.75); TTS (1 month interval): scale ranged from	Parent or other caregiver, with an early high school reading level. Scored and interpreted by a licensed or certified professional

	information gathered from interviews, observations, and other information collected by trained professionals			0.69 to 0.89 (median = 0.81); BSQ (1 month interval): scale ranged from 0.67 to 0.94 (median = 0.81); MCTQ (75-day interval): scale ranged from 0.79 to 0.93 (median = 0.88). Validity: literature on the clinical evidence for validity and appropriate use of temperament data in practice can be found in Coping with Children's Temperament (1995), written by Carey and McDevitt or in Developmental-Behavioral Pediatrics (1992), edited by Levine, Carey, and Crocker. Concerns: lack of diversity of normative sample, which was primarily a White middle-class Eastern US population. Product information: http://harcourtassessment.com/haiweb/cultures/en-us/productdetail.htm?pid=015-8040-015	
Devereaux Early Childhood Assessment Program (DECA)	This screening instrument includes 37 items, which are designed to assess 27 positive and 10 problem behaviors. Behaviors are rated as occurring "never", "rarely", "occasionally", "frequently", or "very frequently". It includes guidelines for supportive interactions and partnerships with families. English and Spanish versions available	2–5 years	10 minutes	Standardized and norm-referenced	National normative sample of 2000 children with adequate validity and reliability studies. Internal reliability = 0.80 for parents, 0.88 for teachers. Test-retest reliability = 0.55–0.80 for parents, 0.68–0.91 for teachers. Inter-rater reliability = 0.59–0.77. Construct validity 0.65; Criterion validity 0.69. Product information: http://www.kaplanco.com/store/trans/productDetailForm.asp?CatID=17%7CEA1000%7C08&CollID=2329	Parent, caregiver; scoring and interpretation completed by a highly trained individual
Early Screening Project	This screening instrument is meant to identify children at-risk for adjustment problems, acting-out, and withdrawn behavior patterns. It comprises 3 successive stages of assessment, combining parent, teacher, and other professional observations. Available in English	3–5 years	At least 10 minutes/stage	Based upon their scores, children may be classified as "at risk", "high risk", or "extreme risk"	Normative sample: not nationally representative. Psychometric studies have supported the technical adequacy (reliability and validity) of the ESP. Test–retest reliability, inter-rater reliability, and concurrent validity: acceptably high to strong results. Predictive validity: moderate results. Concerns: lack of national representation in the normative sample. Product information: http://www.nekesc.k12.ks.us/esp.html	Teachers nominate children for screening who act out or are withdrawn. In the 2nd stage, the teacher completes a behavior checklist; in the 3rd stage a trained professional observes the child for two 10-minute sessions and the parents complete a questionnaire

(Continued)

TABLE 2.1 (Continued)

Name of instrument	Description	Age range	Time frame	Scoring	Psychometric information	May be administered by
Eyberg Child Behavior Inventory (ECBI) and the Sutter–Eyberg Student Behavior Inventory – Revised (SESBI-R)	The 36 items of the ECBI and the 38 items of the SESBI-R focus on oppositional behaviors (e.g. attention, conduct, and oppositional-defiant) at home and in school, for children with and at-risk for these behaviors. Parents complete the ECRI, while teachers complete the SESBI-R. They rank each behavior on two scales: Intensity (frequency of behavior on a 7-point scale from "never" to "always") and Problem (yes/no for whether this behavior is a problem). Available in English, with a number of unofficial translations	2–16 years	10–15 minutes	Yields Total Intensity Score and Total Problem Score	This instrument has adequate validity and reliability studies. Test-retest reliability = 0.87 for intensity; 0.93 for problem. Inter-rater reliability: acceptably high to strong results. Internal consistency = 0.98 for intensity; 0.96 for problem. Concurrent validity: acceptably high to strong results, while predictive validity has moderate results. Discriminant validity = 0.80. Concerns: small normative sample of 798 children (although it was representative of 1992 census). Product information: http://www3.parinc.com/products/product.aspx?Productid=ECBI	Parent or caregiver, requiring 6th grade reading level. Graduate-level clinical training needed to interpret the results
Greenspan Social-Emotional Growth Chart	This individually administered screening instrument utilizes a 35-item questionnaire for parents or other caregivers; the items are presented in the order in which they are typically mastered. It can be used to identify social-emotional deficits, to monitor development of social-emotion capacities, and to establish goals for intervention	Birth–42 months	10 minutes	The items on this instrument are rated using a 5-point scale; results are reported as cut scores	Reliability: 0.83–0.94, depending on age band. Product information: http://harcourtassessment.com/haiweb/cultures/en-us/productdetail.htm?pid=015-8280-229	Parent, caregiver
Infant–Toddler Symptom Checklist	This 21-item general screen is appropriate for clinic use. There are 5 separate age-related checklists, screening the areas of self-regulation, self-care, communication, vision, and attachment. The checklists are for 7–9 months; 10–12 months; 13–18 months; 19–24 months; and 25–30 months. Available in English	7–30 months	10–20 minutes	Most items rate behaviors as "never or sometimes", "most times", or "past"	Adequate validity and reliability. False positive = 0.03–0.13; false negative = 0.0–0.14. Concerns: size (221 children) and diversity (majority, white middle class) of normative sample. Product information: http://harcourtassessment.com/haiweb/cultures/en-us/productdetail.htm?pid=076-1643-559	Parent, with scoring and interpretation by highly trained program staff
Mental Health Screening Tool (MHST)	Developed to determine a child's need for more in-depth mental health evaluation. Intended for use by those in contact with young children, particularly those in out-of-home placements, who do not have extensive experience with or expertise in evaluating mental health	0–5 years	10 minutes	This screening instrument can be used as a resource to identify those children most in need of more intensive mental health screening and/or assessment	Three sites in California pre-tested this instrument as it was being developed. Product information: http://www.cimh.org/downloads/ScreeningTool0-5.pdf	County department of social services or mental health caseworkers, public health nurses, child-care staff and providers, foster parents, early intervention service providers, receiving home/shelter staff, and pediatricians

(Continued)

Instrument	Description	Age	Time	Scoring/Interpretation	Reliability and Validity	Completed by
Pediatric Symptom Checklist (PSC)	The original 35-item checklist is a screening tool for psychosocial dysfunction. It has been validated in other forms and translated into a number of languages. All forms can be downloaded without charge from: http://www.massgeneral.org/allpsych/psc/psc_home.htm	4–16 years	10–15 minutes	Items on this tool are rated as "never", "sometimes", or "often" present and scored 0, 1, and 2, respectively. The examiner calculates the total score by adding together the score for each item. For children ages 4 and 5, the PSC cut-off score is 24 or higher. A positive score on the PSC indicates the need for further evaluation by a qualified health or mental health professional	Validity studies have revealed agreement between the PSC and the Child Behavior Checklist (CBCL) and the Children's Global Assessment Scale (CGAS). The authors report high rates of overall agreement (79%: 92%), sensitivity (95%; 88%) and specificity (68%; 100%) with the CGAS with samples of children drawn from both middle and low SES. Product information: http://www.brightfutures.org/mentalhealth/pdf/professionals/ped_symptom_chklst.pdf	Checklist completed by families. A positive score indicates that additional evaluation is needed by a physical or mental health practitioner
Preschool and Kindergarten Behavior Scales – 2nd Ed. (PBKS-2)	These scales include 34 items in the social skills scale (includes social cooperation, social interaction, and social independence subscales) and 42 in the problem behavior scale (includes externalizing and internalizing subscales). It is specifically designed to screen the preschool through kindergarten population and for intervention planning. Available in English and Spanish	3–6 years	15–20 minutes	Behaviors are rated as occurring "never", "rarely", "sometimes", or "often"	Normative sample of 2855 children. Test-retest reliabilities are 0.69–0.78. Internal consistency is 0.96–0.97. There is high concurrent validity. Inter-rater reliability: moderate results. Concerns: normative sample was not nationally representative. Product information: http://www.proedinc.com/customer/productView.aspx?ID=2285	Parent, teacher, primary caregiver; interpretation requires a professional with training in psychological testing
Social Skills Rating System	This instrument focuses on positive behaviors; ratings produce social skills, problem behaviors, and academic competence scales. There are 49 items on the parent's version, with 40 on the teacher's. Versions available in English and Spanish	3–5 years	10–15 minutes	Scores for this instrument yield 3 scales: Social Skills, Problem Behaviors, and Academic Competence scales. For each scale, standard scores and percentile ranks are available. In addition, scores indicate Behavior Levels (fewer, average, and more) for both the scales and subscales. Frequency and Importance ratings for the items reveal behaviors that may need intervention	Normative sample: not nationally representative. Internal consistency: 0.73–0.95. Test-retest reliability: is 0.85 for teachers and 0.87 for parents. Concurrent validity: moderate results. Concerns: the preschool norms are from a separate sample of 200 children. Reviewers note that additional studies on the preschool version of this system are needed. In addition, normative sample not representative of the nation. Product information: http://ags.pearsonassessments.com/group.asp?nGroupInfoID=a3400	Parent, teacher
Strengths and Difficulties Questionnaire (SDQ)	The SDQ comprises a brief questionnaire, with several versions to meet the needs of researchers, clinicians and education specialists. All versions of the SDQ ask about 25 attributes divided among 5 scales: emotional symptoms, conduct problems,	3–16 years	10 minutes	25 items are divided among 5 scales (Emotional Symptoms Scale, Conduct Problems Scale, Hyperactivity Scale, Peer Problems Scale, and	Normative sample: not nationally representative. Test-retest reliability: acceptably high to strong result; internal consistency and predictive validity: moderate results. In a British study	Parent, teacher, with interpretation by trained program staff

TABLE 2.1 (Continued)

Name of instrument	Description	Age range	Time frame	Scoring	Psychometric information	May be administered by
	hyperactivity/inattention, peer relationship problems, and prosocial behavior. Designed to identify the need for more in-depth assessment. Versions available in English, Spanish, and more than 45 additional languages			Prosocial Scale) of 5 items each, generalizing scores for conduct problems, hyperactivity, emotional symptoms, peer problems, and prosocial behavior; the first four of these can be summed to yield a total difficulties score	published in 2000, multi-informant SDQs (parents, teachers, older children) identified individuals with a psychiatric diagnosis with a specificity of 94.6% (95% VCI 94.1–95.1%) and a sensitivity of 63.3% (59.7–66.9%). Concerns: lack of national representation in normative sample. Product information: http://www.sdqinfo.com/	
Temperament and Atypical Behavior Scale (TABS screener)	Screener consists of a 15-item, single sheet form. Responses are yes/no. Only children whose scores indicate a potential problem need to be assessed with the more extensive TABS Assessment Tool. Areas screened are temperament, attention and activity, attachment and social behavior, neurobehavioral state, sleeping, play, vocal and oral behavior, senses and movement, and self-stimulatory behavior. Available in English	11–71 months	5–30 minutes	Identifies when more extensive assessment is needed (i.e., when one or more of the 15 items is marked "yes"). The more extensive TABS Assessment Tool can be used to qualify a child for early intervention services	Normative sample: not nationally representative. 0.72 agreement with full TABS. Test–retest reliability, internal consistency, and predictive validity: acceptably high to strong results. Concerns: studied only in relationship to full TABS; lack of national representation in normative sample. Product information: http://www.brookespublishing.com/store/books/bagnato-tabs/index.htm	Written at a 3rd grade reading level, this screening instrument is to be completed by parents or other caregivers. Although this could be used by a professional as a screening instrument, using parental responses is preferred

IV. Social-emotional assessment instruments to be completed by professionals

| Achenbach System of Empirically Based Assessment – Preschool Module (ASEBA) | The ASEBA is used to assess adaptive and maladaptive functioning using a set of rating forms and profiles: the Child Behavior Checklist (CBCL/1.5-5) and the Caregiver-Teacher Report Form (C-TRF), revised in 2000. The profiles for the two instruments have the following 6 cross-informant syndromes: Emotionally Reactive, Anxious/Depressed, Somatic Complaints, Withdrawn, Attention Problems, and Aggressive Behavior. The CBCL/1.5-5 also has a Sleep Problems syndrome; while both forms have parallel Internalizing, Externalizing, and Total Problems scales. Examiners use the C-TRF ratings from daycare providers & teachers on 99 items, plus descriptions of problems, disabilities, what concerns the respondent most about the child, & the best things about the child. Similarly, they used the CBCL/1.5-6 | 18–60 months | 20–30 minutes | The preschool profiles feature empirically-based scales and DSM-oriented scales for the following 5 DSM-oriented categories: Affective Problems, Anxiety Problems, Attention Deficit/ Hyperactivity Problems, Oppositional Defiant Problems, and Pervasive Developmental Problems. Scores are available as percentiles and T scores for each DSM-oriented scale in relation to norms for the national sample | Norms are nationally representative, but only of English-speaking parents. Test–retest reliability, inter-rater reliability, internal consistency, concurrent validity, and predictive validity: acceptably high to strong results psychometrically. Concerns: normative sample represents only English-speaking parents. Product information: http://www.assess.nelson.com/aseba/aseba/html | The surveys can be completed by parents, teachers, or caregivers with at least a 5th grade reading level. The interpretation of the materials, according to the publishers, requires graduate training in standardized assessment procedures of at least the Master's degree level, plus thorough knowledge of the |

78

Instrument	Description	Age range	Time	Scoring / Results	Psychometrics & Product Information	Qualifications
	to obtain parents' ratings of 99 problem items; plus descriptions of problems, disabilities, what concerns parents most about their child, & the best things about the child. The CBCL/1.5-5 also includes the Language Development Survey (LDS), which uses parents' reports to assess children's expressive vocabularies and word combinations, as well as risk factors for language delays. This scale indicates whether a child's vocabulary and word combinations are delayed relative to norms for young children from 18 to 35 months of age; it can also be used for older children with language delays, for comparison with norms up to 35 months. Some scales available in Spanish, French and English					relevant manuals and documentation
Behavior Assessment System for Children, 2nd Ed. (BASC-II)	The BASC-II can be used for both assessment and intervention planning. It comprises two rating scales and forms: the Teacher Rating Scales (TRS) and the Parent Rating Scales (PRS). Teachers or other qualified observers complete the TRS to measure adaptive and problem behaviors in the preschool setting. A child's specific behaviors are rated on a four-point scale of frequency, ranging from "never" to "almost always". Similarly, the PRS measures adaptive and problem behaviors in the community and home setting, using a four-choice response format. Results yield two functional scales (functional communication and social skills) and eight clinical scales for children ages 2 to 5. Available in both English and Spanish versions	2.0–21.11 years	10–20 minutes/scale	The scales yield T scores and percentiles, for general and clinical populations	The BASC-II was normed based on current US Census population characteristics. Internal consistency: acceptably high to strong results. Test–retest reliability, inter-rater reliability, and concurrent validity: moderate results. Validity and response set indexes to evaluate the quality of completed forms are available. Product information: http://ags.pearsonassessments.com/group.asp?nGroupInfoID=a30000	Completing the PRS requires approximately a 3rd to 4th grade reading level. School and clinical psychologists to interpret results; training and credentials specified by the test company
Early Coping Inventory	This inventory's 48 items measure behavior in three coping clusters: sensorimotor organization, reactive behavior, and self-initiated behavior. Used for intervention planning. English version only	4–36 months	≈1 hour	Summing the numeric values of scale items yields raw score totals in each of the 3 areas. Using the table provided, the examiner converts the raw scores into Effectiveness scores, which can be plotted on the Coping Profile and used to compare the child's level of effectiveness in the three categories. A second table is provided to convert the sum of the effectiveness scores into an Adaptive Behavior Index score	Test–retest reliability and inter-rater reliability: moderate results. Product information: http://sttesting.com/COPI.html	Observations of the child are completed by someone with knowledge of child development; results should be interpreted by a professional with a background in early childhood development and mental health

(Continued)

TABLE 2.1 (Continued)

Name of instrument	Description	Age range	Time frame	Scoring	Psychometric information	May be administered by
Functional Emotional Assessment Scale	Measures social and emotional functioning, as well as caregivers' capacity to support a child's emotional development. For this instrument, social-emotional development includes regulation and interest in the world; forming relationships; intentional two-way communication; development of a complex sense of self; representational capacity and elaboration of symbolic thinking; and emotional thinking or development and expression of thematic play. Designed to reveal need for additional clinical assessment. English version only	7–48 months	20 minutes	Yields both child and caregiver scores	Normative sample: not nationally representative. Inter-rater reliability: acceptably high to strong results. Predictive validity: moderate results. Product information: http://www.icdl.com/dirFloortime/research/Functional EmotionalAssessmentScales.html	Highly trained individual observes play sessions (live or video) between a child and caregiver
Vineland Social-Emotional Early Childhood Scales (Vineland SEEC)	These scales are based on the popular Vineland Adaptive Behavior Scales and measure early childhood social-emotional development. There are three scales – Interpersonal Relationships, Play and Leisure Time, and Coping Skills – and the Social-Emotional Composite which assess social-emotional. Results identify strengths and weakness in specific areas of social-emotional behavior and can be used for program planning or to monitor progress and evaluate child outcomes, as well as to identify the need for further assessment. Available in English, with a Spanish version of reports for parents	Birth to 5 years 11 months	15–25 minutes	Interviewer-assisted parent report. Yields standard scores (M = 100, SD = 15), percentile ranks, stanines, age equivalents	Normative sample: nationally representative. Test-retest reliability and internal consistency: acceptably high to strong results; inter-rater reliability and concurrent validity: moderate results. Product information: http://ags.pearsonassessments.com/group.asp?nGroupInfoID=a3600	Level 3; Vineland SEEC test users should have a PhD in psychology or be a certified or licensed school psychologist or social worker

Screening Red Flags

The observation of the following behaviors/characteristics or identifying them during a screening may indicate the need for the child to be assessed. Keep in mind that the following may change depending on the age of the child:

- Requires extensive assistance
- Demonstrates lability (quickly escalates from a whimper to intense crying)
- Resists cuddling (pulls away/arches)
- Craves swinging or moving upside down
- Overreaction to light touch
- Easily startled or distressed by normal environmental sounds
- Unusually quiet/passive
- Demonstrates difficulties with transitions/adaptive functioning in coping with physiological needs
- Autonomy demonstrated by progression of independent functioning
- Compliance in following directions/rules
- Difficulty tolerating food textures (such as lumpy or sticky)
- Difficulties with communication/interactions.

An example of outcome information resulting from a screening instrument which would indicate criteria for referral for an assessment is demonstrated by the parent-administered Ages & Stages Questionnaires; Social and Emotional (ASQ-SE; Squires et al., 2002). This screening tool takes 10–15 minutes and is appropriate for 6–60 months of age (and are combined as both appropriate and inappropriate markers):

Behaviorala rea	Associated content
Self-regulation	Can calm down
	Body relaxed
	Has trouble falling asleep
	Calms down within time period
	Cries for long periods of time/screams/has tantrums
	Hurts others
	Has perseverative behaviors
	Is more active than same age peers
	Can settle down after excitement
	Stays with activities
	Moves from one activity to the next
	Destroys and damages things
Compliance	Follows simple directions/routines; follows rules
	Does what you ask
Communication	Listens/turn to look, smiles/looks
	Babbles
	Lets you know/uses words when hungry, sick tired
	Uses words for feelings
	Follows when you point
Adaptivef unctioning	Has trouble sucking
	Stays awake for hour or longer during the day
	Takes longer than 30 minutes to feed
	Is constipated or has diarrhea
	Has eating problems
	Sleeps "x" hours in 24-hour period
	Hurts self on purpose
	Stays away from danger
	Has interest in sex
	Stays dry during the day; is toilet trained

81

(Continued)

Behavioral area	Associated content
Autonomy	Checks when exploring; explores new places
	Clings to you more than you expect
Affect	Likes to be picked up and held; likes to be hugged and cuddled
	Stiffens and arches back
	Is interested in things around her/him
	Seems happy
	Shows concern for others' feelings
Interaction with people Parents	Smiles and laughs
	Watches, listens; plays peek-a-boo; likes stories
	When you leave, cries more than an hour
	Enjoy mealtimes together
	Plays near; greets; talks to adults
	Looks for you; is too friendly with strangers
Peers	Likes to be around other children; plays alongside
	Names a friend; takes turns and shares
	Other children like to play with your child
	Your child likes to play with other children
General concerns and comments	Has anyone expressed concerns about child
	Has concerns about child's eating and sleeping
	Has any worries about child
	Things you enjoy about child

As previously stated, a screening or assessment instrument is chosen based upon the best fit for the child. Therefore, the information elicited and identified will differ from one instrument to another. This example was offered to illuminate one of numerous possibilities.

DeGangi (2000) highlights report measures/scales used in her assessment chapter referred to "the most relevant tools" utilized for the six areas identified for assessment. The areas of assessment she identified:

- Self-regulation, sensory processing and reactivity
- Temperament and behavior
- Sustained attention
- Parent–child interactions
- Development and cognitive
- Communication skills.

The coinciding instruments selected to provide information on regulatory difficulties are as follows:

1   Self-Regulation and Sensory Processing and Reactivity

a. Parent report measures
  i. The Infant–Toddler Symptom Checklist (7–30 months) (DeGangi et al., 1995)
    This is a comprehensive checklist that is structured in a manner making it possible to establish, beyond problems of sensory processing, the degree of a child's regulatory problem in addition to how different behavioral patterns transpire over the course of development.
    There are six versions of the checklist (7–9, 10–12, 13–18, 19–24, and 25–30 months) and a short version for general screening purposes. The checklist may be self-administered or used as part of the interview, especially when parents are unable to complete a questionnaire without assistance due to illiteracy or cultural issues.
    The domains of significance in this instrument are:
    ○ Self-regulation: fussy/difficult behaviors (including crying and tantrums), poor self-calming, inability to delay gratification, difficulty with transitions between activities, and need for regulation (i.e., constant adult supervision)

- ○ Attention: distractibility, difficulty initiating and shifting attention
- ○ Sleep: difficulty falling and staying asleep
- ○ Eating/feeding: gagging, or vomiting possibly related to reflux or other oral–motor problems, food preferences, and behavioral problems during feeding
- ○ Dressing, bathing, touch: tactile hypersensitivities related to dressing or bathing, aversion to exploring through the sense of touch, and intolerance to being confined (e.g., car seat, high chair)
- ○ Movement: high activity level and craving for movement, motor planning and balance problems, and insecurity in movement in space
- ○ Listening, language and sound: hypersensitivities to sound, auditory distractibility, auditory processing problems, and receptive and expressive language problems
- ○ Looking and sight: sensitivities to light, and visual distractibility
- ○ Attachment/emotional functioning: gaze aversion, mood deregulation, flat affect, immaturity in play and interactions, separation problems, difficulty accepting limits, and behavioral problems

*Seventy-eight percent of the infants initially identified as having problems (as per the symptom checklist) were diagnosed as having developmental or behavioral problems at age 3 using standardized measures such as the Child Behavior Checklist (Achenbach, 1989).

ii. The Sensorimotor History Questionnaire for Preschoolers (SHQP) (3–4 years) (DeGangi & Balzer-Martin, 1999)
This instrument may be used as a prescreening tool for 3 and 4 year olds at risk for problems with sensory integration and self-regulation. It includes five subscales that prescreen for problems in self-regulation (attention and activity level), sensory processing of touch, movement, motor planning, emotional maturity, and behavioral control. Additionally, some clinical observations of attention, social interaction, and sensory reactivity

iii. Parent interview about typical behaviors

b. Instruments for direct clinical observation of the child (Tables 2.2–2.4)

i. Text of Sensory Functions in Infants (TSFI) (4–8 months) (DeGangi & Greenspan, 1989)
The TSFI is a 24-item test developed to measure sensory processing and reactivity in infants and is specifically administered by occupational and physical therapists, pediatric psychologists and infant educators, thus requiring a background and training in interpretation of test results in the domain of sensory integration. This instrument fouses on:
- ○ Response to tactile deep pressure: deep touch is applied using a firm stroking pattern to the forearm and hands, soles of feet, abdomen, and around the lips, and cuddling around the shoulder
- ○ Visual tactile integration is examined by the infant's ability to recognize visually and tolerate contact from a tactile stimulus applied to parts of the body (such as masking tape to the back of the hand)
- ○ Adaptive motor skills are observed during administration of the visual–tactile integration items. Responses are observed in the infant's ability to plan and act on the toy or object in an organized manner
- ○ Ocular motor control is measured by (1) the ability to direct the eyes to a bright red yarn ball moving in the periphery toward the central visual field, and (2) the ability to track smoothly a visual target, such as a finger puppet, in all visual fields
- ○ Reactivity to vestibular stimulation is measured by the infant's intolerance to bodily movement in space in different planes (vertical, circular spin, and inverted).

ii. DeGangi–Berk Text of Sensory Integration (TSI) (3–5 years) (Berk & DeGangi, 1983)
This instrument may be used to test children for sensory integration dysfunction once they reach preschool age. It is a criterion referenced test designed either to measure

83

overall sensory integration in 3–5 year olds with delays in sensory, motor, perceptual skills or to evaluate children where there is a suspicion of potential learning problems. It primarily focuses on vestibular-based functions and includes subtests measuring postural control, bilateral motor integration, and reflex integration. It is recommended that the TSI be administered in conjunction with measures of functional performance such as the Peabody Developmental Motor Scales.

iii. The Sensory Integation and Praxis Tests (4–8 years) (Ayers, 1989)
Once a child is 5 years old, more definitive testing of sensory integrative functions is conducted using this instrument instead of the TSI. These tests were designed to identify sensory integrative disorders involving form and space perception, praxis, vestibular–bilateral integration, and tactile discrimination. They demonstrate particular utility delineating areas of treatment for children with sensory integrative disorders. These tests are very helpful in delineating areas of treatment for children with sensory integrative disorders (Fisher et al., 1991)
*Aside from testing, clinical impressions of sensory processing can be directly observed, parents may be interviewed regarding typical behaviors, and observations of play. For example, observations of how a child plays with tactile materials and on moving equipment (slides, swings, etc.) offer information in forming conclusions about sensory processing abilities.

iv. Clinical Observations of Sensory Processing (see Tables 2.2–2.4)

2 Child Temperament and Behavior

a. Parent report measures

i. Parent Stress Index (PSI) (Abindin, 1986)
This is a useful measure of child characterisitcs such as adaptability and demandingness, as well as dimensions of parent stress (i.e., depression and sense of competence). The instrument is parent administered. The Child Domain measures characteristics which impact the parent's response to the child as well as the child's capacity to respond to therapeutic intervention such as adaptability, acceptability, demandingness, mood, distractibility/hyperactivity, and reinforcement to parents. The Parent Domain measures depression, attachment, restrictions of role, sense of competence, social isolation, relationship with spouse, and parent health.

ii. The Infant/Child Characteristics Questionnaire (ICQ) (Bates, 1984)
Provides a good indicator of difficult temperament. The four dimensions the questionnaire assesses are:
- Fussiness/difficult
- Unadaptable
- Dull
- Unpredictable.

iii. Child Behavior Checklist (2–5 years) (Achenbach, 1989)
Used to assess behavior and may be administered by interviewer or by parent. Separate interviews are available for 2, 3, 4 and 5 year olds. Identifies problems in the areas of:
- Social withdrawal
- Depression
- Sleep problems
- Somatic problems
- Aggression
- Destructiveness.

3 Sustained Attention

An important source of information is the quality of the parent–child interaction and the parent–child relationship. The assessment of the parent–child relationship reflects how the infant responds to and copes with their caregiver. Caregivers who are socially responsive, encourage symbolic thinking, and who use elaborated and clear verbal teaching/coaching have children who tend to perform better on standardized intellectual assessment instruments. Likewise, parents who are depressed have children with a higher risk of demonstrating delays in cognitive, language and attentional skills as well as a flatter affect. Thereby indicating the importance of combining an array of measures in assessing emotional development, affect regulation, behavior, and play that engage the participation of both parent and child. Barnard (1979) describes the components of adaptive interactions:

- Social engagement (soothability, attention, and developmental consequence, with caregivers demonstrating the ability to read and respond to the infant/child cues)
- Contingency of responses (capacity to respond to one another's signals appropriately)
- Richness of interactive content (range and content of play)
- Adaptability of the dyad to evolve over time as both the parent and child mature and develop.

a. Parent Report Measures
  i. Parent Interview about Clinical Observations of Attention (Table 2.5)
  ii. Infant–Toddler Symptom Checklist (attentional domain)
  iii. Connors' Rating Scale Revised (CRS-R) (3–17 years) (Connnors, 1997)
     Comprehensive set of scales for parent, teachers or self-report that can be used to measure psychopathology and problem behaviors in children and adolescents. It has both long and short versions of each scale and can be used to assess attention deficit/hyperactivity disorder and other behavioral problems. There are separate scales for males and females.

b. Instruments for Direct Clinical Observation of the Child
  i. Fagan Test of Infant Intelligence (3–7 months) (Fagan & Detterman, 1992)
     This test measures visual recognition memory. It assesses the infant's ability to attend differentially to novel versus familiar stimuli in visual recognition tasks. The infant is presented with a novelty problem consisting of two pictures. The infant is initially exposed to a stimulus in the form of a picture of a woman's face, for a set period of time. The tester sits behind a screen out of view and observes the infant's visual fixations through a peephole. The tester records on a computer the length of time the infant fixates on the picture. After studying the familiar picture, it is withdrawn and a novel picture presented. The two pictures are then presented simultaneously for a test time (generally 3–5 seconds). The computer is programmed to calculate a "novelty score" which represents the amount of fixation on the novel picture divided by the total time of fixation time on both novel and familiar pictures. This test is a confirmation of the relationship between visual recognition memory and later intelligence (Fagan, 1982).
  ii. Test of Attention for Infants (TAI) (7–30 months) (DeGangi, 1995)
     This instrument measures sustained attention reflected by how long an infant remains engaged in various cognitive behaviors such as visual inspection and manipulation. It specifically measures the infant's ability to (1) initiate and sustain attention during novel and moderately complex events, (2) persist and maintain interest in a given task over time, (3) self-initiate organized adaptive motor, visual, and social responses while sustaining attention, and (4) shift attention between stimuli and focus attention when competing stimuli are present. The test's four subtests are visual attention, tactile attention, auditory attention, and multisensory attention. There are five specific age versions, 7–9 months, 10–12 months, 13–18 months, 19–24 months, and 25–30 months.
  iii. Bayley Scales of Infant Development, Infant Behavior Record (IBR) (0–4 years) (qualitative observations) (Bayley, 1995)
     The Bayley is a descriptive measure of behaviors for children which focuses on interpersonal and affective domains, motivational variables, and a child's interest

85

in specific modes of sensory experience. Specifically resulting in ratings in social orientation, cooperativeness, fearfulness, tension, general emotional tone, object orientation, goal directedness, attention span, endurance, activity, reactivity, sensory areas of interest displayed, energy and coordination for age, judgment of test, unusual or deviant behavior, and general evaluation of the child. The IBR offers a convenient form of recording qualitative observations and evaluations and concludes with a general evaluation of the child's overall performance.

4   Parent—Child interactions

a. Parent Report Measures (clinical observations 2.4)
   i. Infant–Toddler Symptom Checklist (emotional domain)

5   Instruments for Direct Clinical Observation

a. Nursing Child Assessment Satellite Training (NCAST) Teaching and Feeding Scales (Barnard, 1979)
Based on essential interactive activities. Observations are made during feeding and during two developmentally taught tasks (one at the child's level and one slightly above their ability). Parent behaviors are scored for sensitivity to the child's cues of distress and fostering of cognitive and emotional growth.

b. Parent–Child Early Relational Assessment (PCERA) (Clark, 1985)
This instrument assesses the quality of the parent–child relationship and serves to evaluate parents and children in families at risk for, or hose who demonstrate, early relational disturbances. Parents are rated on amount, duration, and intensity of positive and negative affective qualities such as sensitivity to infant's cues, visual regard of baby, structuring of the environment, tone of voice, intrusiveness, and inconsistency. The infant is rated for positive and negative affects and interactive behaviors such as mood, attention, social initiative and responsiveness, motor skills, and communication skills. The dyad is rated on the quality of mutual involvement and joint attention to the task along with the amount of reciprocity and pleasure.

c. Functional Emotional Assessment Scale (FEAS) (7 months–4 years) (Greenspan & DeGangi, 2001)
This scale was developed to evaluate parent–child interaction patterns (Figure 2.3). It is based on the assumption that stages of emotional development can be observed via play interactions between the parent and child and that clinically relevant behaviors can be included within each stage. The FEAS focuses on the constitutional and maturational patterns of the child, the parent's capacity to maintain and reinforce the child's interactions and the dynamic interaction between parent and child. The parent is asked to engage the child in symbolic play just as they would at home in different situations. It is suggested to observe the parent and child in several different play situations to observe the child's varying play skills, interactional abilities, and the parent's capacity to facilitate the child's play skills.
The parent–child interaction is observed with each set of toys for 5 minutes with the parent and the child being scored for six levels of emotional development including:
- Regulation and interest in the world
- Forming relationships (attachment)
- Interactional two-way communication
- Complex sense of self
   ○ behavioral organization of sequential circles of communication
   ○ behavioral elaboration of feelings dealing with warmth, pleasure, assertion, exploration, protest and anger
- Emotional ideas: representational capacity and elaboration of feelings and ideas that are expressed symbolically
- Emotional thinking of complex intentions, wishes, and feelings in symbolic communication expressed through logically connected ideas.

Items also measure the infant's/child's regulatory patterns and caregiver responsivity. This instrument is intended for use with children with regulatory disorders, pervasive developmental disorders, emotional and behavioral problems and those who have experienced physical or emotional abuse or neglect. Each level of the scale has at least eight items which serves as a measure of progress and thus developing treatment goals.

d. Transdisciplinary Play-Based Assessment (6 months–6 years) (Linder, 1990)
Described as a naturalistic, functional developmental assessment of the child based on observations of a transdisciplinary team of parents and professionals. The goal of the assessment is to identify service needs, to develop intervention plans, and to evaluate progress in children. Observation guidelines are presented in cognitive, social-emotional, communication and language, and sensorimotor development.

6   Developmental Cognitive and Communication Skills

a. Bayley Scales of Infant Development, Mental Scale (Bayley, 1995)

Developmental Screening Framework

A thorough Developmental Screening should include a review of the following areas:

- A physical examination which includes a vision and hearing exam
- Self-help/daily living skills
- Emotional functioning (temperament)
- Social function parameters
- Fine and gross motor skills

TABLE 2.2 Clinical Observations of Somatosensory Dysfunction

Tactile hypersensitivities

1. Dislikes being touched, cuddled by others; pulls away from being held, arches, grimaces, cries or whines
2. Distressed when people are near, even when they are not touching (i.e., standing nearby, sitting in a circle, etc.)
3. Avoids touching certain textures; hates getting hands messy (i.e. fingerpaints, paste, sand)
4. Likesfi rm touch best (i.e., seeks firm hugs from others)
5. Prefers touch from familiar people
6. Dislikes having face or hair washed; especially dislikes having a haircut
7. Prefers long sleeves and pants even in hot weather, or prefers as little clothing as possible, even when it is cool
8. Touches everything in sight
9. Bumps hard into other people or objects
10. Withdraws from being near others, particularly groups
11. May hit, kick or bite others and is aggressive in play
12. Has a strong preference for certain food textures (i.e., only firm and crunchy, or only soft)
13. Dislikes being dressed or undressed
14. Resists being placed in certain positions

Tactile hyposensitivities

1. Seems unaware of touch unless it is very intense
2. Doesno t react to pain (i.e., shots, scrapes)
3. Biteso r hits self
4. Likes to hang by arms or feet off furniture or people
5. Unaware of messiness around mouth or nose

Poor tactile discrimination (for children over 2)

1. Difficulty with fine motor tasks (i.e., holding a pencil, buttoning)
2. Always looks at hands when they are manipulating objects
3. Usesmo uth to explore objects

TABLE 2.3 Clinical Observation of Vestibular Dysfunction

Vestibular hypersensitivities

1. Easily overwhelmed by movement (i.e., car sick)
2. Strong fear of falling and heights
3. Does not enjoy playground equipment and avoids roughhousing play
4. Is anxious when feet leave ground
5. Dislikes having head upside down
6. Slow in movement such as getting into therapy bench, or walking on uneven surfaces
7. Slow in learning to walk up or down stairs and relies on railing longer than other children same age (for children with mild motor delays)

Underresponsiveness to movement

1. Craves movement and does not feel dizziness when other children do
2. Likes to climb to high, precarious places
3. No sense of limits or controls
4. Is in constant movement, rocking, running about

TABLE 2.4 Clinical Observations of Motor Control and Motor Planning Problems

Motor control

1. Frequently breaks
2. Trips over obstacles
3. Falls frequently (after 18 months)
4. Slumped body
5. Leans head on hand or arm
6. Prefers to lie down
7. Has a loose grip
8. Fatigues easily during physical activities
9. Is loose jointed and floppy; may sit with legs in a "W"
10. Has difficulty manipulating small objects, particularly fasteners
11. Eats in a sloppy manner

Motor planning

1. Fear of trying new motor activities; likes things to be the same and predictable
2. Difficulty making transitions from one activity to the next
3. Must be prepared in advance several times before change is introduced
4. Cannot plan sequences in activities, needing structure from an adult
5. Easily frustrated
6. Is very controlling of activities
7. Difficulty playing with peers
8. Aggressive or destructive in play
9. Temper tantrum easily
10. Did not crawl before starting to walk
11. Difficulty with dressing

- Cognitive functioning
- Language and communication.

While an assessment would be comprised of the same areas as a screening, an assessment differs from a screening in that it explores the infant/child needs in greater depth and is completed by a team of professionals whom integrate their findings into a comprehensive assessment.

A comprehensive assessment will generally include a history, direct observation of functioning of the infant/toddler and family, and a hands-on interactive assessment

TABLE 2.5 Clinical Observations of Attention

1. Vulnerable to distraction such as sights and sounds, distracted at least 3 times during testing by environmental stimuli
2. High activity level, constantly running about and unable to sit still for an activity, attempts to leave the table three or more times during testing; may stand up for parts of the table topt esting
3. Plays only briefly with toy before wanting a new activity
4. Impulsive in handling materials, needing three or more reminders to wait before touching
5. Tunes out from activity, difficult to re-engage; processing of directions is slow; urging needed to respond
6. Can't shift focus easily from one object to another after playing for long period of time
7. Gives up easily; is frustrated and needs urging to persist
8. Prefers only easy tasks
9. Wanders aimlessly without focused exploration
10. Depends on an adult to focus attention during play activities
11. Becomes excited when confronted with crowded, bustling settings such as a crowded supermarket or restaurant

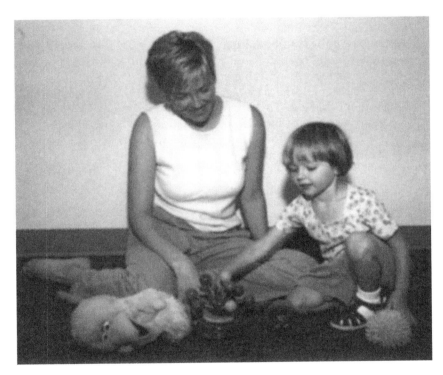

FIGURE 2.3
Child and mother playing with textured toys during administration of the Functional Emotional Assessment Scale.

89

including sensory reactivity and processing, motor tone and planning, language, cognition, and affective expression. Assessment is a thorough process that includes:

- Caregiver/family interview
- Reason for referral
- Developmental history
- Clinical observation
- Infant/toddler Mental Status Exam
- Utilization of instruments best suited to fulfill necessary informational needs for
  - Diagnostic formulation
  - Treatment planning.

Stages of Assessment

A family system assessment needs to be thorough. This requires meeting with the parents/caregivers, meeting with the child, and then meeting with the parent/caregivers with the child. The result is that the family system assessment will take place in 2–3 phases.

PHASE 1

The parent/caregiver is seen first. The purpose of this phase of assessment is to determine:

- Who comprises the household
- Who are the family members who do not reside in the household but significantly impact the child
- Identify non-family members who are significant to the family system
- Obtain a developmental history of the child which includes parental/caregiver perception of the child, knowledge of developmental issues, and parenting skills, are they able to set appropriate boundaries and limits?
- Use the time as an opportunity to explore and identify parental/caregiver issues and obtain an initial mental status exam for each parent/caregiver (do they need a psychological evaluation, referral for medication evaluation, referral to supportive classes, substance abuse evaluation, etc.)
- Assessment of the couple/marital relationship
  - Do they work together (on the same page with views and practices)
  - Do they agree and amicable/supportive in their differences
  - Is there risk of domestic violence (DV), anger management problem/history of criminal behavior
  - Separation/divorce/blended family issues
  - History of mental illness/emotional stability (look for dissociation/PTSD)
  - History of substance abuse
  - Explore family related stressors
    - Living conditions
    - Financial circumstances
    - Supports/resources
    - Health
    - Housing
    - Employment
    - Coping skills
  - Education level/training.

PHASE 2

The child needs to be seen individually (age appropriate):

- The child is seen alone to obtain level of functioning, perception of parents and family, neuropsychological factors, etc. Ascertain the child's strengths and needs
- This phase of the assessment can be included in the individual child assessment and report.

*The structure of this phase of the assessment is dependent upon the age of the child being assessed.

PHASE 3

In various combinations the child and parents/caregivers are assessed. The family must be observed in at least one setting in a structured and unstructured manner. Therefore, a home visit is highly recommended. Examples of the combinations of attendance for this stage of family assessment include:

- Child with parent/caregiver (both)
- Child with one parent/caregiver at a time
- Entire family system
- Gather information from extended family members and other supportive non-family members.

*Family conferencing is a gathering of family members, friends, community specialists and other interested people who meet together to provide strength and support in the development of a care plan.

*It is anticipated the family will be seen together unless it is contraindicated as a safety issue, absence (military service, incarceration, etc.) or other identified issue which would impede the process in some manner.

SUMMARY AND RECOMMENDATIONS

Strives to create a useful dynamic picture of the family system:

- Safety and protection issues
- Strengths
- Areas of relative weakness/limitations/needs
- Resources within the nuclear family, extended family, community resources (formal and informal resources)
- Coping skills and abilities
- Fit between parent(s) and child.

The focus of this report is to integrate the dynamic observational aspect and interactions during the interview assessment with all of the information that has been obtained.

91

Following the evaluation process, a feedback session is scheduled with caregivers, other significant adults in the child's life and all of the professionals involved in the case. A comprehensive treatment or preventive intervention plan is developed to deal with the nature of the child's difficulties (their overall capacity and functioning in major areas of development including social-emotional, sensory and motor abilities in comparison to age expected developmental patterns, etc.), as well as their relative strengths, and the relative contributions of family relationships, interactive patterns, constitutional-maturational patterns, stress, etc. With this baseline of difficulties and competencies there will be a review in the form of multiple assessments over time. This is necessary because infancy/toddlerhood development is a time of rapid changes in response to internal and external stressors.

Depending on what observations have been made or what specific difficulties or deficits are identified by screening or assessment tools, the following are services which may be provided to intervene with regards to a child's behavioral, attentional, learning, and/or social difficulties:

- Consultation and training for the family in ongoing adjustment of the sensory environment
- Training for the family in sensory regulatory interventions
- Behavioral and social interventions provided by a licensed mental health professional, or an early interventionist
- Occupational therapy consultation to other providers involved in the case
- Occupational therapy treatment with the child
- Speech pathologist for consultation and treatment
- All consultation reports are to be sent to the pediatrician.

DIAGNOSIS

An accurate diagnosis is imperative for the recognition and clarification of difficulties affecting a child's learning and behavior that places them at risk of being misunderstood. The diagnosis not only brings understanding to the child's difficulties but aids the family in getting the support necessary for dealing with the identified developmental challenges. Children with undiagnosed learning disabilities, attentional problems, and behavioral problems may be mistakenly labeled and their difficulties misinterpreted. An accurate diagnosis ensures appropriate treatment for the child as well as aiding parents and teachers in understanding a child's learning, thinking, how they see themselves, and how they interact with the world "they see".

Diagnostic systems guide assessment and interventions. Developmental psychopathology is seen from a contextual and transactional perspective which is also dynamic. Two major contributions resulting from the diagnostic frameworks that follow are:

1. Assessment for educational classification, and
2. Assessment for diagnosis mental disorders.

Infant mental health is viewed as their capacity to form close and secure interpersonal relationships along with being compelled to explore the environment and learn within their increasing social context (parents/siblings/other family, community and cultural expectations). Likewise, concerns arise when their behavior is unusual. For instance, if parents/others experience their difficult behavior as it interferes with satisfying interactions, and this is seen across multiple settings by a variety of people and persists. The mental health of young children is seen as the extrapolation of this phenomenon to increased complexity in a wider range of social contexts. The process of diagnosis and case formulation aid in determining the characteristics severity, and cause of presenting problems resulting in a classification (diagnosis) described by a constellation of symptoms. The diagnostic picture for infants and small children is further complicated by regulation of affect and behavior. As a result there are a number of alternative diagnostic classification systems which can be utilized to diagnose presenting difficulties. However, this text offers a summary of the *DSM Axis I* and ICD-10 disorders for children and a summary of *DC:0–3R* Axis I diagnoses with a multi-axial review. Therefore, there will be a brief description of the three central diagnostic systems followed by a summary demonstrating how each system diagnostically defines disorders of childhood. The only diagnostic system which will be outlined per axis is DC:0–3R.

Diagnostic and Statistical Manual (DSM-IV TR) Axis I Disorders

The DSM-IV is well established and recognized as a diagnostic classification system in clinical settings for the purpose of diagnosing behavioral disorders in children. It is divided into five axes for the assessment of multiple domains of information, known as a multi-axial diagnosis. The DSM classification system is challenging for this population because it only offers a small number of child psychiatric disorder categories and lacks developmentally sensitive adaptations. The system generally does not incorporate constructs and criteria that characterize disorder in younger children as viewed and described by intervening professionals outside of the mental health field. It also lacks an integrated emphasis on contextual factors influencing developmental psychopathology (attachment, relationships, behavior). Note: Other diagnoses which are not specific to children but may diagnostically apply to children include anxiety, mood disorders, eating disorders, somatoform disorders, and substance use disorders (DSM IV, 2000; Wolraich et al., 2008).

Another widely recognized and accepted classification of mental and behavioral disorders used to make pediatric diagnoses is the International Classification of Diseases, 10th Edition (ICD-10). The ICD-10 is divided into ten categories of pediatric behavioral and emotional disorders.

The Diagnostic Classification of Disorders of Infancy and Childhood: Zero to Three

The DC:0–3 was developed by variety of professionals specializing in the diagnosis and treatment of infants and small children, specifically the Multidisciplinary Diagnostic Classification Task Force instituted by the Zero to Three National Center for Infants, Toddlers, and Families. This task force recognized the unique challenges presented by this young population who presented with problems which could not be classified utilizing the DSM-IV or ICD-10. The DC:0–3 classification system was designed to offer complementarity in extending the diagnostic classification of the DSM's Axis I, thus facilitating diagnostic clarity and, therefore, clarifying treatment and benefitting research as well. The purpose of the DC:0–3R is to provide a focus on early childhood, provide a developmentally sensitive diagnostic tool for young children (framing diagnosis as a dynamic process) resulting in a comprehensive prevention or treatment plan, and considers the impact of relationships (context of family).

THE 5 AXES OF THE DC:0–3R

AXIS I

Clinical Disorders

Post-traumatic Stress Disorder
Deprivation/Maltreatment Disorder
Disorders of Affect
Prolonged Bereavement/Grief Reaction
Anxiety Disorders of Infancy and Early Childhood
    Separation Anxiety Disorder
    Specific Phobia
    Social Anxiety disorder (Social Phobia)
    Generalized Anxiety Disorder
    Anxiety Disorder NOS
Depression of Infancy and Early Childhood
    Type I: Major Depression
    Type II: Depressive Disorder NOS
Mixed Disorder of Emotional Expressiveness
Adjustment Disorder
Regulation Disorders of Sensory Processing
Hypersensitive
    Type A: Fearful/Cautious
    Type B: Negative Defiant
Hyposensitive
    Sensory Stimulation-Seeking/Impulsive
    Sleep Behavior Disorder
    Sleep-Onset Disorder (Protodyssomnia)
    Night-Waking Disorder (Protodyssomnia)
    Feeding Behavior Disorder
    Feeding Disorder of State Regulation
    Feeding disorder of Caregiver-Infant Reciprocity
    Infantile Anorexia
    Sensory Food Aversions
    Feeding Disorder Associated with Concurrent Medical Conditions
    Feeding Disorder Associated with Insults to the Gastrointestinal Tract
Disorders of Relating and Communicating
Multisystem Development Disorder (MSDD)

AXIS II

Relationship Classification Characterizing the functional level of relationships and interactions (1) of infants and young children, (2) parent's level of distress, conflict, adaptive flexibility, and (3) the effect of the relationship on the child's parents and family. There are two instruments which provide guidance in evaluation relationships (1) Parent–Infant Relationship global Assessment Scale, and (2) Relationships Problems Checklist.

AXIS III

Medical and Developmental Disorders and Conditions Describes physical (medical and neurological), mental health, and/or developmental diagnoses (including other diagnostic classification system, speech/language pathologists, occupational therapists, physical therapists, special educators, etc.). This axis is consistent with other classifications systems (DSM and ICD), indicating any coexisting physical (including medical and neurological) and/or developmental disorders. It is an important component of the diagnostic picture because:

- symptoms of mood disorder may be due to endocrine problems
- irritability, frustration, behavioral dysregulation may be due to hearing/speech/language problems
- abrupt onset irritability, restlessness or motor coordination difficulties may be due to heavy metal toxicity
- abrupt onset obsessions or compulsions may be due to PANDAS (pediatric autoimmune neuropsychiatric disorders associated with streptococcal infections).

AXIS IV

Psychosocial Stressors Describes the nature and severity of psychosocial stressors that influence disorders of infancy and early childhood. Like Axis III, this Axis IV is consistent with other classification systems.

- Identify stressors that influence symptoms and disorders in children
- Impact of a stressor
  - severity = intensity, duration, sudden stress, frequency, unpredictability
  - developmental level of a child = chronological age, endowment, and ego strength
  - availability and capacity of caregiving adults to serve as protective buffer to help child understand and cope with the stressor.

AXIS V

Emotional and Social Functioning Describes emotional and social functioning in the context of interaction with caregivers in accordance with age appropriate expected patterns of development. Dimensions of emotional and social functioning in the DC:0–3R include:

1. Attention and regulation (0–3 months)
2. Forming relationships: mutual engagement (3–6 months)
3. Intentional two-way communication (4–6 months)
4. Complex gestures and problem solving (10–18 months)
5. Use of symbols to communicate (18–30 months)
6. Connecting symbols logically (30–48 months).

   *Each of these rates the child's functioning on the 6-point Capacities for Emotional and Social Functioning Rating Scale.

Assessing infants and young children is challenging. In review, the DC:0–3R

- focuses on the first 3–4 years
- provides a developmentally sensitive diagnostic framework for this population
- considers the impact of relationships
- considers behaviors/problems not identified by other diagnostic classification systems

- complements the DSM and ICD classification systems
- allows for the multidisciplinary range of intervening professionals to speak the same language
- serves as a foundation for the diagnostic process and dynamic formulation which guides clinical treatment
- identifies appropriate family services/interventions
- promotes research.

Frankel et al (2004) report that the DC:0–3R has not been generally used by pediatricians in comparison to the traditional DSM. When they performed extensive chart reviews on newborn to 58 months they described the presentation of symptoms being categorized into 5 groups:

1. Sleep disturbances
2. Oppositional and disruptive behaviors
3. Speech and language/cognitive delays
4. Anxiety and fears
5. Relationship problems.

Their findings verified inter-rater reliability for diagnoses regardless of diagnostic system used.

As previously stated, there are three diagnostic classification systems used in association with young children. Possibly the most useful way for the reader to understand how these classification systems overlap and contribute to the dynamic formulation is to present Figure 2.4. Assessment and diagnosis is an ongoing process in a continual effort to develop a better understanding

Infants and Toddlers Who Require Specialty Services and Supports
(birth to 47 months of age)
Crosswalk between Diagnostic Classifications 0-3, ICD 9 CM and DSM IVR+

DC 0-3 R Diagnosis		ICD 9 CM Diagnosis ** Note: Refer to ICD 9 Coding Manual for Exclusions to this Diagnosis		DSM IVR Diagnosis	
100	Post traumatic Stress Disorder	308	Acute reaction to stress** (requires 4th digit subclassification listed below). Includes: • Catastrophic stress • Gross stress reaction (acute) • Transient disorders in response to exceptional physical or mental stress which usually subside within hours or days		
		308.0	Predominant disturbance of emotions • Anxiety as acute reaction to exceptional (gross) stress		
		308.1	Predominant disturbance of consciousness Fugues as acute reaction to exceptional (gross) stress		
		308.2	Predominant psychomotor disturbance • Agitation states as acute reaction to exceptional (gross) stress • Stupor as acute reaction to exceptional (gross) stress		
		308.3	Other acute reactions to stress** • Acute situational disturbance • Brief or acute posttraumatic stress disorder	308.3	Acute Stress Disorder
		308.4	Mixed disorders as reaction to stress		
		308.9	Unspecified acute reaction to stress		
		309.81	Prolonged posttraumatic stress disorder** • Chronic posttraumatic stress disorder	309.81	Post traumatic Stress Disorder
150	Deprivation/Maltreatment Disorder	313.89	Emotional Disturbance of Childhood NEC**	313.89	Reactive Attachment Disorder of Infancy or Early Childhood
		313.9	Unspecified emotional Disturbance of Childhood or adolescence		

+ To be used as a guide in Clinical Assessment/Diagnosis

FIGURE 2.4
Crosswalk between Diagnostic Classifications 0–3R, ICD-9CM and DSM IVR+.

Infants and Toddlers Who Require Specialty Services and Supports
(birth to 47 months of age)
Crosswalk between Diagnostic Classifications 0-3, ICD 9 CM and DSM IVR+

DC 0-3 R Diagnosis		ICD 9 CM Diagnosis ** Note: Refer to ICD 9 Coding Manual for Exclusions to this Diagnosis		DSM IVR Diagnosis	
200	**Disorder of Affect**				
210	Prolonged Bereavement/Grief Reaction	309.00	Adjustment disorder with depressed mood • Grief reaction	309.0	Adjustment Disorder with Depressed Mood
		309.1	Prolonged depressive reaction**		
220	Anxiety Disorder of Infancy & Early Children	300.00	Anxiety state, unspecified** • Anxiety: neurosis, reaction, state (neurotic) • Atypical anxiety disorder	300.00	Anxiety Disorder NOS
		300.01	Panic disorder. Panic: attack, state	300.01	Panic disorder without
		300.02	Generalized anxiety disorder	300.02	Generalized Anxiety Disorder
		309.21	Separation anxiety disorder	309.21	Separation Anxiety Disorder
		313.0	Overanxious disorder** • Anxiety and fearfulness of childhood and adolescence • Overanxious disorder of childhood and adolescence		
221	Separation Anxiety	309.21	Separation anxiety disorder	309.21	Separation Anxiety Disorder
222	Specific Phobia	300.29	Other isolated or specific phobias	300.29	Specific Phobia
223	Social Anxiety Disorder	300.23	Social Phobia	300.02	Social Phobia
		313.2	Sensitivity, shyness and social withdrawn disorder (requires 5th digit subclassification—listed below)		
		313.21	Shyness disorder of childhood Sensitivity reaction of childhood or adolescence		
		313.22	Introverted disorder of childhood --Social withdrawal of childhood or adolescence --Withdrawal reaction of childhood or adolescence		
224	Generalized Anxiety Disorder			300.02	Generalized Anxiety Disorder
225	Anxiety Disorder NOS			300.0	Anxiety Disorder NOS
230	**Depression of Infancy and Early Childhood**				
231	Type I Major Depression	296.2X	Major Depressive Disorder, Single Episode, Unspecified 5th digit: 0 unspecified 1 mild, 2 moderate, 3 severe without mention of psychotic behavior, 4 severe with specified as with psychotic behavior, 5 in partial or unspecified remission, 6 in full remission	296.20	Major Depressive Disorder, Single Episode, Unspecified
		296.3X	Major Depressive Disorder, Recurrent, Unspecified 5th digit: same as above	296.30	Major Depressive Disorder, Recurrent, Unspecified
232	Type II Depressive Disorder NOS	311	Depressive Disorder, not elsewhere classified --Depressive Disorder NOS --Depressive State NOS--Depression NOS	311	Depressive Disorder NOS
		313.1	Misery and unhappiness disorder		
		300.4	Neurotic Depression --Anxiety depression --Depression with anxiety --Depressive reaction --Dysthymic Disorder --Neurotic depressive State --Reactive Depression	300.4	Dysthymic Disorder
240	**Mixed Disorder of Emotional Expressiveness**	313.9	Unspecified emotional disturbances of childhood or adolescence	313.9	Disorder of Infancy, Childhood, or Adolescence NOS

+ To be used as a guide in Clinical Assessment/Diagnosis

FIGURE 2.4
(Continued)

Infants and Toddlers Who Require Specialty Services and Supports
(birth to 47 months of age)
Crosswalk between Diagnostic Classifications 0-3, ICD 9 CM and DSM IVR+

DC 0-3 R Diagnosis		ICD 9 CM Diagnosis **** Note: Refer to ICD 9 Coding Manual for Exclusions to this Diagnosis**		DSM IVR Diagnosis	
300	Adjustment Disorder	309 309.0	Adjustment Reaction (309.0—309.9) Brief depressive reaction --Adjustment disorder with depressed mood --Grief reaction	309.9	Adjustment Disorder: Unspecified
		309.24	Adjustment reaction with anxious mood	309.24	Adjustment Disorder with Anxiety
		309.28	Adjustment reaction with mixed emotional features	309.28	Adjustment Disorder with Mixed Anxiety and Depressed Mood
		309.3	With predominant disturbance of conduct --conduct disturbance as adjustment reaction --destructiveness as adjustment reaction	309.3	Adjustment Disorder with Disturbance of Conduct
		309.4	With mixed disturbances of emotions and conduct	309.4	Adjustment Disorder with Mixed Disturbance of Emotions and Conduct
		309.29	Other --culture shock	309.9	Adjustment Disorder NOS
		309.82	Adjustment reaction with physical symptoms	309.9	Adjustment Disorder NOS
		309.83	Adjustment reaction with withdrawal --Elective mutism as adjustment reaction --Hospitalism (in children) NOS	313.23 309.9	Selective Mutism Adjustment Disorder NOS
		309.9	Unspecified adjustment reaction --Adaptation reaction NOS --Adjustment reaction NOS	309.9	Adjustment Disorder NOS
400*– Regulation Disorders of Sensory Processing Sensory Processing when coupled with parent/child interaction					
410*	Hypersensitive	312.9	Unspecified disturbance of conduct	312.9	Disruptive Behavior Disorder NOS
411*	Type A: Fearful/Cautious	313.0	Overanxious disorder** --Anxiety and fearfulness of childhood and adolescence --Overanxious disorder of childhood and adolescence (Note: Also see 313.2, 313.21 or 313.22 for Sensitivity, shyness and social withdrawn disorder)	300.02	Generalized Anxiety Disorder
412*	Type B: Negative/Defiant	312.81	Conduct Disorder—Child onset type (Note: for young child over 36 months of age)	312.81	Conduct Disorder—Child onset (Note: for young child over 36 months of age)
		312.9	Unspecified disturbance of conduct	312.9	Disruptive Behavior Disorder NOS
		313.81	Oppositional Defiant Disorder	313.81	Oppositional Defiant Disorder
420*	Hypo/Underresponsive	314.00	Attention deficit disorder Without mention of hyperactivity --Predominantly inattentive type	314.00	Attention Deficit Disorder—Predominately inattentive type
430*	Sensory Stimulation – Seeking/Impulsive	314.0 314.01	Attention Deficit Disorder --Requires 5th digit subclassification-listed below With hyperactivity—combined type --Overactivity NOS --Predominantly hyperactive/impulsive	312.30 314.01	Impulse Control Disorder NOS ADHD-Hyperactive impulsive disorder
		314.9	Unspecified hyperkinetic syndrome --Hyperkinetic reaction of childhood or adolescence NOS --Hyperkinetic syndrome NOS	314.9	Attention Deficit/Hyperactivity Disorder NOS
500*	Sleep Disorder				
510*	Sleep Onset Disorder	307.40	Nonorganic sleep disorder, unspecified	307.47	Dyssomnia NOS or Parasomnia NOS
		307.41	Transient disorder of initiating or maintaining sleep • Hyposomnia associated with acute or intermittent emotional reactions or conflicts • Insomnia associated with acute or intermittent emotional reactions or conflicts • Sleeplessness associated with	327.02	Insomnia Related to….

+ To be used as a guide in Clinical Assessment/Diagnosis

FIGURE 2.4
(Continued)

Infants and Toddlers Who Require Specialty Services and Supports
(birth to 47 months of age)
Crosswalk between Diagnostic Classifications 0-3, ICD 9 CM and DSM IVR+

DC 0-3 R Diagnosis		ICD 9 CM Diagnosis ** Note: Refer to ICD 9 Coding Manual for Exclusions to this Diagnosis		DSM IVR Diagnosis	
		307.42	Persistent disorder of initiating or maintaining wakefulness • Hyposomnia, insomnia, or sleeplessness associated with: anxiety, conditioned arousal, depression (major) (minor), psychosis	307.42 or 327.02	Primary Insomnia Or Insomnia Related to…
		307.43	Transient disorder of initiating or maintaining wakefulness • Hypersomnia associated with acute or intermittent emotional reactions or conflicts	307.15	Hypersomnia Related to….
		307.44	Persistent disorder of initiating or maintaining wakefulness • Hypersomnia associated with depression (major) (minor)	307.44 or 327.15	Primary Hpersomnia or Hypersomnia Related to….
520*	Night –Waking Disorder	307.45	Circadian Rhythm Sleep Disorder of nonorganic origin	307.30 or 327.31	Circadian Rhythm Sleep Disorder, Unspecified type or Delayed Sleep Phase Type
		307.46	Somnambulism or night terrors	307.46	Sleep Terror Disorder or Sleepwalking Disorder
		307.47	Other dysfunctions of sleep stages or arousal from sleep Nightmares: NOS, REM-sleep type, sleep drunkenness	307.47	Dyssomnia NOS, Nightmare Disorder, or Parasomnia NOS
		307.48	Repetitive intrusions of sleep Repetitive intrusions of sleep with: atypical polysomnographic features, environmental disturbances, repeated REM-sleep interruptions	307.47	Parasomnia NOS
		307.49	Other "Short sleeper," subjective insomnia complaint	307.42	Primary Insomnia
600	**Feeding Behavior Disorders**				
601	Feeding Behavior Disorders	307.50 307.59	Eating Disorder, unspecified Other • Infantile feeding disturbances of nonorganic origin • Loss of appetite—of nonorganic origin	307.59	Feeding Disorder of Infancy or Early Childhood
602	Feeding Disorders of Caregivers Caregiver/Infant Reciprocity	307.59	Other • Infantile feeding disturbances of nonorganic origin • Loss of appetite—of nonorganic origin	307.59	Feeding Disorder of Infancy or Early Childhood
603	Infantile Anorexia	307.59	Other • Infantile feeding disturbances of nonorganic origin • Loss of appetite—of nonorganic origin	307.59	Feeding Disorder of Infancy or Early Childhood
800	**Other Disorders**				

* Not Axis I Diagnoses

FIGURE 2.4
(Continued)

of the child and family. Otherwise, the diagnosis is frozen in time and based on limited, aged information, which carries potentially long-term negative consequences for both the child and family. The goal is to diagnose and clarify problems not individuals. The assessment process of the child is an attempt to develop an understanding of their unique strengths and resources, relative weaknesses, and vulnerabilities, always with the ultimate goal of being as informed as possible clinically in order to provide the most beneficial interventions.

In determining a diagnosis it is not the label that carries any benefit, other than to communicate with other intervening professionals, it is the understanding of the impact to the life of the child and their family system and how to intervene effectively and comprehensively to prevent, manage, alleviate or eliminate the associated difficulties. Diagnostic considerations include the primary working diagnoses, the rule/out diagnoses as well as the possibility of comorbid diagnoses. Additionally, more than one primary diagnosis may be identified. Therefore, all diagnoses that meet the specified criteria should be used. Figure 2.5 is a diagnostic decision tree adapted from Wright & Northcutt (2005) from the ZERO TO THREE National Center for Infants, Toddlers and Families (Zero to Three, 2005).

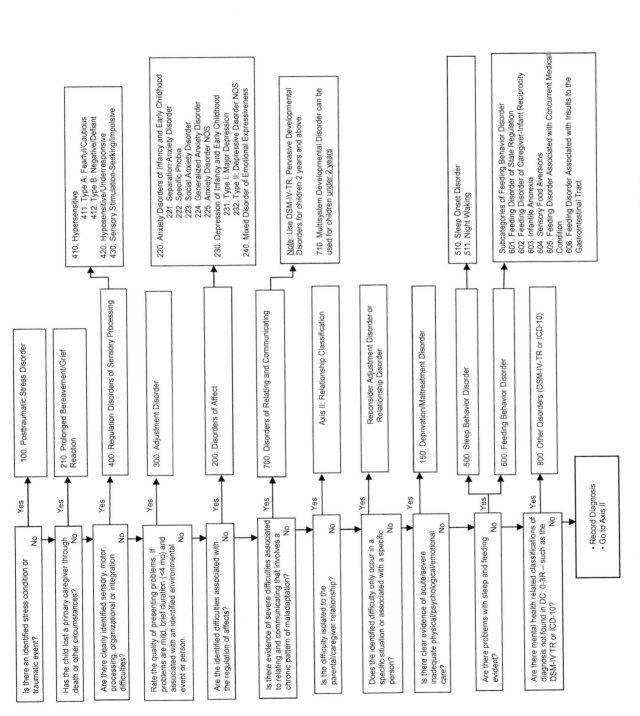

FIGURE 2.5

Diagnostic decision tree adapted from Wright & Northcutt (2005) from the ZERO TO THREE National Center for Infants, Toddlers and Families.

Assessment

↑   ↓

Child

Treatment Plan   Diagnosis

↩

FIGURE 2.6
Individualized Family
Service Plan (IFSP) and/
or an Individualized
Education Plan (IEP).

Completing Assessment and Diagnosis

Once the assessment and diagnostic phases have been concluded, it marks the time of intervention. NECTAC (April 2011 Fact Sheet) clearly states the reasoning behind early intervention in association with children's earliest experiences playing a critical role in brain development. Positive and enriching early experiences are crucial prerequisites for later success in school, workplace, and their social environment:

1. Neural circuits, which lay the foundation for learning, behavior and health are the most flexible (plastic) during the first 3 years of life. As time passes beyond this frame intervention yields less return of benefit for the child
2. Stable relationships enjoyed with caring and responsive adults in safe and supportive environments, along with appropriate nutrition are key factors of healthy brain development
3. Early social and emotional development combined with physical health provide the foundation of effective cognitive and language skills development.

Therefore, it is not a process bringing closure, but rather the opposite. The goals of intervention of the child have been identified and the resources needed by the parents to carry out their role in meeting these goals have also been identified. For the professionals engaged in this work their efforts culminate in an age-related plan of intervention referred to as an Individualized Family Service Plan (IFSP) and/or an Individualized Education Plan (IEP) (Figure 2.6).

What is an IFSP and IEP

(ED.gov http://www.ed.gov/pubs/edpubs.html http://www.cde.ca.gov http://www.cde.ca.gov/sp/se/fp/documents/ecil http://www.ihdi.uky.edu.nectc/idea2004/files/idea2004AndTransition.pdf http://www.ihdi.uky.edu/NECTCNEW/DOCUMENTS/RESOURCES/Regulations_5-03.pdf)

The Individualized Family Service Plan (IFSP) and the Individualized Education Plan (IEP) are legally defined processes with a prescribed developmental basis from which identified deficits with associated interventions are set forth to ensure the providing of necessary resources designed to result in optimal scholastic outcome. Program interventions are to take place for the IFSP and IEP in the least restrictive environment, or the most normalized environment in which the needs of a child with disabilities can be met appropriately. The team of professionals along with the parents (caregivers/guardians) work together to create a comprehensive plan for optimizing a child's learning ability.

DIFFERENCES BETWEEN SERVICES AND OUTCOME

Outcomes are statements outlining or defining what is to be changed. Through the assessment process team members identify a child's strengths as well as relative weaknesses and develop outcomes based upon those relative strengths and weaknesses as well as the ability of the caregiver resources and concerns resulting in a plan of intervention and their priority. According to the California Department of Education (2001) outcomes demonstrate the following characteristics:

• have the potential to be assessed
• are collaboratively developed by the entire team
• provide criteria that measure the expected change(s) identify expected results, procedures to be used and the time frame for achieving the desired outcome.

To the contrary, services describe what/how agencies and/or other team members will provide to assist the child and their families in meeting the outcome or target of change.

Therefore, criteria, procedures and timelines for change refer to the standards, methods, and target dates used to review and determine progress toward meeting the identified outcomes. For example:

1. Criteria: Betty will say 10 new words
2. Procedure: methods of evaluating progress, not the methods used or provided services, such as staff observations, parent reports, checklist measurements, standardized tests
3. Timelines: references specified dates when progress towards accomplishing outcomes will be assessed.

Figure 2.7 is an example, pages 9 and 10 from the California Department of Education, illustrating examples of expressing outcomes of the IFSP, including the aforementioned components.

Early Intervention Outcomes on the IFSP

Outcomes in developmental areas	Criteria (to evaluate progress)	Procedures (to evaluate progress)	Timeline (to evaluate progress)
Cognitive Kalisha will play meaningfully with toys.	Kalisha will stack blocks and place rings on a ring stacker without assistance.	Parent or teacher observation	6/01
Cognitive Susan will look at books.	Susan will turn pages appropriately and point to objects when requested to.	Parent or teacher observation	6/01
Physical movement Maria will first sit supported and then she will sit unsupported.	Maria will sit supported with towel rolls during storytime. Maria will sit unsupported.	Parent, teacher, or therapist observation	6/01 9/01
Physical movement Ping will walk.	Ping will progress from knee-standing to standing and walking with support.	Parent, teacher, or therapist observation	6/01
Physical movement Ben will gain better use of his hand.	Ben will pay with a toy by using both hands at midline.	Parent, teacher, or therapist observation	10/01
Communication Jenny will make more sounds.	Jenny will imitate combinations of /b/, /m/, and /p/ sounds with vowel sounds.	Speech therapist will mark off on a checklist	4/01
Communication (Receptive) Refael will follow spoken one-step directions.	Refael will follow directions, such as "Get the ball" and "Give me the bear."	Speech and language therapist's observation	4/01
Communication (Expressive language) Dan will increase his use of words and signs to indicate his need for food.	Dan will use eight signs to ask for food in a social situation.	Parent or teacher observation at mealtime	8/01
Social-Emotional Corey will improve his attending behavior.	Corey will listen quietly for 25 percent of storytime.	Charting by teacher	6/01

FIGURE 2.7
Illustrating examples of expressing outcomes of the IFSP.

Outcomes in developmental areas	Criteria (to evaluate progress)	Procedures (to evaluate progress)	Timeline (to evaluate progress)
Social-Emotional Justin will improve eye contact.	Justin will maintain eye contact with the speech and language therapist for 15 seconds when told, "Look at me."	Charting by speech and language specialist	6/01
Social-Emotional Wyatt will engage in parallel play.	Wyatt will play next to another child for ten minutes at each group visit.	Parent or teacher observation	6/01
Social-Emotional Peter will imitate social hand motions.	Peter will participate in imitative social games, such as peekaboo and bye-bye, and will clap hands.	Parent or teacher observation	4/01
Self-help and adaptive dressing Jasmin will learn to dress herself by first learning undressing.	Jasmin will remove socks, shoes, and coat with teacher's or parent's physical help and verbal directions. Jasmin will remove (list the item) when asked.	Parent, teacher, or therapist observation	6/01 9/01
Self-help and adaptive feeding Ashley will self-feed.	Ashley will finger-feed herself crackers, peas, and small bits of food.	Parent or teacher observation	5/01
Parental concern Ahmad's parents will learn more about Down syndrome.	Parents will report that they have received information through discussion and books and were notified of support groups.	Parent report	By semiannual review (6/01) or date of genetic clinic appointment
Parental concern Jill's parents will have a break from the demands of providing constant care for Jill.	Parents will report satisfaction with the respite care and family resources they have received.	Parent report	By semiannual review (12/01)
Speech language Brandon's mother wants him to say "Mama."	Brandon will increase vocalization to a minimum of three words, including "Mama."	Parent report and teacher observation	By semiannual review (12/01)
Parental concern Tran's weight and height will be appropriate.	High and weight are within normal limits on infant weight and height chart.	Charting of weight and height	In three months (7/01)
Parental concern The family will have resources to get to out-of-area medical appointments so that Nick's health is maintained	Medical appointments are kept.	Parent report	By semiannual review (12/01)

FIGURE 2.7
(Continued)

The Early Intervention/IFSP Process

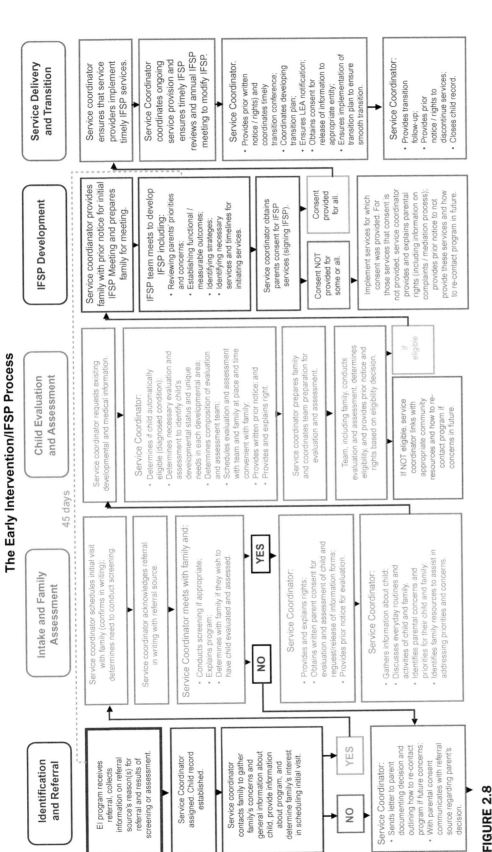

FIGURE 2.8
The Early Intervention/IFSP Process.

THE IFSP

An IFSP is the result of an evolving process that is initiated with the first contact with a child's family. The IFSP is based on the relationship between the family and involved professionals. The relationship needs to be flexible to assure the goal of meeting the child's needs. Therefore, the IFSP is a dynamic process which changes as a function of the changes in the child and family. As stated above, the IFSP is a legally defined process with distinct timelines. There are some circumstances that may interrupt the linear timeline such as:

- Medical needs/the health of the child
- Family crisis
- Diagnostic appointments
- Family work schedules.

Additionally, an interim IPSP may be conducted under two circumstances and must be fully completed within the 45-day timeline from the referral date and include the results from all evaluations/assessments and other required components. Furthermore, when a child with an existing IFSP is referred from another local educational agency (LEA), identified school services must be initiated immediately. The two circumstances are:

1. During the initial evaluation and assessment process if it is determined that the child is eligible before the process is completed. The interim IFSP is allowed to begin when the parents give their consent to meets the identified immediate needs. Local educational agency
2. An interim IFSP is required when the evaluation/assessment has not been completed within the 45-day timeline as a result of exceptional circumstances.

An example offered by the California website for an interim IFSP: a local educational agency is in receipt of a referral of a child with Down's syndrome. The physician making the referral states that occupational and physical therapy services are to be implemented immediately. An Interim IFSP can be written to eliminate any delay in the initiation of services. The school's identified administrator then sets assessments in motion and the IFSP meeting with the parents is held within the 45-day period.

The IFSP is essential to early intervention. The term IFSP is generally used to refer to the planning document in which outcomes, services and timelines are described. However, the document represents a process by means of which the family and early intervention personnel collaborate in identifying the family's resources, concerns and priorities as they relate to the child, gathering information about the child's functioning in daily routines (current level of functioning), and developing outcomes that can be achieved with the family's resources and those provided by early intervention. The process begins as soon as the infant or toddler is identified as being eligible for services. It is a plan of services for infant, toddlers and their families. Such a plan includes statements regarding the

- child's present developmental level (in all areas), the family's strengths and needs
- major outcomes of the plan/goals of the plan
- specific interventions and delivery systems to accomplish the outcomes
- dates of initiation, duration of services, and approximate re-evaluation date
- name of service coordinator
- a plan for transition into public schools.

IMPLEMENTING THE IFSP

The National Association for the Education of Young Children (NAEYC) developed guidelines for educational practices with young children ages birth to 8 years of age called Developmentally Appropriate Practices (DAP). It is essential that all personnel working with young children (with or without disabilities) be familiar with DAP. These guidelines set the standards for personnel, facilities and curricula for young children. Guidelines for infants and toddlers suggest that the most appropriate teaching technique for this group is to offer ample opportunities for children to use self-initiated repetition to practice newly acquired skills and to experience feelings of autonomy and success. An overview of NAEYC is available at http://www.naeyc.org/about/.

IFSP CONSIDERATIONS

The IFSP is a planned program that will benefit the family and the child, outlining what services will be delivered, how they will be delivered, and what skills and areas will be addressed. The IFSP must be reviewed with the family every 6 months at a minimum, unless otherwise prescribed by the state. Reviews may occur more frequently if either the family requests them or they are necessary because of major changes. The review serves to focus on the progress on all outcomes and if modifications or revisions of outcomes are necessary. The service coordinator is responsible for these changes to the parents and to team members. If more frequent meetings are necessary the service coordinator must forward written notice to the family regarding the purpose of the changes and proposed actions. If existing IFSP outcomes are impacted then the service coordinator must contact team member(s) to discuss the proposed changes. All changes to the IFSP must be documented on the IFSP and the parents should initial and date changes.

Outcomes of the IFSP must be measurable, and the team should always strive to develop outcomes using family friendly language to ensure clarity of communicating the goals of the IFSP. Additionally, infants and toddlers with special needs demonstrate frequent fluctuations in their behavior and functioning which results in a need for continuous assessment of monitoring of progress. The fluctuations represent typical developmental patterns in young children and do not signal a need for revising IFSP outcomes. Unless, however, the child's needs appear to have shifted to a degree that modification of existing outcomes is warranted or there is a need for new ones.

Development of the transition plan may be initiated when the child is 2 years 6 months old and completed by age 2 years 9 months. If the child is older than 2 years 9 months when they enter the early intervention program, the information in the plan is integrated into the record of the first IFSP meeting. At the meeting before the child's third birthday, the IFSP is reviewed and closed, and an IEP is written for preschool educational services.

An example of an IFSP is provided below by Sarah Katz.

IFSP

IDEA and Early Intervention:

Since 1975 the Individuals with Disabilities Education Act has been reauthorized to include safeguards for infants and toddlers with disabilities and developmental delays. This reauthorization included a component that provided guidelines for mandatory preschool and federal monies to support early intervention services for infants and/or toddlers with disabilities.

These federal guidelines are left up to individual states to interpret, however at this time all 50 states do participate in providing these services. Although the service model is individualized for each set of state regulations there are a few non-negotiable mandates set forth in IDEA which much be complied with in the implementation. These include:

- Early intervention services for infants and toddlers under the age of 3 years old, who have been diagnosed with developmental delays. These delays must be diagnosed through comprehensive assessment measures and must be global. Global delays are those which affect the child in one or more areas including cognitive development, physical development, communication skills, adaptive behaviors, and/or social emotional development.

105

Connecticut Birth to Three System ● IFSP Handbook ● 07/2011

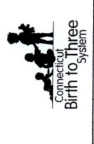

Connecticut
Birth to Three
System

INDIVIDUALIZED FAMILY SERVICE PLAN

*Date: October 2, 2011   *Type of meeting: ☐ Interim IFSP   ☑ Initial IFSP   ☐ Annual   ☐ Review

*Child's Name: Jacob Walker   ***Date of Birth: 6/1/2009**   ☑ *Male   ☐ *Female

*Parent/Foster Parent/Guardian/Family Member (circle one)

Parent/Guardian/Family Member (circle one)

*Name : Tricia and James Walker   *Name

*Address: 2714 10ᵗʰ Ave.   *Address

*City : Elmington   *State   CA   *City   *State   *Zip
*Zip

*Phone (day) : 805-212-1212   (Evening)   *Phone (day)   (Evening)

*Primary Language: English   *Primary Language

*Surrogate Parent: _____   *Phone: _____

*Address: _____

*Service Coordinator/Program: Jane Thompson, Birth to Three Family Services
*Address: 1230 W. Elm Street, Elmington, Ca   *Phone: 805-645-6545

*Physician/Health Care Provider: Dr. Jason Jones   (GP)   *Phone: 805-645-9898

*Address: 237 Main Street, Elmington Ca

*School District: Elmington Unified

Contact Person/Phone: Lucy Jackson, Director, 805-788-9081

*Recommended school district referral date, no later than: 12/1/2011   ☑ *Check if release to LEA (form 3-3) is on file
(Refer the child any time after the 2ⁿᵈ birthday. The decision to refer must be made no later than age 2 1/2)

_____   ☐ *Check if referral to LEA (form 3-8) is on file
date

*Denotes part of the electronic record

Connecticut Birth to Three Form 3-1 (Revised7/1/1)

Confidential Document

Connecticut Birth to Three System ● IFSP Handbook ● 07/2011

Child's Name: Jacob Walker   DOB: 6/1/2009 Date: 10/2/2011

SECTION I. SUMMARY OF CHILD'S PRESENT ABILITIES, STRENGTHS, AND NEEDS

1. Indicate the dates and types of evaluation or assessment report, which were used to develop this plan:

Health Evaluation completed by Dr. Jones, Family Play Therapy assessment completed by Families, INC. and Larry Smith, MSW, Ph.D. Previous medical records and intake forms from West General Hospital

2. Summarize below additional observations by family and other team members of the child's abilities, strengths, and needs in daily routines. Areas to include:

- What are your child's likes and dislikes?
- What are your child's frustrations?
- How does your child spend his/her day?

- Bathing, feeding, dressing, toileting – Adaptive/Self help skills
- Thinking, reasoning and learning – Cognitive skills
- Moving, hearing, vision, health – Physical development
- Feelings, coping, getting along with others – Social/Emotional development
- Understanding, communicating with others and expressing self with others – Communication skills

- Jacob enjoys playing outside, he likes animals, toy trains, and watching Elmo on TV. He seems to want to play with other children but has a very difficult time with respecting personal space and understanding sharing.

- Jacob's frustrations revolve around when he is not immediately gratified or given what he wants. He will throw a tantrum, scream, kick, destroy property, and demonstrate aggression towards others.

- Jacob's day is spent primarily in the home with his mother. His father works 12-14 hour days and is typically out of the home. Jacob's mother has a very difficult time leaving the house because of Jacob's behaviors. She states , "I can't manage him in public." Jacob does not like to be left with a babysitter.

- Adaptive: Jacob is beginning to help dress himself, however fine motor skills are difficult for him. He can feed himself using a spoon or fork but is extremely messy and prefers to use his fingers rather than utensils.

- Cognitive: Jacob has extreme difficulty in reasoning and understanding consequences for his actions and behaviors.

- Physical: Jacob has difficulty with fine motor tasks. His hearing and vision are intact. General health is good. He was seen recently for a bump on his head that occurred while he was having a tantrum and he smacked into a wall.

- Social Emotional: This is the biggest area of concern for Jacob. He is very attached to his mother and does not like to be in the care of anyone else. He throws tantrums and acts up when he is not given what he wants. Jacob will attempt to play with other children, but will quickly become aggressive when he doesn't get what he wants. He has hurt himself and others during tantrums. He seems to have overwhelming feelings of anger and sadness that quickly take over him.

- Communication: Jacob is just beginning to express himself using one or two words including, No, Don't, Mama, Jacob's toy, Eat, Stop, and Mine. He can understand the signs for more, eat, ouch, and stop. Jacob often resorts to screaming and throwing tangible items when he needs to communicate his feelings.

Connecticut Birth to Three Form 3-1 (Revised7/1/11)

107

Connecticut Birth to Three System ● IFSP Handbook ● 07/2011

Child's Name: Jacob Walker DOB: 6/1/2009 Date: 10/2/2011

**SECTION II. SUMMARY OF FAMILY'S CONCERNS, PRIORITIES, AND RESOURCES
AS THEY RELATE TO ENHANCING THEIR CHILD'S DEVELOPMENT - Family Outcome**

1. Information about our family for the IFSP: (Suggestions)
   - ● Things we like to do as a family
   - ● Who is part of our family?
   - ● Important events that have occurred
   - ● People and agencies we find helpful.
   - ● Our family's strengths in meeting our child's needs.
   - ● How our child's special needs affect our family

- Family: Mom (Tricia) and Dad (James). Maternal grandparents and Tricia's sister both live within 20 miles.

-Tricia reports 'their family 'doesn't do much' because of Jacob's behavioral difficulties. They used to like to go to the beach or have friends over

-Important events: Jacob was born 5 weeks early, because of this he has always been in the care of a social worker through West General Hospital. Jacob demonstrated early difficulties with fine motor skills that continue, Tricia reports he had difficulty sleeping and 'would scream all night', Jacobs tantrums began at 1 year of age.

-Jacob has been seen by Larry Smith, MSW . This assessment is ongoing but will most likely result in the recommendation of play therapy for the family. Mr. and Mrs. Walker are not currently involved with any additional agencies.

-Mrs. Walker reports they are having a very difficult time 'controlling and managing' the behaviors. She doesn't know what strengths they have as a family. 'We both love Jacob', she stated, 'but his father is working a lot.'

-Jacob's special needs have changed our lives. We can't go anywhere and we have lost touch with many of our friends.

2. What would be helpful for our family in the months and year ahead? (Family Outcome)

- Mrs. Walker reports the family needs help in understanding Jacob's needs and with controlling his behavior outbursts.

3. What assistance or information will we need to achieve this outcome? (Strategies)

- Further assessment should be conducted to determine Jacob's needs.

-Possible referral to behavioral therapist to conduct at-home evaluation

-Respite care for parents recommended

SECTION III. OTHER SERVICES THAT ARE IN PLACE OR ARE NEEDED

Services such as medical, recreational, religious, social and other child related services, not covered by the CT Birth to Three System, that contribute to this plan.

Resource/Program/Support Service	✓ If Needed	Payment Source
None at this time		

Connecticut Birth to Three System • IFSP Handbook • **07/2011**

Child's Name: Jacob Walker DOB: 6/1/2009 Date: 10/2/2011

SECTION IV. PLAN FOR TRANSITION FROM THE BIRTH TO THREE SYSTEM
TO PRESCHOOL SPECIAL EDUCATION OR OTHER APPROPRIATE SERVICES

Information that would be helpful for our child and family to plan for the future. •Community program options •LEA information •Referral process • Rights and responsibilities •Parent training •Visiting community programs •Adaptive equipment •Transportation •Time with other children • Information sharing.

-At thie time, Jacob has just turned 2. In December 2011, when he is 2.5 years old a referral will be made to the Elmington Unified School District for assessment for special education services and preschool services. These assessments will not take place until Jacob turns 3, but initial contact and referral will be made 12/2011

-Parents are encouraged to take advantage of the Regional Center's program offering respite care.

-A referral will be made though the Regional Center for an in-home behavioral assessment to be conducted

-Family will update team on Dr. Smith's evaluation and the progress of play therapy

-Parents may want to consider individual therapy services to help with coping skills

2. What are the next steps?	Who will be involved:	Date to be completed:
Referral to Elmington Unified School District	Jane Thompson	12/2011
Respite Care Services	Mr. and Mrs. Walker	10/2011
Referral for behavioral assessment	Jane Thompson	10/2011
Play therapy update	Mr. and Mrs. Walker	10/2011

After the initial IFSP meeting, this plan may only be modified at an IFSP periodic review meeting or annual IFSP meeting

Connecticut Birth to Three Form 3-1 (Revised7/1/11)

Confidential Document

110

Connecticut Birth to Three System ● IFSP Handbook ● 07/2011

Child's Name: Jacob Walker DOB: 6/1/2009 Date: 10/2/2011

SECTION V. OUTCOME # 1

What we want is: Help understanding Jacob's aggressive behavior and assistance in helping him stop

What is happening now: Aggression, tantrums, screaming, and destruction of property

What are the next steps (objectives) to reach this outcome?	Expected timeframe for reaching objective
Arrange for in-home behavioral services and support	2 months
Commit to 6 play-therapy sessions	Starting immediately
Arrange for family therapy and individualized therapy	6 months
Sign up for parenting classes though local Regional Center	Starting immediately

Strategies: methods for working on this outcome during your child and family's daily activities and routines	People who will be involved
-Parents will begin taking parenting classes and will complete paperwork for respite care though Regional Center -Assessment with Dr. Smith will continue, play therapy will begin upon completion of this assessment -Parents will begin working with an in-home behavior therapist to gather more information about managing Jacob's behavior	Parents, Dr. Smith, Jane Thompson, behavioral services therapist

(Attach additional pages as needed)

Connecticut Birth to Three Form 3-1 (Revised 7/1/11)

Connecticut Birth to Three System ● IFSP Handbook ● **07/2011**

Child's Name: Jacob Walker DOB: 6/1/2009 Date: 10/2/2011

SECTION V. OUTCOME # 2

What we want is: Assistance with Jacob's weaknesses in fine motor skills and communication

What is happening now: Screaming, using one word demands, and difficulty with fine motor skills i

What are the next steps (objectives) to reach this outcome?	Expected timeframe for reaching objective
Arrange for assessment with occupational therapist	Starting immediately
Arrange for assessment with speech therapist	Starting immediately

Strategies: methods for working on this outcome during your child and family's daily activities and routines	People who will be involved
-Dr. Smith noted there may be some unmet sensory needs that Jacob is struggling with. These needs may be contributing to his negative behaviors. Jane Thompson will arrange for consultations and assessments with the Regional Center's occupational therapist and speech therapist to see if Jacob qualifies to receive therapy in these areas. An update will be given in 90 days.	Parents, Dr. Smith, Jane Thompson

(Attach additional pages as needed)

Connecticut Birth to Three Form 3-1 (Revised7/1/11)

111

112

Connecticut Birth to Three System ● IFSP Handbook ● 07/2011

Child's Name: Jacob Walker DOB: 6/1/2009 Date: 10/2/2011

SECTION VII. IFSP TEAM MEMBERS

The following individuals have participated in the development of the IFSP and/or will assist in its implementation. There will be ongoing verbal communication between the IFSP team members listed below to assist in the implementation of the IFSP.

Name	Relationship	Phone	Method of Participation
Tricia Walker	Mother	805-212-1212	As listed above
James Walker	Father	805-212-1215	As listed above
Jane Thompson	Birth to Three Services Case Manager	805-645-6545	As listed above

Meeting Notes: (discussion, specific scheduling issues, and any other issues)

Connecticut Birth to Three Form 3-1 (Revised7/1/06)

Connecticut Birth to Three System ● IFSP Handbook ● **07/2011**

Child's Name: Jacob Walker DOB: 6/1/2009 Date: 10/2/2011

JUSTIFICATION FOR EARLY INTERVENTION SERVICES THAT CANNOT BE ACHIEVED SATISFACTORILY IN A NATURAL ENVIRONMENT

LOCATION OF SERVICE: _____ **SERVICE:** _____

1. **Explain how and why the child's outcome(s) could not be met if the service were provided in the child's natural environment with supplementary supports. If the child has not made satisfactory progress towards an outcome in a natural environment, include a description of why alternative natural environments have not been selected or outcome not modified.** -At this time, all of Jacob's services are being conducted in the natural setting. Supplementary supports such as play therapy, however, often occur in the therapist's office rather than at home.
2. **Explain how services provided in this location will be generalized to support the child's ability to function in his or her natural environment.**
3. **Describe a plan with timelines and supports necessary to allow the child's outcome(s) to be satisfactorily achieved in his or her natural environment.**

Connecticut Birth to Three Form 3-1a (Revised 7/1/06)

Confidential Document

114

Connecticut Birth to Three System ● IFSP Handbook ● **07/2011**

Child's Name: Jacob Walker DOB: 6/2/2009 Date: 10/2/2011

ADDITIONAL PAGE
INDIVIDUALIZED FAMILY SERVICE PLAN

Connecticut Birth to Three Form 3-1 (Revised7/1/06)

Confidential Document

- States are allowed to determine if they will serve students considered to be 'at-risk' of developmental delay. These 'at-risk' students are conceptualized as those who may experience a developmental delay if they are not provided with early intervention services. Often these children are those who demonstrate atypical development so different from their typically-developing peers or those who have been diagnosed with medical or physical impairments that may be contributory. Often, biological and environmental factors are also considered in the determination of the need for services.

If the need for early intervention services is deemed appropriate, IDEA mandates an Individual Family Service Plan be developed. This plan must be developed by a multidisciplinary team and serves to support both the child and the family in their specific needs. A comprehensive IFSP includes the following components:

- A statement of the child's present levels across all domains
- A statement of the family's concerns regarding development. This statement typically includes documentation of the family's resources and main priorities.
- A set of goals based on the multidisciplinary assessment. These goals, ideally, would address the specific needs of the child in each domain. For example, if the child showed deficiencies in the communicative and adaptive domains but not in the social or self-help domains, the goals would reflect this. A comprehensive set of goals would also include a time line and plan to determine progress.
- A list of the early intervention services which will support the child in reaching these goals. This service plan will include a list of environments in which the services will take place and the specific service providers who will assist with progress towards the goals.

An IFSP must be reviewed annually, however they are often reviewed much more often than that. Typically, a 6-month review is conducted with each family. At this review, the family and service providers determine if the progress towards each goal has been sufficient and if there is a need to reconstruct any portions of the plan.

Once a child reaches the age of 3, they become eligible to receive services under IDEA in the form of preschool with special education support. If a need for these services is found, a multidisciplinary team will reassess the child and the IFSP will be discontinued and an Individual Education Plan (IEP) will be developed. An IEP tends to be more academically based and will follow the child through their academic career as needed.

Source: Heward, W.L., Exceptional Children An Introduction to Special Education 9thEdition, Pearson Education Inc., Upper Saddle, New Jersey.

THE IEP

Eligibility for special education services depends on the presentation of education-related deficits which qualifies a child for special education services when they reach the age of 3. If they are eligible, an individualized education plan (IEP) will be developed. The focus of the IEP is on the child's functioning academically (in school only). Therefore, any problems with sensory processing will only be identified and addressed as they pertain to the child's ability to perform academically (to learn and to function in school). The goal is performance in the school environment. However, sensory issues may still be addressed via specific environmental supports, curriculum modifications, or sensory diet (refer to chapter on treatment), all goal directed toward self-regulation. Even if psychological therapy is directly indicated by the plan, the goal remains focused on performance in the school environment.

IMPLEMENTING THE IEP
Special Education Services

After the age of 3, the child may demonstrate a disability which qualifies them for special education services. If the child is eligible, an Individualized Education Plan (IEP) will

Integrated Outcomes - Individual Education Planning (IEP) Process

Child in Early Intervention - Transition

Provide notification to LEA of child potentially eligible for Part B service (near age 2) With parental consent, schedule transition planning conference for child potentially eligible for Part B
Ensure transfer of records occurs; if not effort must be made to get the info needed.
- IFSP
- assessment reports
- exit COSF (+ related info)

Ensure Part C exit COSF is considered in entry to Part B

Family and team attend transition planning conference;
Part B rights, eligibility, IEP process and possible service options explained to family
Coordinate development of transition plan
Determine family's interest in accessing Part B services

Identification and Referral

Receive referral or paraental request for evaluation. Infuse information about 3 global outcomes into the processes of information gathering throughout child identification and referral.
Provide a written copy of procedural safeguards to parents

Conduct screening, if appropriate (may proceed directly to evaluation)
Explain program in detail. Describe process and purpose of the three outcomes. Clarify the difference between/among other uses of the term 'outcomes' (e.g. IFSP/IEP outcomes).
Determine with family if they wish to have child evaluated for eligibility and services
Gather/use existing assessment information from multiple sources, multiple settings (including preschool classrooms)
Ensure information gathered at this stage is made available for team to use for COSF rating (e.g. Part C info, parent referral to 619, pre-referral into, screening, etc)

Child Evaluation and Assessment

Request and review existing developmental & medical information, including Part C exit COSF

Gather parent concerns. Probe for information on concerns in the three outcome areas.
Determine evaluations and information needed to establish if child is a child with a disability
Determine academic, developmental and functional needs of the child
Schedule evaluation at mutually agreeable time & place with family
Provide prior notice & procedural safeguards upon request

Family provides consent for evaluation (which generally begins evaluation timeline)

Team conducts evaluation/assessment. Embed functional authentic assessment into conversations with families.
Probe family for functional information on child.
Describe present levels of functioning in functional ways so it can be used for IEP development and the COSF rating.
Document supporting evidence of COSF throughout assessment and evaluation process. Consider populating COSF as you go.
Determine eligibility

Provide prior notice/rights on eligibility decision
Ensure COSF is not completed too long after entry to preschool classroom.

IEP Development

Provide family prior notice & procedural safeguards upon request for initial IEP meeting

IEP team, including family, meets to develop IEP including:
Documenting child's strengths and Present Levels of Educational Performance (PLEP)
Finalize COSF as IEP team discusses PLEP, adjusting as needed from earlier in process.
Determine age-anchoring for norm referenced tools; link to early learning standards [age-reference tools]
Parents' priorities & concerns
Establishing functional and measurable goals
Identifying strategies
Determining necessary services

Family provides consent for IEP services

Implement timely services for which consent was provided.

Service Delivery

Ensure that IEP is implemented in a timely manner

Provide IEP services
Monitor progress
Document and share child's progress on the IEP goals and in the three global outcome areas with family regularly

Ensure timely annual IEP meeting (or when requested by family or LEA) to review and modify IEP
Procedural safeguards notice provided annually

*The three outcomes to be measured for federal reporting purposes will be referred to as the "3 global outcomes" throughout, to distinguish them from an individual child's IFSP outcomes.
Text in red font indicates outcomes measurement steps; black font indicates IEP steps

FIGURE 2.9
The Nectac Diagram.

be developed. The focus of the IEP is only on school, therefore, sensory processing will be addressed only in the context of their ability to learn and function in the school environment. The IEP for the preschool child differs from the one for school age children (Kindergarten to age 22). At this level, intervention could be addressed through:

- Environmental supports
- Sensory diet
- Modification of curriculum
- Positive behavior support plan
- Goals for self-regulation.

Present levels of educational functioning, for special education, are assessed for ages of 3 through age 22 and is required only in the areas of suspected disability. The assessment includes information on regarding how the disability impacts the child's participation and/or performance in age-appropriate activities. The assessment is also intended to highlight any expectations of adjustment necessary for the child to participate in the mainstream/regular preschool curriculum. Performance, in the form of strengths and needs, is assessed in the following areas:

- Adaptive skills
- Cognitive ability
- Health (including vision and hearing)
- Gross and fine motor skills
- School readiness or achievement
- Social-emotional interactions
- Speech and language development.

IEP CONSIDERATIONS

The IEP is a program devised to satisfy IDEA's requirements that students with disabilities must receive an educational program based on multidisciplinary assessment designed to meet their "individual" needs. The IEP must consider:

- the student's current levels of functioning
- annual goals
  - long-term goals
  - short-term objectives
- special education and related services
  - specific services to be provided
- time in general education
- timeline for special education services, and
- an annual evaluation.

BASIC IEP PROCESS

The basic process of the IEP is the same as for the IFSP: screen, diagnose, plan program, monitor, and evaluate. The basic special education process under IDEA is the framework from which the IEP is structured. What follows is a brief summary of how a student is identified as having a disability and needing special education and related services, thus, an IEP (ED.gov). An IEP is defined by the following steps:

1. Child is identified as possibly needing special education and related services. Initiated by referral or request (school personnel or parent) for evaluation. Parental consent is required before the child may be evaluated. The evaluation must be completed within a reasonable time following parental consent.
2. The child is evaluated. The evaluation is designed to assess comprehensively all areas related to the child's suspected disability. If parents are not in agreement with the evaluation, they have the right to pursue an IEE (Independent Education Evaluation) and ask the school system to pay for it.

117

3. The child's eligibility is decided based upon the outcome of the evaluation. The parents along with a group of qualified professionals review the evaluation results to make decisions regarding the appropriate education plan for the child. IDEA provides the criteria from which the decision is made, "if the child is a child with a disability". Parents have the right to ask for a hearing to challenge the eligibility decision.

4. If the child is found to be a "child with a disability", as defined by IDEA, they are eligible for special education and related services. Within 30 days following this determination, the IEP team must meet and compose an IEP for the child.

5. A meeting is scheduled by the school system to conduct an IEP meeting. Designated school staff must:
   a. Contact the participants, which includes the parents
   b. Notification of parents must be early enough to ensure they are able to attend
   c. Schedule the meeting time/place agreeable to all parties
   d. Inform the parents as to the purpose, time and location of the meeting
   e. Inform the parents regarding who will be attending the meeting
   f. Inform the parents that they have the right to invite anyone to the meeting that they believe is able to offer knowledge or special expertise about the child.

6. The IEP meeting is held and the IEP is documented following a discussion about the needs of the child. Parents and the child (when appropriate) are a part of the team. The parents must give consent before special education can be provided to the child. As soon as possible following this meeting the child begins to receive special education. If the parents do not agree with the IEP, they can discuss their concerns with the other members of the team to find a resolution. If they are still not satisfied they can file a complaint with the state education agency/department and request a due process hearing.

7. The school executes the IEP as written. Parents are given a copy of the IEP and all school personnel have access to the document. The IEP includes recommendations, accommodations and supports that must be provided.

8. The child's progress toward the annual goals are measured and reported to the parents as outlined by the IEP. The parents are informed regularly of the child's progress. Progress reports must be made at least as often as the parents are designated to be notified of progress.

9. The IEP is reviewed by the IEP team at a minimum of once per year. If necessary the IEP is revised. Parents can offer suggestions for changes as well. At this point, if the parents do not agree with the IEP or placement they can express their concerns and an effort will be made to resolve their concerns. If an agreement cannot be achieved between the parents and other IEP team members, additional options include:
   a. additional testing
   b. an independent evaluation
   c. asking for mediation as part of a due process hearing
   d. filing a complaint with the state education agency/department.

10. At a minimum of every 3 years, the child is required to be re-evaluated, which may be referred to as a "triennial". The purpose of this evaluation is to determine if the child still meets the criteria of being a "child with a disability" and what their specific educational needs are. If warranted, the child must be re-evaluated more often, or if a teacher or parent requests a new evaluation.

Some of the related services under the IDEA provision include (but are not limited to):

- Audiology services
- Counseling services.
- Early identification and assessment of disabilities in children
- Medical services
- Occupational services
  Orientation and mobility services

- Parent counseling and training
- Physical therapy
- Psychological services
- Recreation
- Rehabilitation counseling services
- School health services
  Social work services in schools
- Speech language pathology services
- Transportation.

*If the child requires a specific related service in order to benefit from special education as provided by the IEP, the associated professional(s) should be involved in the development of the IEP.

A child struggling in school may be eligible for support services, allowing for the special education needs, for reasons such as:

- Learning disabilities
- Attention deficit hyperactivity disorder (ADHD)
- Emotional disorders
- Cognitive challenges
- Autism
- Hearing impairment
- Visual impairment
- Speech or language impairment
- Developmental delay.

+Strategies may be implemented by a teacher, occupational therapist or mental health therapist, behavioral specialist or other specialist identified by the IEP. Regardless of the recommended intervention, the goal(s) associated with the IEP is always performance in the school environment (class, cafeteria, playground, etc). An example of the framework that encompasses a referral for an Individualized Education Plan (IEP) is provided below by Sarah Katz and Jamie Mise.

119

CONDUCTING AN EDUCATIONAL ASSESSMENT – BEHAVIORAL DYSREGULATION

Referral for Assessment and Legal

Prior to conducting an assessment, all members of the IEP team should be familiar and comfortable with the regulations set forth in the 2004 reauthorization of the Individuals with Disabilities Education Act (IDEA) as follows:

> The team should explore the need for strategies and support systems to address any behavior that may impede the learning of the child with the disability or the learning of his or her peers (614(d)(3)(B)(i));

> In response to disciplinary actions by school personnel, the IEP team should, within 10 days, meet to formulate a functional behavioral assessment plan to collect data for developing a behavior intervention plan, or if a behavior intervention plan already exists, the team must review and revise it (as necessary), to ensure that it addresses the behavior upon which disciplinary action is predicated (615(k)(i)(B)); and

> States shall address the needs of in-service and pre-service personnel (including professionals and paraprofessionals who provide special education, general education, related services, or early intervention services) as they relate to developing and implementing positive intervention strategies (653(c)(3)(D)(vi).

IDEA also requires the IEP team to address "behavior that impedes his or her learning or that of others" (IDEA Section 614(d)(2)(B)), and the Federal Regulations further point out that "positive behavior interventions, strategies and supports" are to be considered supplementary aids and supports.

Generally, in the educational setting, an assessment referral will come only after a series of Student Team meetings, informal behavior planning, and observations. At this point, a generous amount of data collection will have been conducted and, ideally, the IEP team and/or behavior specialists will have began to determine the function of the student's behavior in order to address them correctly during the assessment. Since the reauthorization of IDEA in 2004, many schools have begun utilization of a Responsiveness to Intervention model (RTI) to address academic and behavior concerns prior to a Special Education assessment. If the student has been enrolled in RTI to address behavior, the IEP team conducting the assessment may want to consider the following:

- Does the student have a suspected disability? Will the IEP team be collecting new data on the behaviors in order to determine eligibility for special education?
- Will the IEP team be reviewing previous academic records and/or data? These data may come from previous Student Study Team plans, Section 504 evaluations, informal behavior charting, previous Behavior Support Plans, Positive Behavior Interventions, and/or tier one and two RTI programs.

If the IEP team agrees the student has a suspected disability that impedes his or her learning (and quite possibly the learning of others), an assessment plan can be developed and presented to the parents. The multidisciplinary team conducting the assessment should include experts who can address all areas of disability including behavioral dysregulation. Commonly, a multidisciplinary team will include the following members:

- *Special Education Teacher* – to address the component of 'impact on learning', review previous educational records, mastery of grade-level standards, and overall progress on standardized curriculum. Special Education teacher may also collect data regarding classroom performance, on-task behaviors, and administer norm-referenced, standardized assessments based on academic achievements of same-aged peers.
- *Speech Language Pathologist* – to assess and determine whether the student demonstrates difficulty understanding or using spoken language (due to any of the following disorders: articulation, voice, fluency, language, or hearing loss) to such an extent that it adversely affects his or her educational performance *(2.5)(c) (56333)*.
- *School Psychologist* – to address global cognitive functioning and any discrepancies between standardized academic achievement and assumed intellectual functioning. School Psychologists may also conduct normative assessments with the purpose of comparing an individual student to a norm-referenced group in the areas of suspected disability. During an assessment concerning a student with behavior difficulties, the most common category of disabilities are Emotional Disturbance and/or Other Health Impairment, however, others may be considered depending on the individual needs of the students.
- *School Nurse* – to address any health and/or medical needs of the students. School nurses often conduct basic hearing and vision screenings but are also a critical component in the assessment of students with co-morbid behavior, medical, and educational needs. This may include conducting a parent interview to discuss family history of behavioral disorders, learning disabilities, and/or mood disorders, developmental history, and medical history. The school nurse is also responsible for understanding which, if any, medications the student is taking and to discuss their potential impact on learning and behavior.
- *Behavior Specialist* (many school districts have an on staff Board Certified Behavior Analyst BCBA) – to address specific behavioral needs. Often the BCBA will conduct a Functional Behavioral Analysis to determine the specific function, antecedent, and consequences of

any given behavior. The BCBA will work to determine why certain behaviors are occurring and to work in conjunction with the multidisciplinary team to integrate the student with behavior difficulties into the educational setting as best possible.

- *Occupational Therapist* – to address any fine motor, gross motor, or sensory processing needs. Current literature and scholarship in the area of behavioral difficulties indicate that students who engage in task-avoidance and/or attention seeking behaviors may, in fact, be doing so as a result of sensory processing disorders. This is especially important if the student has co-morbid disabilities on the Autism Spectrum.

Pre-Assessment Planning

Since the reauthorization of IDEA 2004, a shift in accountability has led to teachers and other professionals in education becoming responsible for students with disabilities. In previous years, only special educators provided classroom instruction and support for students with disabilities.

This shift in accountability has placed an increased emphasis upon teaching, instructional strategies, and placement of students with disabilities in the general education curriculum, but also in assessing their progress using appropriate instruments and procedures. The demand to collaborate with all relevant education personnel in the resolution of behavior problems in the light of increasing academic progress has increased. As members of IEP teams, general educators play an increasing critical role in conceptualizing the needs of students with behavioral disorders.

Keeping this in mind, the IEP team must consider all appropriate environments in which to conduct the assessment. In order for a student's needs to be accurately measured and identified, observations and data collection must occur in all impacted environments including recess, co- and extra-curricular activities, and during academic instruction in the general education setting. If the student being assessed is not currently enrolled in public school, is enrolled in public or private preschool, or is being home-schooled, the multidisciplinary team must do everything to ensure the assessment occurs in all settings. This may mean conducting the assessment in the home and/or outside the school environment as necessary.

Once an assessment plan is developed by the multidisciplinary team, it will be sent home for parent consent to assess. If a written request for assessment is the catalyst for the assessment, the IEP team has 14 days to develop an assessment plan and send it home for consent. Once consent for assessment is received by the educational professionals on the IEP team, they have 60 calendar days to conduct and complete the assessment and determine eligibility. This assessment may also include a thorough review of previous medical, psychological, and other relevant records. Commonly, when an assessment plan is signed a release of information is also signed. This will allow the IEP team to garner access to any or all relevant previous medical and psychological history.

Assessment Tools

In addition to a thorough review of the student's educational and health history, classroom observations, teacher interview, and informal measures, the multidisciplinary team may choose to utilize a series of criterion-referenced and norm-referenced measures as part of the assessment. Criterion-referenced assessments are informal measures in which a teacher/team member will take data on which skills the student has mastered and which are still a challenge. This may also include data on on-task behaviors, compliance, work completion, and off-task behaviors as compared to same-age peers within the educational setting. Norm-referenced measures of achievement serve to establish both standard scores and percentile rankings to a state, national, or standardized norm group as a measurement of progress. These measures serve to assist the team in both determining strengths and weaknesses and in conceptualizing educational programming for the student being assessed. These formal assessment tools may include (but are not limited to) the following:

EDUCATION

- Hawaii Early Learning Profile (HELP) – Curriculum-based assessment covering 5 domains including cognitive, language, social emotional, self-help, and gross/fine motor. HELP can be conducted with students 0–3 or 3–6 years of age and is scored in age equivalent, developmental scores.
- Psycho-Educational Profile (PEP 3) – Assess the skills and behaviors of children with developmental disabilities, especially communication disorders and/or autism spectrum disorders. The PEP 3 is normed for students between developmental ages 6 months and 7 years. Resulting scores from the PEP-3 charts strengths and weaknesses, idiosyncratic development, emerging skills, and autistic behavioral characteristics.
- Kaufman Test of Educational Achievement (KTEA 2) – Diagnostic educational achievement assessment across the domains of reading, comprehension, mathematics, and written language.
- Woodcock Johnson Test of Achievement (WJT-III) – Diagnostic educational achievement assessment across the domains of reading, comprehension, mathematics, and written language.
- Wechlser Individual Achievement Test (WIAT) – Diagnostic educational achievement assessment across the domains of reading, comprehension, mathematics, and written language.

SPEECH

- Clinical Evaluation of Language Fundamentals – Fourth Edition (CELF-4) – A standardized, norm-referenced test that evaluates general language ability through multiple subtests, for ages 5 through 21.
- Comprehensive Assessment of Spoken Language (CASL) – A standardized, norm-referenced test that measures language processing skills – comprehension, expression, and retrieval – in four language structure categories: Lexical/Semantic, Syntactic, Supralinguistic, and Pragmatic, for ages 3 through 21.
- Expressive Picture Vocabulary Test – Second Edition (EVT-2) – A standardized, norm-referenced test that evaluates expressive vocabulary knowledge through a picture identification task, for ages 2 years 6 months through 90 years plus. Goldman-Fristoe Test of Articulation (GFTA-2)/Khan-Lewis Phonological Assessment (KLPA-2) – A standardized, norm-referenced test that evaluates a student's articulation of the consonant sounds of Standard American English, for ages 2 through 21.
- Peabody Picture Vocabulary Test – Fourth Edition (PPVT-4) – A standardized, norm-referenced test that evaluates receptive vocabulary knowledge through a point-to-picture task, for ages 2 years 6 months through 90 years plus.
- Preschool Language Scale – Fifth Edition (PLS-5) – A standardized, norm-referenced test that evaluates auditory comprehension and expressive communication in a comprehensive developmental language assessment, for ages birth through 7 years 11 months.

PSYCHOLOGY

- Connors Rating Scale (CRS-2) – Uses observer ratings and self-reported ratings to determine and evaluate ADHD and problem behaviors in children.
- Behavior Assessment System for Children (BASC 3) – Uses a multidimensional approach to problem behaviors and social emotional needs in children.
- Achenbach System of Empirically Based Assessment (ASEBA) – Uses a comprehensive approach to addressing adaptive and maladaptive behaviors in children.

- Adaptive Behavior Assessment System (ABAS) – Behavior rating format that measures adaptive behavior and related skills.
- Cognitive ability measures including: WISC, Stanford Binet, Woodcock, WIAT, or WRAML.

Determining Eligibility

Once all assessment measures have been completed and a records review has been conducted, members of the multidisciplinary team must meet to determine eligibility criteria. Often, when a student is exhibiting behavioral dysregulation in the educational setting, they will qualify to receive services under the categories of Other Health Impairment (OHI) or Emotional Disturbance (ED). However, if the student is of preschool age and the behavioral difficulties are conceptualized as part of communication difficulties, the student may qualify for services under the category of Speech and Language Impairment (SLI). Please note, category of eligibility is determined individually based on each student's cognitive, academic, language, and psychological profile. While these categories most commonly "fit" the needs of students with behavioral dysfunction, all categories must be looked at as part of the multidisciplinary assessment.

The 2004 reauthorization includes the following parameters regarding eligibility criteria:

OTHER HEALTH IMPAIRMENT (OHI)

Other health impairment means having limited strength, vitality, or alertness, including a heightened alertness to environmental stimuli, that results in limited alertness with respect to the educational environment, that

Is due to chronic or acute health problems such as asthma, attention deficit disorder or attention deficit hyperactivity disorder, diabetes, epilepsy, a heart condition, hemophilia, lead poisoning, leukemia, nephritis, rheumatic fever, sickle cell anemia, and Tourette syndrome; and

Adversely affects a child's educational performance. [§300.8(c)(9)]

SPEECH LANGUAGE IMPAIRMENT (SLI)

Speech or language impairment means a communication disorder, such as stuttering, impaired articulation, a language impairment, or a voice impairment, that adversely affects a child's educational performance.

EMOTIONAL DISTURBANCE (ED)

Emotional disturbance means a condition exhibiting one or more of the following characteristics over a long period of time and to a marked degree that adversely affects a child's educational performance:

An inability to learn that cannot be explained by intellectual, sensory, or health factors.

An inability to build or maintain satisfactory interpersonal relationships with peers and teachers.

Inappropriate types of behavior or feelings under normal circumstances.

A general pervasive mood of unhappiness or depression.

A tendency to develop physical symptoms or fears associated with personal or school problems.

Emotional disturbance includes schizophrenia. The term does not apply to children who are socially maladjusted, unless it is determined that they have an emotional disturbance under paragraph (c)(4)(i) of this section.

If the IEP team determines the student is eligible for Special Education, an Individual Education Plan (IEP) will be developed and will address all assessed areas of need. The IEP should include goals and objectives focused on all the areas that are found to be impacting within the educational setting. If the student is found to have needs that cannot be supported with only goals and objectives directed at behavior and compliance, a Behavior Support Plan can be developed. This Behavior Support Plan should address specific target behaviors addressed by the IEP team and will include an individualized series of goals and objectives to be addressed every 6 weeks by the multidisciplinary team.

CASE EXAMPLE

This case example of a young child, provided by Sarah Katz, demonstrates the continuity of assessment and intervention plan that takes place when a child has been identified as eligible for special services.

Case Example of the Assessment Process

The following assessment example involves a 4-year 4-month old child. Previous assessment at age 3 indicated a possible diagnosis of developmental childhood apraxia of speech, however, at age 4.4 a multidisciplinary assessment was conducted to determine present levels of performance, educational growth, eligibility for continued special education services, and recommendations for educational programming needs. This example depicts how a multidisciplinary team might evaluate a child who demonstrates delays across all domains using various assessment tools.

Background History

Kate is a 4.4-year-old (52 month) female. She is currently enrolled in private preschool which she attends 5 days a week in the mornings. Kate lives at home with her mother, father, and older twin brothers who are in 5th grade. Family history is significant for speech delays, learning disabilities, autism spectrum disorders, and seizure disorder. Kate's mother obtained prenatal care beginning at 7 weeks. Exposure to drugs, tobacco, or alcohol was denied during the pregnancy. Kate was born full-term via vaginal delivery. She was 7lbs 8 ounces at birth. Two days after birth, Kate returned to the hospital and was treated for jaundice. She was hospitalized for 6 days.

Developmental milestones were delayed. Kate sat at 11 months, crawled at 14 months and walked at 2 years. At the age of 2.11 she had approximately 10 words in her vocabulary. Health was significant for reoccurring ear infections and trouble breathing. Kate had an adenoidectomy and PE tubes placed in January 2008. Kate was referred for a multidisciplinary assessment as a result of a parent request for speech-language assessment. Kate's educational history is as follows:

Tests Administered

In accordance with Ed. Code 56320, the following considerations have been made with regard to procedures and materials to ensure compliance with all federal and state requirements:

All test materials were administered in the pupil's primary language or through the use of an interpreter. All test materials have been validated for the specific purpose for which they were used and were administered by trained personnel in conformance with the instructions provided by the producers of the test. Tests and other assessment materials include those tailored to assess the specific areas of educational need and not merely those which were designed to provide a single general intelligence quotient. Assessment materials were selected so as to not be racially, sexually, or culturally discriminating. Tests were selected and administered to best insure that when a test is administered to a pupil with impaired sensory, manual, or speaking skills, it produces test results that accurately reflect the pupil's aptitude, achievement level, or any factors that the test purports to measure and not the pupil's impaired sensory manual or speaking skills unless those skills are the factors the test purports to measure.

Orofacial Examination
- Goldman Fristoe Test of Articulation – Second Edition (GFTA-2)
- Kahn-Lewis Phonological Analysis-2 (KLPA-2)

- Verbal Motor Production Assessment for Children (VMPAC)
- Peabody Picture Vocabulary Test – Fourth Edition (PPVT-4)
- Expressive Vocabulary Test – Second Edition (EVT-2)
- Clinical Evaluation of Language Fundamentals Preschool – Second Edition (CELF Preschool-2)
- HawaiiEa rly Learning Profile Strands (HELP)
- Vineland Adaptive Rating Scale

GeneralO bservations

Kate willingly participated in the evaluation sessions. Two sessions were observations at her preschool, three sessions were completed at the elementary school located closest to her home. Kate was pleasant and cooperative during the evaluation. She appeared to put forth appropriate effort with all tasks presented. Results were perceived as valid.

ClassroomO bservations

Kate was observed in the educational setting at her private preschool classroom. She was observed during recess/outside play and in the classroom setting during center time.

Observation #1 Kate was observed for a 45-minute play period outside. Kate was active, climbing on the play structure and bouncing a ball. She was friendly and approached the observers on many occasions. It appeared she preferred to engage in play and interact with adults rather than peers from her class. Kate followed simple directions given to her by the observers and her teachers ("go play in the house", "get some water", and "time to ride your bike"). Although she is liked by her peers, Kate rarely initiates spontaneous play. Kate's gross motor skills appeared to be intact during this observation. She was able to pedal a tricycle, climb stairs, drink from a water fountain, and bounce and throw a ball.

Observation #2 Kate was observed during "center-time" in her preschool class. During this observation, Kate was responsible for completing the work at three stations: making a hand print with paint (turkey hand), decorating and gluing feathers on an Indian headdress, and tracing her name on a laminated piece of sentence strip.

Kate began at the Indian headdress station. She followed directions given by her teacher, and decorated the headband with markers. On multiple occasions she looked back at the observers, smiled, waved, and showed her marker. On the first occasion, she held up the brown marker and stated, "black", on the second occasion, she held up the green marker and stated, "yellow". Kate was given a bottle of glue and directed to glue paper "feathers" to the headdress. She attempted to glue on her own, but when she was unsuccessful at getting the glue to come out of the bottle, she handed it to a peer at her table and said, "bock" (broken). Kate was then given assistance with gluing and completing her headdress.

In the second station, Kate was directed to find her name in a group of nametags and trace over it with a marker. Kate successfully found her name after two attempts and held up the name tag to show the observers. She sat for the remainder of the center, and scribbled with dry-erase marker on the name tag.

During the third station, Kate's hand was painted by a teacher and she was instructed to make a handprint on a blank piece of paper. Kate followed directions and completed the project with ease. After the handprint was completed, Kate was instructed to "go wash your hands" by her teacher. As she was given this direction, Kate turned towards her teacher, looked down at her hands, and complied by walking to the bathroom to wash her hands. She was observed in the bathroom independently to use soap, wash and scrub her hands under the tap in the sink, and to get a paper towel to dry her hands. As she was completing this task, Kate looked up at the observer standing in the door and said, "Hi Sarah".

It should be noted, as in the outdoor observation, during the academic observation, Kate did not initiate peer interaction or play. She stayed close to her teachers and chose to sit and work on her center work quietly rather than play with her peers in the kitchen or dress-up station. Kate seems to be able to imitate and engage in reciprocal play with adults very comfortably, however, she is not yet engaging her peers in imaginary play or with independent social interactions. When directed to do so, or when demonstrated a simple task, Kate will engage her peers (i.e., "give the ball to Kate").

125

TestResu lts

Academic/Cognitive/Behavioral Please note – According to the HELP for Preschoolers Assessment and Curriculum Guide: No child is expected to display all HELP for Preschoolers skills listed, nor display all skills for an age range. The age ranges in HELP for Preschoolers are the ages at which a skill or behavior (for children who do not have disabilities) typically begins according to the literature. These age ranges are not when a skill begins and ends. Some skills are time-limited and emerge into more complex skills, while others are lifetime skills.

Cognitive Kate demonstrates cognitive development in the 20–36-month range with emerging skills and upward scatter ranging from 36 to 45 month level. Kate is able to: understand the concept of one (24 months), sort shapes (30 months), point to and identify body parts (30 months), count orally to three (36 months), and march and clap to music (40 months). She does not yet demonstrate understanding of sequencing illustrations (44 months), sort according to shape, size, and length (45 months), or count orally to 10 (48 months). Within her age range (4.4 years), Kate is not yet able to: locate first, middle, and last in a group, match coins, tell or draw a picture to provide a solution, and color within the lines of a circle.

Adaptive scores on the Vineland Adaptive Behavior Scale II indicate Kate is performing in the deficient range. Standard scores fell in the high 60s to mid 70s (average standard scores 100) in all areas with some upward scatter. These scores are as indicated by multiple raters (teachers and parents) and across multiple settings (at school and home).

Gross Motor Kate demonstrates developmental skills in the 36–52 month range with some emerging and upward scatter to 60-month range. Gross motor skills are a relative strength for Kate. At this time she is able to: alternate standing on one foot (36 months), stand on tiptoes (38 months), run a 20-foot distance (44 months), complete a forward roll (45 months), throw a ball 10 feet overhead (53 months), and hang from a bar using an overhand grip (54 months). Emerging skills include skipping, galloping, and walking down stairs carrying an object.

Fine Motor Kate demonstrates fine motor skills range between the developmental level of 20–36-month range with scattered and emerging skills ranging from 36 to 42 months. Kate is able to: imitate a circular scribble (20 months), build a tower using more than 6 blocks (22 months), and uses an appropriate adult-like grasp on her pencil (36 months). She will snip with scissors (28 months), but is not yet cutting on a line. At her age level, Kate is not yet: drawing a square following a model (48 months), completing a picture of a stick-person (48 months), cutting out small square/triangle shapes (48 months), or tracing around her hand (53 months).

Social Kate demonstrates social skills ranging at the developmental level 40–48 months, with emerging skills and upward scatter at the 48–52-month level. She says hello, good bye, please, and thank you at correct times (40–41 months), follows directions given by an authority figure (42 months), shares toys with other children (46 months), participates in cooperative play (48 months), and sits in seat without excess moving during an activity (49 months). It should be noted that many of the emerging skills or skills at Kate's age range that are not mastered at this time are social skills requiring the use of language she has not yet developed.

Self-Help Kate demonstrates adaptive living skills ranging from 48 to 55 months with emerging skills and upward scatter ranging from 55 to 65 months. Per parent report, Kate eats different types of food (48 months), goes to the toilet without frequent accidents (48 months), uses a towel after washing (48 months), washes face with soap when requested (54 months), and covers mouth with a tissue when sneezing or coughing (54 months).

Speech An orofacial examination was completed to assess structure and function of Kate's oral mechanism. Facial features were symmetrical at rest. Breathing and respiration were coordinated and adequate for phonation. Kate's lips were within normal limits for appearance at rest, rounding her lips, drawing the corners back and biting her lower lip. Kate demonstrated adequate intra-oral pressure and labial strength when she closed her lips and puffed her cheeks without allowing air to escape. The surface of Kate's tongue appeared to be within normal limits. She demonstrated the ability to protrude her tongue and move the tongue tip up, down, left and right. Kate pushed her tongue against a tongue depressor both anteriorly (forward) and laterally (left/right) to demonstrate adequate strength. Kate demonstrated difficulty for following complex auditory directions for putting her tongue tip on the alveolar ridge and drawing it back along the hard palate. Kate's teeth were in good condition and adequate for speech production. No concerns regarding the occlusion and alignment between Kate's maxilla and mandible (upper and lower jaws) were noted. The hard palate was within normal appearance for height and vault. The soft palate and pharynx including the uvula, faucial arches, and palatine tonsils were also within normal limits for appearance at rest. Adequate vertical and lateral velopharyngeal movement and symmetry were noted during sustained productions and repeated productions of "ah". Nasal occlusion revealed no change in vocal quality or hypernasality.

During the 172-utterance spontaneous speech sample, Kate's overall speech intelligibility was judged to be 71% on an utterance-by-utterance level to the familiar listener when context was known. Errors noted during the sample were consistent with the errors noted in the *GFTA-2* and *KLPA-2* (e.g., *duck* for stuck; *bish* for fish). Kate also exhibited several vowel substitution errors (e.g., *buck* for broke; *not* for night; *wet* for wait).

The *Goldman Fristoe Test of Articulation – Second Edition (GFTA-2)* was administered to evaluate Kate's production of various speech sounds in fixed word positions. Standardized scores were not provided because some target items on the test were not presented in a standardized manner. Kate often required a verbal model when she did not independently label the picture presented. "Any modifications made to standardized procedures may invalidate the use of normative scores for Sounds-in-Words…In these situations, professionals who review the results must rely on clinical judgment to maximize interpretation of the speech samples obtained" (Taken from GFTA-2 Manual, 2000).

The *Verbal Motor Production Assessment for Children (VMPAC)* was a step-by-step assessment of the neuromotor speech production system at rest and when engaged in vegetative and volitional non-speech and speech tasks. The test was divided into three main areas: Global Motor Control, Focal Oromotor Control, and Sequencing.

Based on this standardized measure, Kate exhibited deficits in Focal Oromotor Control, Sequencing, and Connected Speech and Language Control. Additionally, the test indicated Kate would benefit from visual and tactile cues when training targets in speech production. Kate's performance on the *VMPAC* was consistent with assessment findings throughout the evaluation sessions.

Language The *Peabody Picture Vocabulary Test – Fourth Edition (PPVT-4)* was administered to assess Kate's receptive vocabulary skills through a point-to-picture task. Kate was asked to select the appropriate picture in a field of four which best represented the word presented orally. No sentence or contextual cues were allowed. Kate's raw score of 41 converted to a standard score of 79 and reflected overall receptive vocabulary at or better than 8 percent of peers her age. A test-age equivalency of 3 years 0 months was obtained based on the raw score.

The *Expressive Vocabulary Test – Second Edition (EVT-2)* was administered to assess Kate's expressive vocabulary skills through a picture identification task. Kate was asked to name pictures or provide a single category label for groups of pictures presented. Kate's performance on the test was in the low average range. Kate's raw score of 16 converted to a standard score of 67 and reflected overall expressive vocabulary at or better than 1 percent of peers her age. A test-age equivalency of 2 years 0 months was obtained based on the raw score.

The *Clinical Evaluation of Language Fundamentals Preschool – Second Edition (CELF Preschool–2)* was administered to evaluate Kate's general language ability using three subtests (Sentence Structure, Word Structure, and Expressive Vocabulary) that were used to determine a Core Language Score. The Core Language standard score has a mean of 100 and a standard deviation of 15. A standard score of 100 on this scale represents the performance of the typical child of a given age. Because Kate's performance on the core language subtests fell below the average range, further sub-tests were administered to gain more information about how her language modalities were affected. Kate's sum of Core Language subtest scaled scores of 10 converted to a standard score of 61 and reflected Core Language (general language ability) at or better than 0.5 percent of peers her age. The following subtests were administered.

Recommendations Qualified personnel conducted this evaluation and should be considered to be a valid assessment of learning needs and that the results are defensible. Based on the assessment findings, including standardized articulation and language assessments, informal speech and language sample, and parent and teacher input, observations, and the developmental Hawaii Early Learning Profile, Kate continues to meet eligibility requirements for Special Education Services at this time. Kate demonstrated articulation errors, phonological processes, and difficulties in motor sequencing that significantly impacted her intelligibility with listeners in all contexts and deficits in receptive and expressive language as well as cognitive, language, and social delays. The following targets are recommended for specialized instruction to address Kate's assessed needs:

- Follow 1-step verbal directions containing basic concepts (e.g. dimension/size, direction/location/position, number/quantity, equality, etc.)
- Increase Mean Length of Utterance (MLU) to 4–5 words
- Identify, recognize, and count numbers 1–10
- Identify, recognize, and match colors
- Identify, recognize, and write 26 letters
- Identify, recognize, and write her first name
- Demonstrate understanding of sequence (2 or 3 pictures).

Bibliography

Abidin, R. R. (1986). *Parenting stress index*. Charlottesville, VA: Pediatric Psychology Press.

Achenbach, T. M. (1989). *Child behavior checklist*. Burlington: University of Vermont Press.

Achenbach, T. M. (2000). Assessment of psychopathology. In A. J. Sameroff, M. Lewis, & S. M. Miller (Eds.), *Handbook of developmental psychopathology* (2nd ed.). New York: Plenum Publishers.

Ayers, A. J. (1989). *Sensory integration and praxis tests*. Los Angeles: Western Psychological Services.

Barnard, K. E. (1979). *Instructor's learning resource manual*. Seattle: NCAST Publications, University of Washington.

Bates, J. E. (1984). *Infant characteristics questionnaire* (Revised). Bloomington: Indiana University Press.

Bayley, N. (1995). *Bayley scales of infant development*. New York: Psychological Corporation.

Benson, J. B., & Haith, M. M. (2009). *Social and emotional development in infancy and early childhood*. San Diego: Academic Press.

Berk, R. A., & DeGangi, G. A. (1983). *DeGangi-Berk tst of snsory itegration*. Los Angeles: Western Pychological Services.

Caldwell, B., & Bradley, R. (1984). *HOME observation for measurement of the eEnvironment (HOME)* (Revised ed.). Little Rock: University of Arkansas.

California Department of Education (2001). Handbook on developing individualized family service plans and individualized education programs in early childhood and special education <http://www.cde.ca.gov/sp/se/fp/documents/ecii>.

Clark, R. (1985). *The parent-child relational assessment*. Madison: Department of Psychiatry, University of Wisconsin Medical School.

Connors, C. K. (1997). *Connors' rating scales* (Revised). North Tonawanda, NJ: Multi-Health Systems.

DeGangi, G. A. (1995). *Test of attention in infants*. Dayton, OH: Southpaw.

DeGangi, G. E., & Balzer-Martin, L. (1999). The sensory history questionnaire for preschoolers. *Journal of Developmental and Learning Disorders, 3*(1), 59–83.

DeGangi, G. A., Breinbauer, C., Roosevelt, J. D., Porges, S., & Greenspan, S. I. (2000). Predictions of childhood problems at three years in children experiencing disorders of regulations during infancy. *Infant Mental Health Journal, 21*(3), 156–175.

DeGangi, G. A., & Greenspan, S. I. (1989). *The test of sensory functions in infants*. Los Angeles: Western Psychological Services.

DeGangi, G. A., Poisson, S., Sickel, R. Z., & Wiener, A. S. (1995). *Infant-toddler symptom checklist*. Tucson: Therapy Skill Builders.

Early Childhood Training Center's Media Center Website <http://etc.education.ne.gov> Online catalog <http://ectc-library.education.ne.gov>

Fagan, J. F. (1982). New evidence for the prediction of intelligence from infancy. *Infancy Mental Health Journal, 3*(4), 219–228.

Fagan, J. F., & Detterman, D. K. (1992). The Fagan test of infant intelligence: a technical summary. *Journal of Applied Developmental Psychology, 13*, 173–193.

Fisher, A. G., Murray, E. A., & Bundy, A. C. (1991). *Sensory integration theory and practice*. Philadelphia: FA Davis.

Frankel, K. A., Boyum, L. A., & Harmon, R. J. (2004). Diagnoses and presenting symptoms in an infant psychiatry clinic: comparison of two diagnostic systems. *Journal of the American Academy of Child and Adolescent Psychiatry, 43*, 578–587.

Frankel K., & Harmon R. (2006). Overview of DC:0-3R Diagnostic classification of infants and young children. ZERO TO THREE. Publications office: 1-800-899-4301 <www.zerotothree.org>.

Glascoe F.P. (2006). Commonly used screening tools. Developmental Pediatrics Online. Available online at: <http://www.dbpeds.org/articles/detail.cfm?textid=539>.

ICD-10, International Classification of Diseases, (10th ed.). Geneva: World Health Organization.

Individuals with Disabilities Education Improvement Act of 2004 (Public Law 108-446), 20 U.S.C. 1400.

Johnson, S. L. (2005). *Therapist guide to clinical intervention*. San Diego: Academic Press.

Linder, T. W. (1990). *Transdisciplinary play based assessment*. Baltimore: Paul H. Brooks.

Meschan, J., & Perrin, J. (2010). Enhancing pediatric mental health care: Strategies for preparing for a community. *Pediatrics, 125*(3), 575–586.

Miller, W., & Rollnick, S. (1991). *Motivational interviewing: preparing people to change behavior*. New York: Guilford Press.

Reebye, P., & Stalker, A. (2007). Regulation disorders of sensory processing in infants and young children. *BC Medical Journal, 49*(4), 194–200.

Ringwalt, S. (2008). *Developmental screening and assessment instruments with an emphasis on social and emotional development for young children ages birth through five*. Chapel Hill: The University of North Carolina, FPG Child Development Institute, National Early Childhood Technical Assistance Center. Available at <http://www.nectac.org/~pdfs/pubs/screening.pdf> At the end of this document is a list of web sources used for compilation of testing instruments.

Rosenberg, S. A., Zhang, D., & Robinson, C. C. (2008). Prevalence of developmental delays and participation in early intervention services for young children. *Pediatrics, 121*, e1503–e1509.

Shavell, M. I., Mahnemer, A., Rosenbaum, P., & Abrahamowicz, M. (2001). Profile of referrals for early childhood developmental delay to ambulatory subspecialty clinics. *Journal of Child Neurology, 16*, 645–650.

Sosna, T., & Mastergeorge, A. (2005). *Compendium of screening tools for early childhoodsocial-emotional development*. Sacramento, CA: The California Institute for Mental Health. at <http://www.firts5caspecialneeds.org/documents/IPFMHI-compendiumofScreeningTools.pdf>.

Squires, J., Bricker, D., & Twombly, E. (2002). *Ages & Stages Questionnaire; Social-Emotional (SSQ-SE)*. Brookes Publishing Company. PO Box 10624 Baltimore, MD 21285-0624.

Wolraich, M. L., Drotar, D. D., Dworkin, P. H., & Perrin, E. C. (2008). *Developmental-behavioral pediatrics. evidence and practice*. Philidephia: Mosby, Inc..

Wright, C., & Northcutt, C. Decision guidelines for Axis I, II, V. In consultation with Zero to Three's DC:0-3R training task force. Retrieved 4/6/12. <http://www.zerotothree.org/child-development/early-childhood-mental-health/diagnostic-guidelines.html>.

Further Reading

American Psychiatric Association <http://www.psych.org>.

Caldwell, B., & Bradley, R. (1978). *Manual for the home observation for measurement of the environment*. Little Rock: University of Arkansas Press.

Center for Social and Emotional Foundations for Early learning. <http://www.vanderbilt.edu/csefel/>.

Crosswalk between Diagnostic Classification 0–3, ICD 9 CM and DSM IVR+. Department of Community Health-Mental Health Services to Children and Families <http://www.miaimh.org/.../crosswalkaccess_eligibilitywithdch_title_121807.pdf>.

DC: 0-3R (2005). Diagnostic classification of mental health and developmental disorders of infancy and early childhood (Revised ed.). Washington, DC: Zero to Three Press. Available at <http://www.zerotothree.org/>.

DC: 0-3R (2007). Department of Community Health-Mental Services to Children and Families. December 18, 2007. <http://www.miaimh.org/documents/crosswalkaccess_elegibilitywithdch_title_121807.pdf>

DeGangi, G. A. (1991). Regulatory disordered infants: assessment of sensory, emotional, and attentional problems. *Infants Young Child, 3*(3), 1–8.

DeGangi, G. A. (2000). *Pediatric disorders of regulation in affect and behavior*. San Diego: Academic Press.

Diagnostic Classification of Mental Health and Developmental Disorders of Infancy and Early Childhood, Revised 0-3 DC:0-3R (2005). Washington, DC: National Center for Infants, Toddlers and Families.

Diagnostic and Statistical Manual of Mental Disorders (2000), *Text Revision (DSM_IV_TR)* (4th ed.). Washington, DC: American Psychiatric Association. Available at <www.psych.org> and <http:www.psych.org> and <http://www.psych.org/Resources/MentalHealthResources.aspx>

Gealson, M. M., & Zeanah, C. H. (2005). Infant mental health. In M. Hersen & J. Thomas (Eds.), *The comprehensive handbook of personality and psychopathology* (vol. 3). New York: Wiley & Sons.

Georgetown University Center for Child and Human Development (2009). Contemporary practices in early childhood intervention: early childhood social and emotional development and mental health primer. Available online at <http://www.gucchdgeorgetown.net/CPEI>.

Greenspan, S. I. (2003). Childcare research: a clinical perspective. *Child Development, 74*(4), 1064–1068.

Greenspan S.I. The basic course on the Greenspan Floortime Approach <www.stanleygreenspan.com>.

Greenspan, S. I., & DeGangi, G. A. (2001). Research on the FEAS: test development, reliability and validity studies. In S. Greenspan, G. DeGangi, & S. Wieder (Eds.), *The Functional Emotional Assessment Scale (FEAS) for infancy andea rlyc hildhood.c linicala ndr esearcha pplications(pp. 167–247)*. Bethesda: Interdisciplinary Council on Development and Learning Disorders (ICDL). <www.icdl.com>

Gross, D., Conrad, B., Fogg, L., Willis, L., & Garvey, C. (1993). What does the NCATS (Nursing Child Assessment Teaching Scale) measure? *Nursing Research, 42*(5), 260–265.

HOME Observation for Measurement of the Environment (HOME). Information from University of Arkansas at Little Rock. <http://www.ualr.edu/coedept/case/ent/home.html> To obtain materials for administering and scoring the HOME inventories, contact Lorraine Coulson at 501-565-7627 lrcoulson@ualr.edu

National Information Center for Children and Youth with Disabilities. Transition planning: a team effort. NICHY, P.O. Box 1492. Washington, DC, 20013. (202) 884-8200 or (800) 695-0285 or web <http://www.nichy.org/pubs/transum/ts10txt.htm>.

National Institute of Child Health and Human Development (NICHD). <http://www.nichd.nih.gov>.

National institutes of Mental Health. <http://nimh.nih.gov/health/topics/autism-spectrum-disorders-pervasive-developmental-disorders/index.shtml>

National Mental Health Information Center. <http://mentalhealth.samsa.gov/child/childhealth.asp>.

NECTAC. State examples of IFSP forms and guidelines, <http://www.nectac.org/topics/families/stateifsp.asp>.

US Education Department Office of Special Education Programs (OSEP), (2007). Infants and toddlers receiving early intervention services under IDEA, Part C, by age and state: Fall 2007. Part C Child Count. Table 8-1. Available at <http://www.ideadata.org/arc-toc9asp#partcCC>.

Wieder, S., & Greenspan, S. I. (2001). The DIR (developmental, individual-difference, relationship-based) approach to assessment and intervention planning. *Bull Zero to Three, 21*(4), 11–19. National Center for Infants, Toddlers, and Families

Zero to Three, Early Childhood Mental Health and Social Emotional Development <http://www.zerotothree.org/site/PageServer?pagename=key-mental>, <http://www.zerotothree.org/site/PageServer?pagename=key-social>.

Zero to Three (2005). Diagnostic Classification of Mental Health and Developmental disorders of Infancy and childhood: Revised Edition (DC; 0-3R).

CHAPTER 3

Treatment Planning

PREPARING FOR TREATMENT PLANNING
Developing Individualized Early Childhood Treatment Plans

Working with children requires individualized plans of intervention based upon case-specific needs and carried out by a multidisciplinary treatment team. No pediatric case is exactly like another, whether it is child characteristics or associated influencing characteristics such as factors associated with caregivers (socioeconomic status, education, life experiences, etc.), sibling complications, family systems issues, contributions of pos/neg by extended family members and/or cultural expectations. Thus, as with all treatment planning endeavors, it is imperative that the working model or dynamic/developmental formulation be correct so that effective interventions can be employed.

The parameters of intervention are incorporated into a plan or program of interventions designed for infants, toddlers, preschoolers and kindergarteners. In addition to the team of intervening professionals is the role of parents in the change process. The theoretical foundation of parent–child interventions is a flexible integration of attachment theory (relationship based), social-learning theory and cognitive-behavioral therapy (CBT) necessary for basic skill building. The seasoned professional team members function utilizing a framework which is updated according to changes, issues targeted for change and unplanned circumstances which impact the effectiveness of the treatment plan. Their functional framework is derived from sources of developmental information previously identified, the foundation of emotion and the most useful treatment plan format (which is generally driven by the intervention environment). Two examples of the influence of intervening environment upon treatment plan format are the IEP and IFSP of the educational environment and the dynamic formulation of a clinical environment.

Parent–child intervention supports and reinforces the development of perceptions, attitudes, and behaviors that express positive affect, age-appropriate discipline and management, reciprocal play, shared exploration of their environment, and constructive resolution to differences and conflicts. Not only the children in many of these circumstances are presenting with difficulties and deficits, the parent may demonstrate a lack of interest or an inability to soothe which negatively impacts attachment, offer negative or punitive discipline, unmodulated or dysregulated behavior of their own, violent or coercive behaviors, significant relationships or environmental circumstances. The aforementioned parental deficits in skill coupled with environmental problems negatively impact a child's feelings of safety, nurturance, encouragement, mentoring, learning and overall age-appropriate development. Because of the interest of intervening in the lives of young children to remediate difficulties/challenges and promote healthy development, numerous programs and recommendations for intervention are available.

131

Therapist's Guide to Pediatric Affect and Behavior Regulation. DOI: http://dx.doi.org/10.1016/B978-0-12-386884-8.00003-3

According to the UCSF-San Francisco General Hospital program for pediatric intervention referred to as The Child Trauma Research Project, young children exposed to severe interpersonal violence are at risk for interference with mastery of age-appropriate development as well as numerous psychiatric and behavioral problems. In their program, the parent and child attend weekly therapy sessions. The integration of these modalities in a flexible network are to be used in accordance with the family's needs and promoting a sense of competence for both the parent and the child. As can be seen below, the foundation of their program is a useful conceptualization of parent–child intervention which can be modified for use in non-trauma intervention. The program highlights the use of six core intervention modalities for parent–child therapy.

Core Intervention Modalities for Children Exposed to Trauma

- Guided parent-child interaction
  Utilizes play, physical contact, and language to encourage health exploration, manage overwhelming affect, clarify feelings, and correct misperceptions and distortions. The facilitator promotes the parent's sensitive responsiveness to the child's signals, safe and supportive physical contact, age-appropriate playful interactions, age-appropriate use of language to explain real situations and express feelings appropriately "using their words".
- Unstructured developmental guidance
  An intervention modality that provides the parent with age-appropriate information about the child's feelings and needs as they come up during the course of the therapy sessions.
- Modeling appropriate protective behavior
  A modality which involves taking action to intervene and stop the escalation of dangerous behavior, self-endangering behavior or intervening to prevent a child from harming another child. The focus is on the mutual reflection of care between a parent and child and the importance of being safe from danger.
- Affective interpretation
  A modified psychoanalytic technique which emphasizes linking the parent's affective responses to life experiences coupled with current parenting practices.
- Emotional support and empathic communication
  Supportive and empathic interventions utilized through both words and actions the belief of accomplishing treatment goals which may seem overwhelming and out of reach. Emphasizing and reinforcing the satisfaction experienced in achieving personal goals and in meeting developmental milestones, reinforcing the use of effective coping strategies (and the reinforcing aspect of success) and giving feedback about progress.
- Concrete assistance dealing with daily problems
  A modality serving to take appropriate action to prevent or resolve the consequences associated with family crisis/stressful circumstances. Additionally, obtaining assistance of necessary resources and services that enhance and improve the family's quality of life.

DeGangi (2000) promotes a family-centered approach that addresses parental concerns and offers parent guidance along with the use of child-centered activities. Dr DeGangi's work with regulatory disordered young children and their families offers first hand experience associated with her years of work in the field. The family is recognized as a constant in the child's life versus professionals who provide services being a potentially fluctuating factor. Additionally, there is full acknowledgement and use of the aspects of the dyadic relationship:

1. Behavioral quality of the interaction
2. Affective tone
3. Psychological involvement

The dyadic relationship is critical to development and adjustment. Therefore, the mother should be referred to a mental health provider/psychiatrist as well if (she):

- Lacks empathy, makes hostile comments, or attributes persecutory intent to her baby

- There is a lack of bonding or other mother–baby relationship problem
- Is unable to follow advice
- Feels persistently angry, or continues to report anxiety or depression symptoms even when any baby or child problem is improved.

*The father's role is an invaluable source of practical and emotional support in the family-centered approach. The role of the father is often neglected, and they need to be actively engaged in all aspects of assessment and intervention (including appointments). Fathers are often concerned about how their partner is coping and is interested in being educated and developing their own tools to help their family. However, if a father presents as emotionally distant or other psychological/emotional problems are evident, he should be referred to treatment. If the marriage/union is unstable or there are concerns of domestic violence or severe/chronic acrimony, the couple should be referred for an evaluation and treatment if identified as necessary.

When an intervening professional hears from a mother that she cannot stand another minute of listening to her baby crying because it is driving her crazy, it is a direct indication of the significant impact an irritable child can have upon a caregiver and may reflect their own cry for help. Interestingly, most people who hear of this type of scenario are filled with the concerns of the "emotional" state of the caregiver. Although there are numerous reasons to be concerned about how the caregiver is responding warranting support/intervention, what is central to the case is the underlying emotional experience of the child. While the entire family system may be assessed for determining adequate support and intervention, it is the understanding of the internal experience of the infant/child that needs to be a clinical focus. If intervention ensues without a working hypothesis with associated understanding of what the infant/child is emotionally experiencing, the goal of soothing, reinforcing adjustment and resilience, and the longer term goal of maximal benefit will be fraught with missed opportunities.

Greenspan (1998, 2002; Casenhiser et al, 2007), an icon in the field of child development and intervention, felt it was crucial to conceptualize the child's emotional and developmental needs and translate the identified needs into treatment. This translation is accomplished by answering questions like:

1. Is the child engaged or not engaged, in what situations does this occur, and how do they engage or disengage?
2. How does the child communicate, gesturally, by affective expressions, words?
3. Does the child organize affective experiences symbolically?
4. By observing the child along dimensions of engagement, intentional behavioral patterns, and representational elaboration, how are their difficulties conceptualized?

Cohen et al (2005) offer an integrative continuum to improve early childhood social and emotional development as well as behavioral concerns which includes:

- *Promotion*
  - ○ Services designed to maintain social emotional well-being
  - ○ Might include public/direct family education to increase awareness of factors which increase risk and how to minimize or alleviate risk, home visits, family support programs (educate primary caregivers on development, healthy relationships, environment and experiences)
- *Prevention*
  - ○ Focus on children at risk of poor developmental outcomes
  - ○ Early identification and intervention strategies that decrease the risk of social and emotional development associated with mental health problems
  - ○ Carried out via screenings provided through child-care setting, pediatrician office, home visit, comprehensive child development programs/child abuse programs (may address exposure to environmental toxins such as lead/mercury, quality of care of child, addressing domestic violence, etc.)

- *Treatment*
  - Targets and develops individualized treatment for young children and their families currently exhibiting symptoms of mental health problems
  - Generally comprised of a skilled multidisciplinary team offering different points of intervention (therapeutic day care, child–parent psychotherapy, parent education, child occupational therapy, speech therapy, etc.)

BEHAVIORS THAT WARRANT CONCERN
Infant and Toddlers Age 0–3

- Chronic feeding or sleeping difficulties
- Inconsolable fussiness/irritability
- Incessant crying with little ability to be consoled
- Extreme upset when left with another adult
- Inability to adapt/adjust to new situations
- Easily startled/alarmed even by routine activities
- Inability to establish relationships with children or adults
- Excessive hitting/biting/pushing of other children
- Excessive withdrawn behavior/flat affect

Preschoolers Age 3–5

- Engages in compulsive activities (head banging or other repetitive self-destructive behaviors)
- Out of control tantrums
- Withdrawn behavior/demonstrates little interest in social interaction
- Demonstrates repetitive aggressive/impulsive behavior
- Difficulty playing with others
- Little or no communication/lack of language
- Loss of earlier developmental achievement

Reviewing a summary of developmental milestones is beneficial for contrasting observed concerns. To obtain a factsheet on milestones: http://www.cdc.gov/ncbddd/actearly/milestones/milestones-3mo.html http://www.cdc/ncbddd/actearly/milestones-5yhtml

While diagnostic nomenclature provides numerous and obvious points of value clinically, it is the identification of symptoms which impact the quality of life, relationships and learning which is central to intervention by the treatment plan, not the diagnostic label. Therefore, it is highly important that a therapist and/or treatment team be diligent in clarifying an accurate clinical picture so that a consistent treatment plan can be developed for cognitive-behavioral interventions. Treatment plan goals should focus on facilitating the child in developing self-soothing, problem-solving skills, increased ability to tolerate stress and frustration, and beginning to understand the association between choices and consequences (age appropriate). This requires parental intervention to aid them in an increased understanding of their child's experience, expectation of age-appropriate responding, how to set limits and redirect behavior, mechanisms to reinforce/encourage, and how the team (including parents at this level) works together to help the child develop skills and resolve issues. *In other words, when working with young children the realization that each and every behavior has a purpose, and the underlying reason why it occurs is the target of interventions.* Prevention strategies decrease the likelihood that a child will have problem behavior. This could include environmental changes, changes in activities, establishing routines, personal support, new ways to prompt a child, developing realistic expectations and limitations.

Replacement skills to replace a problem behavior with a functional, resourceful and positive behavior. The more efficient (easier) and effective (outcome) the replacement behavior the increased likelihood of a child adopting it. For this to take place, the replacement behavior must produce or approximate a positive effect as good as or better than the replaced behavior, i.e. the same function as the challenging behavior. A replacement skill needs to be relevant to the situation/environment, abilities of the child, and produce an immediate desired outcome for the child (meeting the wants and needs of the child).

<u>Caregiver guidance and responsibility</u> in responding to challenging child behaviors in a manner that does not maintain problem behavior, but instead facilitates and reinforces desired behavior. The caregiver must provide reinforcement to encourage the use of socially-appropriate replacement skills. This is accomplished by redirecting a child to use the replacement skill, reinforcement, and providing adequate practice.

Case examples have been adapted from DeGangi (2000) to increase the facilitation of conceptualizing the types of issues focused on by the intervening professional(s). Each treatment frame will offer a case example with varying range of complexity as well as variation in the depth of treatment planning. There may also be additional information outlined for some diagnoses and not for others, and the overlap of treatment objectives will not be duplicated. For example, the sensory processing issues discussed in the ADHD section will not be duplicated in the (following) RDSP section. However, the outline of treatment goals and associated focus of intervention is a consistent format across diagnoses. Below are two case examples indicative of the child presenting problems seen in the next section. Dr DeGangi's rich case presentations were drawn upon for the case examples in this section. A few case examples will serve to illustrate.

Case Examples
CASE EXAMPLE #1

Matti is a 3½ year old experiencing difficulties at preschool. His difficulties are a demonstration of how cognitive appraisal could impact mood regulation. He is described as an intelligent and competent child, but as often being irritable when instructed to make transitions from one activity to another, when other children intrude upon his personal space, activities were physical and unstructured, and when classroom noise escalated. It was not uncommon that when, after several hours of school, the children were asked to pick things up and get ready for snack time he would get overwhelmed by distress and hit or bite his peers or totally withdraw. The teacher could not predict what events might cause a good or bad day for Matti. Every time he bit one of the other children he was sent home and, for a time, his parents kept him at home for a break hoping to figure out how to deal with their son's behavior. At one point, a full-time aid was assigned to him to support him making transitions, not bite others, and to reorganize when distressed. Matti seemed even more upset and did not want to go to school – it had become a negative experience and he wanted to avoid it. A treatment plan was devised to change his cognitive appraisal of himself and school, and how behaviorally to create an emotionally manageable foundation which could be expanded toward mastering the regular schedule. This was accomplished by reintroducing Matti to school, but for only for a few hours (since that had seemed to be his limit of tolerance) and his aid would use positive reinforcement for task completion. Scheduled breaks were provided allowing him the opportunity, without demands, to reorganize himself. Breaks consisted of the choices of sitting in a cocoon chair and looking at books, sucking on a popcicle, building a fort that would allow him a quiet separate space to retreat to, etc. This was combined with a home program for behavioral reinforcement and compliance for good/friendly play (not biting or hitting), making transitions (picking up toys and art supplies), and self-calming when agitated (appropriately asking for time alone so that he could organize himself). After practicing these changes for about two months his compliance at home and school was greatly improved and he was starting to express a more positive outlook about himself and school as evidenced by wanting to go to school, and often remarking that he liked something. The teacher and parents continued to collaborate on providing him practice to reinforce the self-management skills he had learned.

135

CASE EXAMPLE #2

Lindsay, a 5 year old, had difficulty with the perceptual aspects of facial expression, reading and interpreting social and affective cues, and would become overwhelmed by environmental demands. She liked playing dress-up and had a special outfit she always selected for playtime. It appeared that the focus of her dress-up play was on things going wrong (cookies getting burned) and disasters (dolly getting lost in the park, etc.). It seemed as if she was looking for the therapist to appear stunned, surprised or alarmed by what she was doing. In this theme of playing, Lindsay was the hero always coming to the rescue. Initially, the therapist used a repetitious script for Lindsay to play in an effort to predict and understand her affective expression. Over time, the range of script was from predictable to less predictable and, in fact, might be silly or novel situations. The focus of the intervention was skill building moving from more expressive emotions to subtle ones. This range of practice was helping Lindsay to learn effectively how to read social cues.

TREATMENT PLANNING FORMAT

The format utilized to demonstrate identified problems will vary depending on the need of the environment. For example, private practitioners will create and utilize a format that is more in keeping with their practice structure along with the professional collateral contacts and treatment team they work with. However, a school, other formal program or agency might utilize a number of different forms, such as the one shown in Figure 3.1 used by an education specialist which rates evidence of behavior characteristics.

136

CHILD _____

PERSON RATING _____ DATE _____

CHARACTERISTIC	SCORE	E D INDICATOR	S M INDICATOR
Conscience Development		Self-critical, pervasively poor self-concept Unable to enjoy life	Self-critical, pleasure seeking, lack remorse over norm violations, little care for others' rights/feelings
Reality Orientation		Naive, gullible, fantasy base, denial and confusion, distorts reality without regard to self interest	Sweet-wise, not easily duped, often lies but is reality oriented
Adaptive Behavior		Cautious, inhibited, dependent, less inclined to explore, consistently poor adapting any setting	Self-reliant, "on their own", adjustment more situationally dependent
Domain		Affective disorder - anxiety, guilt, depression Mood swaings, frequent inappropriate affect	Character disorder – maladaptive behavioral pattern disturbing to others but not to the individual
Aggression		Hostile aggression to inflict pain, sole purpose of hurting others or self	Aggression as a means to an end, hurt others to acquire something, protect turf, attain status
Ego Strength		Hypersensitive, feelings easily hurt, overly dependent	Acts tough, more of a survivor, independent, self-assured
Anxiety		More anxious and fearful, appears tense	Appears relaxed and "cool", minimal aexiety over wrong doing shown
Peer Relations		Often ignored or rejected, poor relations, others alienated by individual's need for attention or bizarre behavir/thoughts, wants to trust, insecure	Accepted by sociocultural group, intact relations with other term alliances for self=serving purposes, manipulative

FIGURE 3.1

Form to rate evidence of behavior characteristics.

Types of Friends		No really close friends, often younger (level of social maturity) children, law abiding	Own age or older, attracted to those who habitually break rules (similar wayward tendencies)
School Behaviour		Psychological problems interfere, do poorly in school, unable to comply, inconsistent achievement, attention and concentration impaired, responds to structure, good attendance record	Unwilling to comply, dislikes school except as place for social contacts, generally low achievement, avoids achievement even in areas of competency, excessive absences
Locus of Control		Blames self, owns responsibility	Blames others, projects

Note: Please indicate in the score column whether each characteristic most closely matches E D or S M. if neither designation applies or you are unsure of closest match, do not mark that characteristic's score box.
ED = emotionally disturbed
SM = socially maladjusted
*In California only ED is protected by special education. Be sure to know the laws of the state in which yoy practice

FIGURE 3.1
(Continued)

Before embarking on treatment planning, it is important to enter into that conceptual frame with a developmental perspective of the skill of inhibitory control and its connection to self-regulation. The ability to exert conscious control over behaviors emerges gradually over the first several years of life with a rather prompt increase in the ability to follow rules to shape behaviors and to inhibit undesirable responses between 3 and 5 years of age. Response inhibition occurring between the ages of 3–5 provides children with an important source of regulation over their tendencies to approach and respond to situations. Therefore, bear in mind that the age range may be protracted in some instances and not in others or protracted across the board in some instances. Thus, requiring the "best fit" intervention based upon need, skill level and support required to reinforce the shaping of change.

TREATMENT PLANNING
Crying
CASE EXAMPLE

Bonnie, age 1½ months, is described as crying for hours. Her parents feel frustrated that they cannot soothe their baby, extremely fatigued, and concerned that something more serious is wrong with Bonnie. She is bottle fed using a common formula.

Treatment

Bonnie's pediatrician asked her parents numerous questions about feeding time, parental/caregiver practices, and environment to determine what course to proceed. He determined that Bonnie had colic and that her mother was experiencing post-partum depression. Bonnie's father was involved in her care, but lacked the skills to be supportive to his wife during this distressful time. The pediatrician initiated intervention in the following manner:

1. Educating the parents about colic. Colic generally starts at 2 weeks, ends at 3 months and demonstrates a peak in the evening. Time is taken to reinforce all of the caring efforts of the parents and to alleviate their concerns. The pediatrician offered several other recommendations he thought were worthy of trying and gave them instructions for additional resources in the community they could access for support
2. Referring the mother to a psychiatrist and psychologist who specialize in treating post-partum issues with the recommendation of the father participating adjunctively in therapy.

All infants, whether or not they are identified as having colic, cry more during the first 3 months of life than any other time (Figure 3.2). In order to clarify patterns parents/caregivers will offer the most accurate information by keeping a diary. One problem in dealing with this issue is that few people agree as to how much crying is considered

FIGURE 3.2
A mother comforts her crying baby through her loving touch.

excessive. The etiology of crying ranges from benign to life threatening. A thorough history and physical examination remains the cornerstone of the evaluation of the crying infant and should drive the decision tree of what to investigate. Three major areas are reviewed in brief with further considerations (Chatoor et al, 1984, 1985, 2004; DeGangi 2000; Karp, 2005).

GASTROINTESTINAL

- Problems with formula/cow's milk
- Lactose intolerance
- Reflux
- Immaturity
- Intestinal motility
- Fecal microflora

BIOLOGICAL FACTORS

- Feeding technique
- Motor regulation
- Increased serotonin
- Tobacco smoke exposure

PSYCHOSOCIAL

- Temperament
- Hypersensitivity
- Parental variables
  - Depression/mental illness
  - Low intellect
  - Substance abuse
  - Environmental instability

For most irritable infants there is no underlying medical cause. In some cases it may be attributed to food allergies (such as cow's milk), lactose intolerance, bowel spasms or gas, and only if there is frequent vomiting is gastroesophageal reflux a possible cause. Both feeding and sleeping are associated to crying. The duration of baby crying tends to peak at about 6 months, and most disappears at 3–4 months. A baby that cries persistently may not have yet learned to self-soothe and regulate their own crying, thus becoming persistent criers.

While the case example was rather straightforward and was used to demonstrate common issues, such is not always the situation. Fussiness and crying with its association to feeding offers the additional complexity of emotional and feeding development. *Therefore, when evaluating, diagnosing and formulating a treatment plan in the pediatric forum in general, to be thorough, it is imperative to take into consideration the multifaceted possibilities associated with homeostasis, attachment, separation, sensory processing, emotional growth and development, along with biological/neurological and family systems issues.

GOALS

1. Decrease or eliminate crying
2. Identify environmental needs

TREATMENT FOCUS AND OBJECTIVES

1. R/O medical problems. Examples of when babies should be referred for medical assessment:
   - excessive vomiting (more than 5 times/day)
   - continues to have feeding problems beyond 3 months of age
   - avoids gaze
   - withdraws emotionally and does not respond to parents when not crying
   - does not enjoy play

2. Identify environmental needs
   a. Assess the mother–infant relationship and maternal fatigue, anxiety and depression. Maternal psychosocial state. Invite the mother to talk about how stressful it is to care for a baby who cries a lot. Inquire if she has pleasurable time with her baby (if not, mom may be depressed). Discuss the relationship between depression, fatigue and decreased frustration tolerance. Possible referrals for mother:
      i. primary care physician
      ii. mental health provider/psychiatrist

Assess stress in the home environment in particular parental relationship stress/acrimony
   b. Assess stress in the home environment, in particular parental relationship stress/acrimony. Family psychosocial state
   c. Fathers are a valuable resource. The father's way of interacting with the baby may be different and beneficial. Educate the father on how to be more supportive of the mother and how important it is to share child-rearing tasks
   d. Parenting skills
   e. Support. All families with a crying infant are tired. Practical support is greatly needed to help families through this time. Parents are encouraged to:
      i. elicit support from family and friends
      ii. rest once a day when the baby is asleep
      iii. plan ahead for the baby's most difficult time of the day (such as preparing dinner in advance, etc)

*It is common to feel frustration, anxiety, even anger when chronic or inconsolable crying takes place. Just as frustrating is a baby who seems indifferent, won't cuddle or make eye contact. In these situations (possible attachment problem/pervasive developmental disorders), caregivers need to find ways to get their own stress in check so that they can get into a calm and balanced state. That will allow for more effective use of resources and problem solving to determine what is going on with the child and how to soothe them.

   f. Educate caregivers
      i. explain babies normal crying and sleeping patterns
      ii. normal physical sensations. Explain to parents that some babies may struggle to cope with normal physical sensations, such as digestion, elimination, normal reflux, tiredness and hunger. When babies find these sensations to be overwhelming/distressing/frightening they become irritable and cry
      iii. helping caregivers better to deal with discomfort and distress through a baby-centered approach
      iv. helping caregivers recognize when their baby is tired and apply a consistent approach to settling their baby
      v. encouraging parents to accept help from friends and family, and to simplify housekeeping demands
      vi. if they are unable to manage baby crying, inquire into available parenting center programs, infant social worker visits etc.
   g. Settling techniques. Refer to sleep interventions
   h. Behavior diary. Caregivers can use a simple diary to record crying, feeding, and sleeping patterns on a daily basis. In some cases, a diary can help them solve the problem. For example, recognizing that the baby/child cries less if sleep is increased and they sleeps better if napping during the day is decreased
   i. Establish a predictable routine. The more predictable (without rigidity) the less chaotic is the child's experience. Keeping in mind how the routines of feeding and settling work together (demonstrating their importance), the following may be appropriate
      i. plan for routine of feeding, playtime, and then letting the baby sleep when tired (not just after a set amount of time).

*The case of the baby who wants to be carried all of the time or seems to need their caregiver all of the time: if they are left alone they will cry persistently and not even respond to the settling technique described above. Caregivers are encouraged to minimize separations by remaining in sight. They can also carry the baby in a sling or move the baby via a carrier from

139

FIGURE 3.3
Irritable, cranky, over-stimulated child.

room to room. It will not spoil the baby to fall asleep in the parents' bedroom at night until fully settled enough to tolerate being moved back to their own room. This can be aided by providing a transitional object like a teddy bear or other soft/baby safe object in case they wake during sleep, that can gradually come to represent maternal care and support the baby to self-soothe.

Irritability and Other Mood Regulation Problems (Figure 3.3)

CASE EXAMPLE

Garrett, a 4½ year old, is described as a verbal, imaginative, charming boy who enjoys dramatic play – often dressing up in character. He is challenged by being hypersensitive with associated overreactivity (such as screaming at his parents not to touch him as if they were abusing him and calling them names, and they are unable to calm him), easily angered, bullying others to get his way, no longer wanting to go outside to play, overwhelmed by affective cues, difficulty reading facial cues, experiences difficulty with unexpected movement (fear of being high/falling), and dislikes/tries to avoid any new activities with unfamiliar movement routines. Generally, always striving to be in control and the center of attention. Additionally, there is tactile defensiveness with problems related to food textures, clothing labels, only wearing certain clothes no matter what the weather is, etc. Garrett demonstrated signs of difficulty with self-soothing and mood control. There was a challenging dichotomy of distinct need to create excitement and discharge energy through physical play, but also becoming overwhelmed and overstimulated. One of the ways he tried to calm himself was to retreat to a play tent in the living room where he was away from almost all stimuli. While exploring Garrett's behavior with his parents, they noted that until 6–8 months ago they would not have identified any significant problems with their son. The only identified change or stressor had been the elimination of a pacifier used to go to sleep at night. The parents described this as a challenging change. At first Garrett seemed ready to give up the pacifier, but when it came time actually to do it, he did, but he experienced it as a traumatic event.

Treatment

1. Parent intervention: Garrett's parents received counseling to help them manage/improve Garrett's
   a. problems associated with self-calming
   b. non-compliance
   c. ability to read social cues
   d. problem solving social situations
   e. anticipate and predict acting out and tantrums
2. Behavioral management
   a. ignore his name calling
   b. time out for tantrums
   c. reinforce positive responses
      i. play well with others
      ii. eye contact
   d. using pictures of events that are scheduled for his participation
   e. games like charades to improve his ability to read facial cues
3. Developmentally based individual CBT to improve
   a. problem solving
   b. impulse control
   c. coping with anxiety and stress
   d. complying with situational demands

   e. reading and response to social cues

   f. to identify the signs of becoming disorganized and how to alert others about what to do

4. To deal with his high need of tactile-proprioceptive input

   a. objects selected for play incorporated this sensory component (resulting in improved physical organization)

5. Occupational therapy

   a. sensory integration therapy to deal with the underlying relationship to mood and behavioral problems

   b. activities focused on proprioceptive input (resulted in decreased need for aggression and withdrawal in social situations)

GOALS

1. Rule out medical problems

2. Rule out parental issues

3. Address sensory hyperactivity contributing to irritability

4. Avoid overstimulation

5. Soothe both parents and child

6. Create opportunities for child skill development to self-calm

7. Facilitate learning how to make the transition from one activity to another

8. Provide clear limits/boundaries

9. Facilitate increased self-reliance

10. Develop frustration tolerance and a sense of mastery

11. Validate parents feelings of isolation and provide respite

12. Address parental anxiety about child's behavior

13. Facilitate parental understanding to differentiate what the crying or irritability means

TREATMENT FOCUS AND OBJECTIVES

1. Rule out medical problems

   a. Colic, ear infection, reflux, severe allergies, urinary tract infection

   b. Milk intolerance or a diet heavy in gluten

   c. Referral to a nutritionist can be beneficial for diet management and education

2. Rule out parental issues

   a. If marital discord is present refer for conjoint therapy

   b. If individual problems are present refer to a mental health provider and, if necessary, refer to a psychiatrist as well

3. Address sensory hyperactivity contributing to irritability

   a. Address hypersensitivity in play

      i. Activities that provide deep pressure or proprioception are beneficial. For example, sitting in a bean bag chair with a heavy blanket on them, rolling up like a pig in a blanket

   b. If hypersensitive to sound, encourage them to participate in activities that allows them to make their own sounds, banging objects on different surface to elicit a variance of sound at their will, elemental musical instruments such as different types of drums, cymbals etc.

   c. Forward and back rocking normalizes vestibular responses by providing linear movement

   d. For further treatment intervention associated with sensory processing difficulties refer to Regulatory Disorders of Sensory Processing

4. Avoid overstimulation

   a. Caregivers to remain calm and reassuring. When a child is inconsolable caregivers often become frantic and overwhelmed themselves

   b. Try certain calming techniques for a long enough period of time for a thorough effort and to avoid overstimulation (i.e., rocking and then switching to swinging in the air)

   c. The therapist may need to model several different techniques for soothing the child. One strategy that may help is taking a pillow and holding it securely/firmly behind the infant's back and hugging the child

5. Soothe both parents and child

   a. Create environments that are soothing to both parents and child such as a chaise/day bed for two with soft thick quilts, or a tent lined with big comfortable pillows. Such an environment provides a physical and emotional embrace to them both

6. Create opportunities for child skill development to self-calm

   a. Infants under 6–8 months of age need to be soothed by caregivers, but from ages 6–9 months they should be given the opportunity to soothe themselves. Facilitate learning to problem solve frustrating situations (with caregiver support)

   b. If crying persists longer than 5–10 minutes (even with caregiver encouragement to self-soothe), the caregiver needs to hold the infant and rock them, etc.

   c. For older children, caregivers need to support self-calming first and if they are not successful redirect them toward a calming activity/distraction

   d. Over time, the caregiver may immediately direct the child toward the self-calming activity, gradually withdrawing the child's dependence on the caregiver

   e. Self-calming can be introduced through (1) modifying the environment via introducing different objects, interactions, and play which promotes calming, (2) looking or listening to something novel, or (3) helping them to organize their own movements

   f. Provide sensory inhibition through firm deep pressure and linear movement. For example, bringing the hands to front center, touching the palms to body parts, or facilitating the infant to suck on their own fingers

   g. For older children, they may learn a number of "heavy work" activities such as pushing a chair or heavy box across the room

   *It is beneficial to combine a self-soothing activity with a purposeful activity

   h. Have parents create a "calm corner" or calm room" for the child. For example, might be a play tent or a sheet over a card table. The space can be filled with soft pillows making it comfortable. There might also be a box of activities such as books, puzzles, squeeze balls or other similar things which serve to calm and distract the child

   *Since a child may exhibit difficulty making transitions, it is useful to have several boxes or backpacks of self-calming materials

7. Facilitate learning how to make the transition from one activity to another

   a. Facilitate the shifting of attention from one activity to another without difficulty. This requires that the child be helped to anticipate and plan the next activity, make changes in activity and, eventually, be able to accomplish it without the support of parent/caregiver/ or other adult

   b. Facilitate an increased sense of autonomy and capacity to tolerate separations from the parent. Give the child a warning of the transition to help them prepare

   c. Provide objects that help the child to self-organize in order to transition from one activity to the next (but also represent the connection between the parent and the child for internalization)

     i. parent may carry a keychain with a picture of the child and themself

     ii. blanket or stuffed animal which is comforting to the child

     iii. if traveling in the car to the next activity give them a pad and colors to keep them busy until they arrive

     iv. using photos or cards which represent the activity (this would require the parent to take photos of the child involved in the variety of activities they want to facilitate improved adjustment with for practice and self-efficacy)

     v. the parent or caregiver can signal, "don't forget your cuddle bear" (stuffed animal)

8. Provide clear limits/boundaries
   a. Work with parent to establish a problem-solving approach to setting limits and how to go about it
      i. when the child challenges the parent, the parent is instructed firmly to assert "no" coupled with a gesture
      ii. if the child doesn't comply, they are calmly removed from the room or the object is taken away from them even if it results in a tantrum
      iii. it is useful for the parent/caregiver and the child to acknowledge the child's anger and frustration. Hopefully, the child can be redirected to another activity to circumvent an escalation
      iv. if the child becomes inconsolable, they are to be moved to a time out corner to calm down. As soon as they are calm, then redirect them to another activity
      v. parents need to plan for consistency in how they will set limits with a variety of repetitive circumstances such as a when they are in a hurry, and other public situations.*Keep in mind that children have limits too.* Therefore, keep visits short to mall, grocery store, restaurant, etc., so that the outcome is positive and there is a feeling of success for all
      vi. reinforce the child for all of their positive efforts to calm themselves in situations which are challenging for them, "I like how you calmed yourself"
   b. Define appropriate consequences that can be consistent and help the child to learn that every choice has a consequence. For instance, when a child acts out at a restaurant what is the plan. If this is done by the parent for their routine activities, it will become more predictable for the child and help them comply
   c. Suggest that the parents pick a few selected behaviors to work on such as sitting at the table for mealtime, turning off the television when it is time to go to daycare/school, getting dressed for bedtime. De-emphasize the behaviors that are not currently targeted – you can't work on everything at once
      i. a parent may not like the clothing choices made but, instead of making it an issue at the moment, praise and reinforce their compliance. Clothing choices can be worked on later by offering choices of several outfits
      ii. praise can be coupled with a tangible object sometimes such as stickers, stars on a chart, a visit to the reward box to pick something, etc.
9. Facilitate increased self-reliance
   a. If a child demands attention, modify their behavior by playing with them for 10–15 minutes. Once the child is playing well, the parent encourages the child to continue playing while they do a small chore/activity in the same room. Every few minutes, the parent is to reassure and praise the child "good playing alone – good job!" If necessary, the connection can be maintained while child and parent participate in separate activities in the same room, by singing a song, etc.
   b. If the parent is engaged in meal preparation, provide the child with their own utensils so that they can imitate the parent activity. If the child complains take the time to redirect them verbally or physically
   c. Parents need to be clear about when it is an appropriate time to pick them up and when it isn't. This is followed up by a parent when they are free to pick the child up to hold them and participate in a brief activity with them, like reading a story
   d. For a preschool or school-aged child, teach them to label emotions and read bodily signals so that they can initiate self-soothing strategies independently
      i. use the concept of a traffic light to identify the intensity of an emotion like a mood meter. Red means that they need to put on the brakes (mad/angry feelings), green is for focused or calm feelings, yellow denotes frustration
      ii. the incredible 5-point scale (Dunn-Buron & Curtis, 2003) could be adapted as a behavioral rating scale for emotional management (range: happy = 1, Angry = 5)
      iii. may ask the child how their engine is running: fine, fast, running rough, etc.

143

10. Develop frustration tolerance and a sense of mastery
    a. Use child-centered play to develop the capacity to tolerate frustration
        i. validate and encourage continued effort. For example, a child is trying to put an object into a container which is proving difficult. Validate them with, "I can see it doesn't fit" instead of jumping in to fix the situation. Parents may help by repositioning the container or offer a larger container. However, do not take the object from the child – the idea is for them to struggle with it until they succeed
        ii. if the parent can tell that the child is struggling, instead of identifying it, wait for the child to look to the parent for help. This allows the child to learn to coordinate communication with others when frustrated and increase their resources
        iii. the parent can reassure the child first when they recognize that the child is becoming frustrated, and then encourage them, "you can do it, just keep trying", "good job – I knew you could do it!"
        iv. the parent could help the child solve the problem if the above (i–iii) do not work but using physical or verbal guidance and then praising the child for what they have learned. This could be reinforced by having the child show the parent what they just learned so that they can do it on their own next time
    b. Developing a sense of mastery facilitates a feeling of self-efficacy that helps the child who feels irritable that they can overcome their frustration and be left with a self-pleasing feeling for their accomplishment
        i. give the child small jobs like turning off the light, turning off the television, closing the door, etc. These are all tasks that the child can do and doing them daily will leave them with a sense of mastery
        ii. encourage the child to do age-appropriate activities that they can master such as playing with Lego, stirring with a spoon when helping mom to make pudding, etc.
11. Validate parents' feelings of isolation and provide respite
    a. When parents express their feelings of frustration and isolation encourage them to express all of the associated situations for how they feel and validate them. They may actually feel so frustrated that they fear that other caregivers might experience the same level of frustration and abuse their child
    b. If (a above) is a parental experience, it is likely that they never get a break and are emotionally exhausted. In that case, they are in need of respite. An example could be the parent of a baby who cries for hours or is highly irritable. In this situation, respite needs to be explored with the parents to restore or refuel their capacity to deal with the level of distress. They need to give themselves a break. It could prevent their own explosion or decompensation
12. Address parental anxiety about child's behavior
    a. Parents should be encouraged to talk about their own anxieties and perceptions with regard to their child's crying and/or irritability. What do they think the problem is? Sometimes they could be accurate and other times it could be a reflection of their own issue. For example, parental belief that their baby crying was due to the baby feeling abandoned. The therapist explored this belief with the parents and it was discovered that both parents had abandonment issues from their childhood. Therefore, they had to be instructed on how to maintain healthy connections with their baby to avoid over dependency and the stunting of other child skill development
    b. Increase parental awareness for their own reaction to their child's irritability. Sometimes a parent/caregiver finds that they have the same emotion or are responding in the same way as their child (resonance). For example, they both get stressed or anxious and the result is an escalation in emotionality. Once parents become aware of the "contagious" mood that takes over their environment, they generally are better able to manage it
13. Facilitate parental understanding to differentiate what the crying or irritability means
    a. Facilitate the parents/caregivers to observe the child crying when it is a cry of frustration and then continue to the observation to recognize when and how the

child self-soothes. Encourage them to listen so that they can understand what the child is trying to tell them

b. Validate the parents for the distress they experience when hearing their child cry and educate them about the different reasons for crying and how it also plays a role in healthy developmental processes

c. Sometimes parents need to be validated that they have a difficult child that will continue to be more demanding and irritable than a child who is seen as easy or cooperative

Sleep

CASE EXAMPLES WITH ASSOCIATED INFORMATION ARE OFFERED BELOW

The need for feeding and diaper changes are common reasons for night-time awakening for infants/babies. No defined threshold age was identified whereby night-time awakening is automatically considered abnormal or problematic. The perception of caregivers largely rules whether a child's night-time waking is considered to be a problem. It is estimated that up to one-third of toddlers and preschoolers awaken at night to the degree of being considered a problem by parents. However, in many cases, parents are contributors to sleep difficulties exhibited by young children. The duration that an infant experiences inconsistent parental care and non-circadian environmental conditions may result in the detrimental lack of development of their own rhythmic patterns. In other words, parental and environmental entraining factors are likely contributors to disturbances in both sleep and feeding. Clearly, sleep is a dynamic and regulated set of behaviors and physiological states and stages. Two distinct processes determine the timing of sleep and waking: (1) a sleep–wake dependent *homeostatic process* that interacts with a sleep–wake independent, (2) clock-like *circadian process*. Both mechanisms undergo significant modifications during development. Sleep is restorative for brain metabolism, as well as serving a role in memory consolidation and learning. Therefore, sleep is associated to developmental tasks and, in order for a child to fall asleep and to remain asleep requires:

145

- Regulation of sleep–wake/arousal states
- Internalizing daily routine: caregivers facilitate regulation of sleep–wake cycles by establishing scheduled times for naps, bedtime rituals (bath, read a story, etc.), reinforcing self-soothing
- Transitioning from active→quiet alert→calm state
- Accommodating or screening out environmental noise when falling asleep
- Self-soothing when distressed or awakened at night (able to go back to sleep)
- Bonding. Feeling attached to the caregiver and secure in separating from caregiver to acquiesce to sleep.

*Sleep and feeding disorders in infancy and early childhood are very common. However, if they extend beyond infancy they constitute a specific disorder. For example, if a baby has a sleeping disturbance but no behavioral, sensory or motor difficulties, then this infant is not considered to have a regulatory disorder. However, if the baby is fussy and difficult to soothe (behavioral response) and seldom goes to sleep unless rocked or jiggled (motor response) and needs auditory input such as white noise (sensory response) to settle, then these three responses, not just the sleep disturbance, may result in the diagnosis of a regulatory disorder.

By age 2–3 years, sleep has acquired new meaning. It is not uncommon that the 2 year old without a history of sleep problems is now demonstrating difficulties. This is related to tasks challenging to the toddler such as:

- The need to calm down following a full day of activity
- Balanced sensory movement stimulation and calming activities
- Dealing with fears of darkness and being alone
- Learning to tolerate limits/boundaries set by parent/caregivers associated with imposed bedtime rituals

- Bonding, feeling secure and attached to the parents/caregivers allowing for the acquiesce to sleep
- Developing autonomy.

*Toddlers need support, guidance and reinforcement in the negotiation of these tasks

In addition to the various types of sleep disorders there can be complexities associated with regulatory disorders. For example:

1. THE HYPERSENSITIVE CHILD/SENSORY INTEGRATION DYSFUNCTION TO TOUCH, SOUND/TACTILE DEFENSIVENESS

Potential types of problems:

a. Agitated with bed-sheets laying on their body or how pajamas feel. They may fall asleep more easily if a parent is laying down beside them (which is unfortunately reinforcing of this arrangement)
b. Difficulty screening out environmental noise. The slightest noise agitates them. The problem is aggravated if it is a noisy household, i.e., numerous children, parent doing shift work, etc.

Case Examples

Bobby, a 4-year-old boy, has parents who structured bedtime rituals beginning in infancy consisting of 15 minutes of massage and then he would be dressed for bed. He would change his bed clothes several times every night to determine the "right ones", then needed his father to read several stories, followed by having his mother lay down by him, sing songs, turn on the flashlight and eventually he would fall asleep. This nightly routine took about 2 hours. Intervention with sensory integration activities along with a series of pictures offering a stepwise progressive view of what he was to anticipate for changing this enduring night-time struggle helped Bobby to anticipate and appropriately adjust to the steps of his routine. His parents were also educated about the consistent role they would play in increasing his sense of security, prediction and self-soothing.

An 11 month old was sleeping 16–18 hours/day. It was determined that he was delayed in developmental milestones and severely hyperactive to all stimulation. The intervention was to construct a calm and soothing environment and use a sound machine to block out all environmental noises.

Kelly, a 3 year old, would take a three-hour nap every day after six hours of day care, going to bed by 5 pm and sleeping through to 6 am. She was hypersensitive to touch and was shutting down when she came home, but aggressive at day care (biting and hitting). Intervention was sensory integration activities to address tactile defensiveness, creating a calm down area for her at day care and at home, and to decrease the number of activities at daycare.

2. CRAVING MOVEMENT/VESTIBULAR STIMULATION

The child becomes hyperaroused by movement. Infants with this dysfunction wish to be held, carried and bounced continuously, like being in a swing, and/or fall asleep most consistently when riding in a car.

Case Example

Jesse, a 9-month-old baby boy, would only fall asleep for his mom when placed in his carrier on top of a dryer (no heat). Vestibular stimulation is a double-edged issue. On one hand it seems to soothe, but it may also cause overstimulation. As children who crave vestibular movement grow older they tend to demonstrate a proclivity toward high proprioceptive input and engage in actions like wresting with siblings/dad, climbing high, pushing heavy objects, etc.

3. PROBLEMS WITH ATTACHMENT AND SEPARATION/INDIVIDUATION

There may be several reasons which explain why attachment issues are an underlying cause for a child's struggle to fall asleep. Insecure attachment/disorganized attachments result in anxiety when there is separation from the parents (day or night). The reason for the insecure attachment needs to be explored and understood. For instance, do the parents struggle with their own interpretation of separation fear conveying to the child that the world is an unsafe place by their overprotectiveness (such as not allowing them to play at a friend's house or go to a birthday party, etc.).

Case Example

Lucy at age 4 presented as anxious and hyperactive. She was a demanding child whose parents needed to be constantly involved with her as the center of attention. She did not independently organize any play activities. At the age of 5, her parents finally came to terms with her sleeping in her own bed. The parents checked in on her constantly – to the point of taking turns sleeping in a sleeping bag by her bed to make sure she was alright. Intervention included facilitating autonomy through developmentally appropriate activities and addressing the parents' difficulties in encouraging and reinforcing these necessary changes.

DeGangi (2000) sets forth the following process for evaluating pediatric sleep difficulties:

1. What is the morning awakening time?
   a. Describe the morning routine
   b. What is the child's mood when they wake up?
   c. Do the parents have a special ritual for arousing the child for their morning routine (singing, massage, loud alarm clock, etc.)?
2. What are the daily activities of the child?
   a. How much time is spent in each activity daily?
3. In what ways is the child stressed by separating from the parents/caregivers during the day?
   a. Do both parents work? If yes, both full time?
   b. How is the child cared for during the day (daycare, babysitter, family member)?
   c. How does the child generally manage separation from the parent?
   d. How do the parents feel about leaving their child for work, for couple's time/date, etc.)?
   e. How do the parents deal with leaving the child (sneak out, talk to the child, etc.)?
4. How does the child manage all of their challenging points of transition and limits set during the day?
   a. Whether at home or some other setting, does the child have regular routines and scheduled activities?
   b. Does the child do well with the routines/activities and appear to like them?
   c. Are the parents/caregivers comfortable with the routines and lifestyle organization?
   d. Is the child dependent on the routines and experiencing obvious difficulty adjusting to a change in their routine and/or activities?
5. How much intrinsic stimulation is the child exposed to in their daily setting(s) (home, daycare, additional caregivers, etc.)?
   a. How does the child demonstrate their management of stimulation (follow the caregiver around, have to be in the same room at all times, retreat to a corner or calming place, etc.)?
6. Does the child nap daily, how long, and if so is it a scheduled time?
   a. How long does the child typically nap?
   b. If the child takes a long nap does it interfere with night-time sleep?
   c. Do they nap in a different place than they sleep at night?
   d. Does the child need any assistance to help them fall asleep for a nap (bottle, rocking, being held, etc.)?

7. Describe the evening routine/close of the day?
   a. Describe the evening wind-down and bedtime ritual.
   b. Do they have a snack? (If yes, what?)
   c. When is the child put to bed and when do they fall asleep?
   d. Where do they fall asleep?
   e. Describe the sleeping environment and noises?
   f. How does the child fall asleep (self-soothing, rocking, etc.)?
   g. Is the child's behavior consistent regardless of who carries out the night-time routine?
   h. Does the child's bedtime have an impact on the entire family?
8. What is the child's sleep pattern, i.e., once asleep do they awaken, how often, and how do the parents respond?
   a. How do the parents know the child is awake (loud crying, baby monitor, etc.)?
   b. What does the child do when they wake up (make noises, talk to themselves, cry, etc.)?
   c. If the child cries, how do the parents interpret it?
   d. How does the parent feel when the child awakens (engaged, empathic, frustrated, angry, irritated)?
   e. How do the parents respond to the awakened child?
   f. Do the parents wake up to find the child in their bed?
9. What are the sleeping arrangements (does the child sleep in their own bed, in their parent's bed, start out in one bed and move to another, etc)?
   a. How much time does the child spend asleep at night (fall asleep time to wake up time $= x$h)?
   b. Does the child wet their bed, get up to eat, or get up to use the bathroom at night?
   c. Do the parents give the child a bottle in the middle of the night while they are sleeping?
10. Do the child's night-time behaviors disturb their family sleeping patterns or neighbors?
   a. Are there any special circumstances to be considered while resolving the child's sleep problem (parental medical issue, living environment/neighbor proximity, etc.)?
   b. Does the child's sleep problem interfere with social activities (peer socialization/activities, family activities, etc.)?
11. Does the child experience bad dreams or other sleep disturbances (nightmares, night terrors, sleep walking)?
   a. Has the child ever engaged in something considered an emotional or physical safety issue at night (leaving the house, watching x-rated TV, cook, etc.)?
   b. Does the child use the TV to fall asleep? Are the TV programs they watch to fall asleep stimulating or do they provoke fear?
   c. Has the child ever watched a scary movie that has interfered with sleep?
12. Explore parent(s) sleep history. Did they sleep with their parents, etc.?
   a. What is their belief about how a child learns to fall asleep and sleep through the night?
13. Do either of the parents present significant issues of loss/grief (death of parent, child, etc.)?
   a. Ask parents to share their first memory of being separated from their parents. How did they manage it?
   b. Do they experience any sleep problems? If so, what do they think is underlying it?
   c. If the parents experience sleep difficulties what do they do to manage it?
14. Are the parents well adjusted, do they enjoy alone time/solitude, and what do they do with their alone free time?
   a. Is the child ever left to play/occupy themselves with the parents close by? Is the child capable of doing this or requiring constant connection/attention of the parents?
   b. Has the child ever been left with someone else (family member, babysitter)? If so, how does the child manage it?
15. Has the child's sleep difficulties changed over time? If so how?
   a. What has been tried for helping the child sleep that has worked? What has been tried that has not worked?
   b. What do the parents think will help their child's sleep problem now, and what are they willing to do?

Treatment of sleep disorders in infants and young children begins with effective bedtime management defined by establishing a regular sleep schedule, an appropriate sleep environment, and consistent limit setting for dealing with bedtime struggles (Figure 3.4). Major influences associated with sleeplessness in young children include:

1. Persistent night-time feedings
2. Separation issues
3. Temperament
4. Co-sleeping
5. Bedtime routines and environment
6. Fears and anxieties

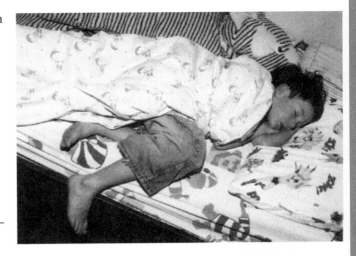

FIGURE 3.4
A child finds comfort sleeping in his own bed with a stuffed tiger and stimulating bed sheets.

GOALS

1. Rule out medical problems
2. Improve and regulate sleep pattern
3. Eliminate night-time fears

TREATMENT FOCUS AND OBJECTIVES

1. Rule out medical problems
   a. Identify if milk intolerance or other food allergy interfere with sleep. If the child is breast fed, explore mother's dietary choices which may have a negative influence on the infant
2. Regulate sleep patterns
   a. Infants. Newborn sleep cycles may take about 6 months to become established. While newborns sleep 16–17 hours on average, it is for short periods of time and, as they get older, the numbers of hours of sleep decrease. Suggestions for improved infant sleep:
       i. when feeding or changing during the night try to keep the infant as calm and quiet as possible
      ii. do not allow the infant to sleep long during the day
     iii. put the infant in the crib at the first signs of drowsiness so they learn to relax in their crib as part of preparing for sleep. If rocking them to sleep becomes a habit they may need you to help them get back to sleep when they awaken at night versus being able to get themselves back to sleep
      iv. avoid putting the infant/baby to sleep with a pacifier because it will be difficult for them to fall asleep without it. A pacifier should only be used to satisfy an infant/baby's need to suck
       v. begin to delay a reaction to fussiness at 4–6 months of age. Waiting for a few minutes gives them the opportunity to settle themselves and go back to sleep. Once they realize that the caretaker is not going to run in and comfort them, they will begin to fuss less and return to sleep
   b. Establish and follow a bedtime routine. A regular and well-structured set of pre-bedtime activities usually helps settle children and promotes sleep onset. Keeping the routine quiet and consistent supports and reinforces children to achieve a quiet, relaxed state more conducive to sleep onset. A routine happens at about the same time every day (predictable) and in the same order of sequence that signals a close to the day and transition to sleep might include:
       i. a bath and getting ready for bed
      ii. reading a bedtime story
     iii. playing a quiet game
      iv. singing a lullaby
       v. being tucked in
      vi. kiss goodnight

149

   c. Sleep environment is more supportive and reinforcing of falling asleep if it is quiet, dimly lit/dark, use of a night light for kids that are afraid of the dark. Put the child down to sleep without the parent remaining present (staying conditions the child to expect the parent to stay) allowing the child the opportunity to fall asleep independently and minimize dependence on caregiver presence

   d. Making sure that the child has plenty of opportunities to fall asleep on their own. Maintain a consistent bedtime and waking time throughout the week. Eliminate late sleeping and daytime napping that is age inappropriate. Additionally, a regular sleep schedule promoting entrainment and stabilization of biological rhythms improves sleep onset and regular bedtime

   e. Limit setting. Children who cry or leave the room at bedtime in an attempt to stay up later sometimes repeat this behavior to the degree of being a nightly problem. When caregivers give in, the result is consistent delay and disruption of sleep onset. Limits must be reinforced consistently by all caregivers (possibly for days or even weeks) for maladaptive bedtime behavior to be eliminated

     i. talk with parents/caregivers about how to cope with the child's crying when it occurs at night and what crying is about

     ii. by allowing the child to cry the parents help the child learn that this is the time to rest not play, etc.

     iii. discourage parents from projecting their feelings of distress on the child

   f. Extinction (systematic ignoring) involves placing a child in bed and ignoring agitation or inappropriate behavior until morning. The only exclusion is legitimate concerns regarding illness or safety

   g. Graduated extinction. Parents ignore bedtime tantrums or night-time waking for a prescribed period of time before re-entering the child's room and briefly calming the child before leaving. The specified time of ignoring the child's resistance progressively increases over time

   h. Scheduled awakenings. This unusual intervention for young children with night-time waking occurring at predictive intervals requires the caregiver to pre-emptively waken the child and then resettle them 15–30 minutes before their normal/spontaneous night waking episodes. The scheduled wakenings are gradually spaced out or delayed systematically. It is important to review with parents ways in which they may be inadvertently reinforcing sleep difficulties by staying in the room, not allowing the child time to self-soothe, etc.

   i. Bedtime fading initially delays a child's bedtime by about 30 minutes. If rapid sleep onset does not occur, the child is removed from bed and kept awake for 30–60 minutes, with repeating of the process until the child falls asleep easily. On successive nights, the initial bedtime is set 30 minutes before the time of rapid onset of sleep being achieved the prior night. The rules are applied on subsequent nights until the child's sleep onset is faded toward a predetermined bedtime goal

   j. Settling technique. The goal of this technique is to teach babies to fall asleep on their own and to ensure caregivers have a consistent approach to settling. Consistency is important in a baby-centered approach. In other words, the irritable baby requires a consistent message about how to fall asleep. There are numerous variations of setting. Most techniques recommend that the caregiver pats or rocks the baby until they are quiet but not asleep. The caregiver then leaves the room. If the baby starts crying, the caregiver re-enters the room after a moment, and if the baby has not ceased crying, begins to resettle the baby. The process continues until the baby falls asleep

   k. Discourage allowing the child to have a bottle to fall asleep or to have a middle of the night feeding (after 4 months of age)

   l. Behavior diary. Caregivers can create a simple diary to record basic behaviors such as crying, feeding, and sleeping patterns. The diary will demonstrate actual amount ingested during feeding, amount of time crying, and time slept in a 24-hour period of time

m. Give the child a security object at bedtime to provide them with comfort should they awaken in the middle of the night. This transitional object can be used in the daytime as well. Sometimes, if the object smells like mother's perfume, it is desirable. Another scent option is for the parents to sleep with the object for several nights prior to giving it to the child so that it smells like them

n. If the child has motor issues which interfere with them being able to position comfortably in bed, it may be useful to use a waterbed, crib cradle (similar to a suspended hammock) or vibrating crib attachment. *These are only to be initiated if the child is completely healthy and there is no risk of neck compression which could cut off air flow (suffocate)

o. Provide opportunity for play about sleep, like nesting in pillows or cubbies during child-centered play. Preschoolers often enjoy pretending to put their parents to sleep and giving them bedtime rules. It can be a fun rehearsal

p. The time frame between dinner and bedtime should be organized, relaxed and enjoyable for child and parents. If the parents feel pressured or stressed that is the environmental influence a child will pick up on. Therefore, the parents must get adequate rest themselves

q. Provide emotional support to parents/caregivers to address their feelings of frustration, guilt or anger associated with parenting stressors. It can be a challenging and difficult time and if success is evading them negative emotions can arise – even emotional distancing from the child

r. Separation games may be useful to support sleep. Sleep is a time of separation of the child from the parents. As such, both need to become comfortable with the process of sleep and separation in general

   i. playing disappearing games with objects. Now you see it now you don't. This is a good game because it is not emotionally associated. Toys can be hidden under a table or sofa/chair cushion. The child is encouraged to find a specific object. Take turns so that they can see the parent running and excited to find the toy. It is a shared pleasurable time

   ii. play peek-a-boo. This can be done relatively close with a dishtowel, under a blanket or around the corner. Another concept is the rolling of an object, like a ball, from one room to the next and encouraging the child to retrieve it

   iii. play magic carpet. Using a towel as the magic carpet, pull it around from one place in the house to another, or create spaces to crawl through, like a big box. Enhance creativity and a fun sharing time with points of separation

   iv. make a goodbye book with pictures of mother, father, and child. Use the book to read to the child offering a positive rehearsal of the real thing

   v. when it is time for goodbye let the child see the parents leave. Ritualize goodbyes so that they are predictable and have a reunion ritual upon return. The parents could practice saying goodbye and leaving for a brief period of time while they do a small chore, and gradually increase the separation aspect of the goodbye-return sequence

   vi. instruct the parents to leave a transitional object with the child when they leave. The parents should carry this object with them when going places to attach meaning to the object

*Once the child reaches 6–7 months, the Ferber method can be used to address awakening at night with increments of parental waiting to intervene prior to entering the nursery to assure the child. The program requires that the child be engaged in a full blown cry before a parental visit, wait 5 minutes, then go in and reassure, but don't pick them up, rock them or play with them. After the baby has settled, the parents should leave the room. The following night the parents are to wait 10 minutes prior to reassuring the child. Each night 5 minutes is added to the time to intervene. If necessary, the increments of time can be a smaller progression to help them adjust.

3. Eliminate night-time fears
   a. Nightmares may actually highlight something that is really bothering a child. If a caregiver's ears and heart are open they can hear a child's unconscious asking for help out loud. Most nightmares are a normal part of coping with changes/challenges of daily life
      i. use role-playing and fantasy rehearsals to coach a child to see how they can control the fear of the night
      ii. create a new ending to the nightmare, thus changing it so that it is no longer scary
      iii. reassure and encourage a child to explore creative solutions to a dream, "what would feel better", "how would you like it to turn out?". If a nightmare is recurring seek to understand the elements
         - three stage of nightmare resolution. Changes within a dream suggest the onset of resolving a psychological challenge
            1. threat – the main character is threatened and unable to defend themselves
            2. struggle in an attempt to confront the adversary to ward off danger
            3. resolution is the vanquishing of the threat
         - the "R"s of nightmare relief and closure
            1. reassurance soothes the nightmare fear, encouraging the view of trying to understand what is bothering/concerning the child
            2. rescripting is a way to guide a child's imagination to rewrite the ending of the nightmare. Make it fun, brainstorming what changes to make. Rescripting is akin to assertiveness where challenging solutions are generated which builds confidence in facing the dilemma
            3. rehearsal is practicing the solutions to the nightmare. It involves repeating the dream and its solutions until a feeling of mastery has been achieved. It is the "working-through" where insight is gained
            4. resolution, the last step, can only come after a child feels secure enough to explore new solutions through other creative forms such as writing, drama, and talking about it (rescripting)
      *If nightmares continue and there are no evident stressors identified, then consult with the child's pediatrician to rule out physical causes
   b. Night terrors, more severe/frightening than nightmares, occur most often in toddlers and preschoolers during the deepest stages of sleep. Handle night terrors by:
      i. remain calm. Night terrors are usually more upsetting for the caregiver than for the child
      ii. don't try to wake the child
      iii. make sure the child does not harm/injure themselves. If they try to get out of bed gently restrain them
      iv. just be soothing, after a short time the child will probably relax and go back to sleep
      v. if a child has night terrors, it is important that all caregivers understand what happens and what to do
   c. Sleep walking/talking. Similar to night terrors, sleep walking/talking takes place during deep sleep. When sleep walking, the child may have a blank stare and not be responsive. When they do awake they are not likely to remember it. Sleepwalkers will often return to bed on their own. Ways to handle it include:
      i. make sure the child doesn't hurt themselves when sleep walking. Make sure their space is relatively clear and free of things to trip over, etc.
      ii. lock outside doors so that they cannot leave the house
      iii. block stairways to avoid an accident
      iv. don't try to awaken them, instead gently guide them back to bed and they will probably settle back to sleep on their own

Feeding Disorders (Figure 3.5)

CASE EXAMPLE

Austin, a 3-year-old boy, was admitted to the hospital after failing to maintain his growth curve. He lives with his parents and two older siblings, neither of whom has had an eating disorder. However, his mother comes from a family with a longstanding history of Crohn's disease. She describes herself as always having had a small appetite, being a fussy eater, and experiencing struggles with her own mother over eating. The mother states that she still experiences some difficulties with food and clothing textures.

Austin's gestation and delivery were normal. However, his mother always found him difficult to feed. He had a systemic infection when he was approximately 6 months of age which required a change in his formula, which he refused to take. Aside from this, he did make a successful transition to table food. He didn't like jarred baby food and his mother did question if he had difficulty with the texture. When Austin was age 1½, he was making regular doctor visits. His mother was very concerned that Austin did not eat very much, but he did maintain his growth curve. Not long after this he began to experience gagging episodes, was diagnosed with reflux, and placed on thickened fluids. Over the next year and a half his Mom became increasingly worried about his low food intake and nutritional status. Austin was allowed to eat anytime and his Mom employed numerous coaxing strategies. At this point, mealtime had become a stressful time for both Austin and his mother. He was admitted to the hospital, lethargic and exhibiting evidence of micronutrient deficiency.

The assessment team found that Austin was able to achieve basic cycles of feeding, elimination, and satiety cues. He also demonstrated evidence of regulatory disorder of sensory processing (formula refusal and fussiness about textures and tastes). His mother's numerous attempts to help him may have been influenced by her own challenging history with food. The interviews with Mom revealed a high level of anxiety. Her making food continuously available to Austin likely contributed to his own food intake. Additionally, when he was diagnosed with reflux, it not only identified his experience of increased discomfort with eating, but his mother felt even more compelled, out of concern, to coax him to eat.

Treatment

1. Involved a multidisciplinary team
2. Family therapy sessions
   - Impact to the family members, and their interpretation
   - Encouraged and reinforced Dad's support to Mom and increased engagement in the family system
   - Addressing the behavior of one of the siblings who demonstrated coercive behavior toward Austin
3. Sessions for Mom to help her understand the reasons for the problem
4. Nutritional supplementation for Austin
5. Treatment for Austin's reflux
6. Parent–child therapy to address the feeding process
7. Occupational therapy assessment to determine the extent of Austin's regulatory disorder of sensory processing and strategies to work on his sensitivities

As Austin began to thrive, Mom was able to address her own rigidity in other areas of her relationship with Austin. One year after treatment, their relationship was much healthier and Austin continued to thrive. The family system was healthier, Dad was taking a more supportive role to Mom and more engaged in family activities/demands. Additionally, Austin was on task with other normal developmental expectations.

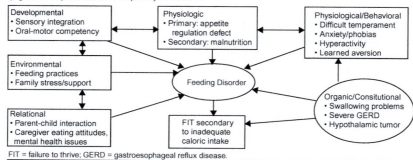

FIGURE 3.5
Etiological factors in feeding disorders. Printed with permission from Winters NC (2003). Primary Psychiatry 10(6).

DEVELOPMENT AND FEEDING SKILLS

Like other functional and developmental skills, feeding is influenced by cultural norms. As a result, the feeding behavior of an infant/child is impacted by:

- How they are taught to self-feed
- What they are fed/eat
- What comprises family mealtime.

Because self-feeding is a complex task with the potential for a multitude of negative outcomes, the range of constitutional, biological and emotional aspects that can interfere with the process must be considered:

1. Mechanical problem
   a. sucking
   b. swallowing
2. Reflux (GERD)
   a. makes eating a painful process
3. Tactile hypersensitivities (present in the mouth, face, body), resulting in
   a. pulling away from the nipple
   b. rejecting food textures
   c. gagging on certain foods
   d. difficulty being held and fed
4. Medical problems
   a. maladsorption, resulting in
   b. failure to thrive

Failure to thrive (FTT) is a constellation of symptoms representing severe growth disturbance often associated with maladaptive feeding behaviors. Therefore, a multifaceted treatment approach is needed encompassing medical and behavioral modification interventions. Emotional problems associated with the development of homeostasis, attachment, and separation/autonomy impacting the infant/child feeling safe, secure, and bonded may also result in a feeding problem.

Eating problems which initiate early in life may continue as the child ages. Additionally, the mothers of FTT children may be struggling with their own psychosocial issues. The etiology of FTT disorders may be:

- organic/biological
  medical problems interfering with eating, normal digestion and/or oral motor problems (drooling, uncoordinated sucking, swallowing)
- non-organic
  emotional issues between parent–child, family stress such as marital problems, domestic violence, substance abuse, parental depression, and any other factors contributing to environmental instability

- mixed types (combination or organic/non-organic issues) for example, oral-tactile hypersensitivities resulting in rejection of food (association of eating to discomfort) combined with parent–child relationship stress

Using Greenspan's model of emotional development (Chatoor et al, 1984, 1985; DeGangi, 2000; Casenheiser et al, 2007), three stages of feeding development are derived taking into consideration both adaptive and maladaptive patterns which can emerge in association with the mother child dyad.

1. HOMEOSTASIS

During homeostasis the infant develops self-regulating calming, rhythms of sleep, feeding and elimination cycles. Successful feeding requires of the infant:

- Coordinated suck and swallow
- Maintenance of a calm–alert state during feeding
- Ability to signal hunger and satiety
- Ability to orient body/mouth toward breast
- Tolerate contact of the nipple in the mouth
- Be held in a fitting position for feeding by the caregiver

Parents must be

- Able to differentiate the different types of crying related to hunger, bodily discomfort, wishing to be comforted/held, etc.
- High on empathy, efficiency and mood control

*All of these factors are associated with babies feeding well (if no organic issues). The more skilled the parent at interpreting the needs of the infant the more relaxed the process proceeds.

Problems with Homeostasis

The FTT infant has not mastered basic tasks of homeostasis. For instance, identifying and expressing their feelings of hunger and satiety or confusing these feelings with needing to eliminate. These types of problems are often combined with parental expression of their own difficulties in helping their child to establish states of hunger, satiety, or being confused by the baby's signals. Often, the consequence is that the distressed parent tries to apply feeding as the tool to console the infant resulting in the infant/baby expecting to be consoled by feeding whenever they are in distress. Another situation whereby the infant/baby is not on a good feeding schedule may be associated to:

- Parental neglect, depression, mental illness, substance abuse, poverty (affecting food availability), stressful family circumstances which interfere with appropriately and effectively attending to the infant/baby needs
- Fussy or colicky infant/baby experiencing difficulty regulating sleep–wake and feeding schedules. These babies are often overstimulated and may respond by not sleeping enough or shutting down for long periods of time. For the child who remains awake and is inconsolable (crying constantly), the parents may overuse the pacifier or feedings throughout the day. The result is that with multiple feedings the infant/baby develops a grazing routine and never feels satiated (never experiencing hunger or satiety) thus prolonging dysregulation. Additionally, if the infant/baby is feeling overstimulated due to hypersensitivities they may shut down and sleep for long periods of time (to shut out noise and other sensory confusion). Added to the FTT there are likely to be significant developmental delays.

2. ATTACHMENT

The dyadic relationship offers powerful reinforcement for the mother at about 6 weeks. At this time, a baby begins to gaze back at her, reach for her face and cuddle toward the breast when being fed. Holding her baby close while the baby suckles is a time of tremendous intimacy thus highlighting the importance of developing the bond of attachment.

When the dyadic relationship is fraught with avoidance and insecurity as a result of a rejecting mother not able to nurture and support their child's attachment, there is a marked inhibition of affect, decreased mother–infant reciprocity, a lack of mutual/shared pleasure and less physical closeness with a mother lacking empathy and not reading the child's cues associated with feeding or play, FTT is the likely outcome. This is an example of non-organic FTT. The infant/child with poor attachment may demonstrate:

- Avoidance of gaze with caretakers and others
- Appear listless or apathetic
- Doesn't cuddle when needs help
- Lacks pleasure in feeding time
- Lack of pleasure in play
- Lack of appetite (possibly underlying depression in baby or signaling problem between parent and child)

*There may be developmental delays as a result of lacking the motivation or drive to explore their environment, which is an important factor in progressing normal development.

3. SEPARATION AND INDIVIDUATION

An important aspect of the foundation in the ability to separate and develop a sense of self from the caregiver takes place between 6 months and 3 years. A notable hallmark is when the baby crawls away from its mother and then experiences the "aha" experience of both delight and fear that they have wandered away from their point of security. The child begins to develop a cause and effect understanding and awareness that links their actions to a given response. For example, the repetition of sitting in the highchair at mealtime and dropping their cup or utensils onto the floor which are retrieved by the parent.

The time frame of 7–9 months is marked by the baby's interest in finger foods, using a spoon, and experimenting with new food textures. Self-feeding requires a modicum of separation from the parent along with a feeling of competence to self-nurture/soothe. It is a sense of control. They are choosing what they eat.

At 12–18 months, the baby expresses themselves through feeding (choices of food and behavior) and play. They may even refuse to eat their favorite food to the consternation of the parent. If there is not a power struggle (granting of autonomy) with the parent, this behavior is generally short lived. Many behavioral demonstrations of separation and individuation along with associated boundaries are exhibited. One example is the baby biting down on their mother's nipple during feeding. There is also increased clarity in their signals of distress, hunger, or being tired whereby the attentive caregiver appropriately responds.

Feeding behaviors progress through toddlerhood commensurate with the development of the child's competence in self-feeding. The family experience of mealtime contextually changes. Now the family joins together in mealtime rituals to socialize. If the parent is uncomfortable with messes, this stage will be challenging. Generally, a child likes putting their hands in their food, feeling the textures and often making a mess of themselves and their highchair/floor. This tactile experimentation may or may not be a pleasurable experience depending on their tactile system. The child is a focal point of pleasure and encouragement demonstrating their language development with an array of new words as well as gestures. They enjoy the attention and may become somewhat of a comic learning the ability to make others laugh at their antics, definitely being a participating member of the family in this group setting. The preschool years reveal increased competence in the form of sharing (give and take) of food and taking turns during an episode of conversation.

Separation and individuation are manifested in the struggle of autonomy versus dependency. There is the obvious refusal of food and possibly extreme food selectivity. "Infantile anorexia nervosa" is entrenched in the infant's declaration for autonomy, thus a power struggle between mother and child around food. This is critical. What is taking place is a disallowing of the child's own body/being to regulate what and how they eat, and the main emphasis becomes the emotions that are associated with eating – anger, control, non-compliance, the mother's intrusiveness/assertion of will, and decreased dyadic reciprocity (negative emotions are experienced by both parent and child). The excessive worry about baby's growth/ development and their eating, and insecurity experienced by the parents may have roots in their own childhood experience.

Typically feeding skills evolve so that infants become increasingly independent as they advance commensurate with aging. The caregiver–infant relationship, particularly involving premature infants with continuing health problems, can complicate an infant's feeding. Influencing factors include length of hospitalization, maternal confidence, ability of parents to cope as a resourceful team with one another, degree of social support, postnatal complications (including aspiration, reflux, aversion to food, and resistance to eating) and infant temperament. Additional complicating factors such as lung disease or congenital heart disease may cause fatigue resulting in the infant not having the necessary energy to feed. Zerzan (2007) identifies then following factors of influence upon feeding.

Factors Influencing Feeding

Very low birth weight infants (VLBW) generally experience difficulties with the feeding relationship for a variety of reasons:

- experience of prolonged airway intubation or tube feeding may perceive any effort to approach their mouth/face as a potential discomfort
- infants fed by nasogastric tubes may have little exposure to oral stimulation (lack of early oral sensory input) and their perception can result in hypersensitivity and hyperirritability during feeding
- infant control over their arousal level may affect the parent–child relationship. Sucking can improve/achieve infant state organization as well as a stress reliever for the infant
- preterm infants exhibit developmental immaturity that may influence alterations in feeding patterns and ability to communicate with caregivers. They also have increased incidence of difficult temperament in the first few months following birth, thus, negatively impacting parent–child interactions

Maternal attitude and behavior negatively impacting feeding/growth

- caregiver–child interaction along with the availability of appropriate foods determine that the developing child successfully obtains food. *This is important because a hungry infant being consoled by a parent providing them with food is one of the ways in which the parent–child bond is strengthened
- premature infants are generally perceived as fragile which can lead to a new mother feeling insecure about her ability appropriately and effectively to handle her infant, thus resulting in unfavorable handling of the infant. This may lead to a mother withdrawing as a result of depression and anxiety. Overall, the result is decreased maternal encouragement during feeding

Potential impact of the parent–child relationship on feeding and growth

- the parent–child relationship can be positive or negative for the parent and the child
- strengths of either the parent or the child can compensate for the deficiencies/difficulties of the other

157

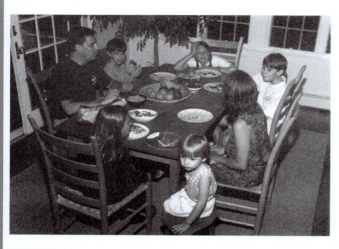

FIGURE 3.6
Observing the family
mealtime is important in
the assessment process.

- therefore, the development of the infant is not only influenced by biological risk factors but by the maternal compensating abilities to make modifications that benefit the feeding experience accordingly
- the child's food aversion may lead to parental anxiety and result in pressure on the child to eat

*Failure to thrive and poor feeding are associated with emotional deprivation of infants. A lack of nurturing leads to decreased food intake which may be linked to a lack of appetite.

ASSESSING THE EATING PROCESS

Assessments are important in that they require all professionals to speak the same language. This is especially invaluable with a multidisciplinary team (which needs to include the primary pediatrician). A comprehensive set of assessments is utilized in order to describe and explain the nature of the feeding disorder (Figure 3.6). An example of an assessment of the eating process:

- A mental health provider conducts an intake interview. To identify:
  - parental concerns
  - a complete medical history
  - a complete family history
  - previous treatment history
  - determining the meaning of the eating problem to both parents/family and child
  - food intake history to be completed by parents
  - presence of supplemental feeding procedures (nasogastric tube or gastostomy tube feedings)
  *The child should be weighed and measured for height and measure the head circumference
- Second and third visit follow ups allow for a developmental assessment and feeding observation (including developmental, sensory, motor, oral-motor, feeding, and language functions). Observations are made of the parent–child interactions using the Functional Emotional Assessment Scale providing an index of the child's emotional development in the context of dyadic interactions. It is recommended that this assessment be done by an occupational therapist, speech and language pathologist, and a clinical psychologist (as per DeGangi, 2000). The evaluation process is concluded with a parent conference to discuss the assessment findings, review treatment recommendations, and goal setting with the parents/family.

The treatment of feeding recognizes the emotional development of the child, associated sensory dysfunction, the impact that problems of feeding negatively impact the family and the parent–child relationship. This requires an integrated, multidisciplinary treatment approach, individualized identified needs, and a child-centered focus on unresolved emotional issues combined to resolve oral-motor and sensory problems.

Goals

1. Rule out medical problems
2. Interview parent(s)
3. Determine quality of feeding experience/observe and assess
4. Resolve attachment issues
5. Resolve issues of separation
6. Address sensory processing needs

7. Resolve issues of homeostasis
8. Improve feeding

Treatment Focus and Objectives

1. Consult with primary pediatrician to review medical history associated with feeding. If infant is currently in the hospital:
  a. Preparing for discharge (D/C) from hospital. Preparing for D/C begins way ahead of the actual D/C psychologically to improve the transition from hospital to home. The planning should be given in writing after being given verbally. This will allow for questions and further notation if necessary and having the written form reinforces parental feelings of security and being in control of a difficult situation. It is also beneficial to provide any books (or recommend them in a timely fashion so that they can be purchased prior to D/C) that are reinforcing, encouraging and offer practical advice. It is also beneficial to provide a practice "rooming in" opportunity for parental practice with available support in a safe environment prior to D/C as a means to enhance parental feelings of competency and to decrease anxiety
  b. Medical management. The primary pediatrician is an integral member of the treatment team and is consulted regularly. If the infant/child suffers with reflux or other medical problems which negatively impact eating consider the following:
    i. positioning needs during and after feeding (promoting digestion in the presence of reflux)
    ii. semi-inclining position for feeding and a period of time after may prevent vomiting
    iii. regular weekly weight checks whenever FTT is an issue; nutritional consult is valuable in addressing dietary needs
2. Interview and educate
  a. Interview parents about their concerns, their own feeding and attachment history, and about the details (and interpretation) of the experience that they are having with their child around feeding and how it has impacted family life
  b. Outline for parents the importance of establishing a routine around mealtime, such as washing hands, setting the table, and clean-up before and after mealtime to help in making the transition to the table, and the associated rationale
  c. Establish food rules during mealtime (i.e., no throwing of food or utensils, no standing up in the high chair, one warning and remove food
  d. Put on the plate or in the bowl only what can be reasonably finished. Avoid giving too much food due to the potential of overwhelming the child
  e. Provide a rationale for a mealtime schedule for parents (the goal is to improve the child's appetite)
  f. Acknowledge and respect cultural issues related to feeding and mealtime
3. Determine the quality of the feeding relationship/observe and assess
  a. Observe feeding
    i. quality of interactions
    ii. facial expressions of caregiver and child
    iii. body language associated with positioning as well as interactions
  b. Assess factors influencing the feeding relationship
    i. feeding skills
    ii. medications
    iii. diseases of prematurity with nutritional associations
    iv. GERD and aspiration, and stressful trauma to the mouth, nose, throat, or esophagus (such as intubation and traumatic suctioning)
    v. Identify the mother–infant interactions to be targeted for intervention
      - Family centered interventions (FCI); FCIs can improve mother–infant interactions. Professionals work closely with the family collaboratively to find solutions that the parent(s) are willing to implement

    -   Family support. Feeding does not take place in a vacuum, isolated from numerous other challenges associated w/VLBW infants. Family support for families with a preterm infant is beneficial to improving parent–child and family interactions which can also result in improved feeding. For mothers, offer validation, knowledge and skills, time for rest and self-care, general support, professional resources, and written information which validates and answers questions.

4. Resolve attachment issues

    a. Engage in rituals associated with mealtime with age-appropriate parent–child contact

    b. Oral-motor needs related to improving sucking, swallowing, and chewing should be practiced at a time other than mealtimes. This stimulation of the mouth can be done during toothbrushing, or playtime focusing on oral motor games. It is a time of encouragement and play between parent and child which is reassuring to the child

    c. Socialize the mealtime experience, incorporating it as a time of sharing with points of appropriate separation/autonomy

    d. Provide opportunities for the child to play appropriately in association with feeding/ mealtime, separation, and control

    e. Parent–infant/child interactions serve as the conduit to reinforce attachment, expression of needs, reciprocal communication, and separation/autonomy

5. Resolve issues of separation

    a. Establish food rules associated with mealtime, as well as opportunities for appropriate choices (such as food exchanges)

    b. Provide opportunities for the child to play appropriately in association with nurturing, feeding, separation, control, or other emotional needs underlying the feeding problem

    c. Parent–infant/child interactions serve as the conduit to reinforce separation/ individuation

    d. Educate and reinforce the parent's ability to read the child's cues and give signals of nurturance and independence/autonomy

    e. Educate and reinforce the child's initiation of adaptive emotional responses within the parent–child interaction

    f. Nurturing the parent is the key to nurturing the infant/child. Therefore, address their issues of loss and deprivation

    g. Educate the parents regarding the developmental stage of separation (explain the emotional and developmental tasks) to enhance their understanding of the developmental conflicts that they are experiencing associated with eating (such as control)

    h. Utilize child-centered activities designed to illuminate and create discovery about the dynamics influencing their interactions and how to respond effectively to the child's emotional needs through play

    i. Child-centered play creates opportunities to provide play about nurturing, feeding, filling, and dumping. Some examples of play materials could be

        i. beans or water and containers that can be filled and emptied

        ii. the use of dolls to nurture and feed

        iii. tableware to practice with

        iv. tunnels to crawl through

        v. obstacles to peak around

6. Address sensory processing needs

Activities designed for sensory exploration are employed to normalize hypersensitivities to touch and movement that affect the infant/child's ability to feed. An example would be the child who demonstrates an inability to tolerate food textures as a result of hypersensitivy to touch in the mouth. To deal with this, introduce a variety of non-threatening tactile experiences to the face (face paint, stickers on the cheek, puppet play on the face, etc.) and functional self-help activities (brushing teeth and gums, wiping nose, lip protector while at the beach, sunscreen cloths, etc.). Addressing tactile problems at times other than mealtime is beneficial

   a. Tooth brushing with a firm toothbrush can be used to desensitize the inside of the mouth

   b. Scrubbing the face and gums gently with a soft scrub brush or terry towel

   c. Firm food textures should be introduced first (easier for the child with hypersensitivities with a progression to smooth, soft textured and uneven textured foods)

   d. Work with the parents to establish food rules that are useful in structuring behavior during mealtime

   e. Address motor needs in holding utensils. Practice could be holding a toothbrush or a breadstick as a spoon (they are easier to hold than a spoon). Use sticky foods for the spoon, such as melted cheese on peas or mashed potatoes. It is best to start with foods that the child is capable of eating on their own (create a list with the parents)

   f. For messy meals use a drop cloth or not wear a shirt so that it is not an issue if food spills on their body (desensitizes to hypersensitivity)

   g. Avoid wiping the child's mouth during the course of mealtime. Clean the face at the end of the meal

7. Resolve issues of homeostasis

   a. Provide a mealtime schedule to improve the child's appetite

   b. Put only enough food on the plate or in the bowl that can be reasonably finished

   c. Label being hungry and full before and after meals to help the child recognize these states

8. Improve feeding

Specific interventions. Take the time to become acquainted with the specific issues experienced in the mother–infant feeding experience. Then offer specific plans for altering the caregiver–child feeding. There also needs to be consideration for the time and commitment to other family activities. This is an opportunity to reinforce parental sense of control over the infant's condition. Educate parents regarding recommended changes and give adequate support for success. Additionally, any intervention which supports caregiver–infant interaction will improve the quality of the infant–caregiver relationship.

   a. Teach parenting skills

   b. Improve observational skills and associated interpretation of child responses

   c. Set up a mealtime schedule, including scheduled snacks. Instruct the parents to not give the child a middle of the night bottle. This sabotages the program

   d. Establish food rules during mealtime (no throwing food or utensils, no standing up in high chair, one warning then remove food

   e. Food should not be given as a reward for doing other behaviors

   f. Everyone should eat at mealtime to model eating. If the parents are not hungry or are dieting, they should schedule that as a snack or small meal

   g. Socialize the mealtime experience (encourage conversation, eating and enjoying the mealtime)

   h. Encourage the parents to take the child to child-friendly restaurants/fast food where the child can see other children eat

   i. Provide caregiver–child enrichment exercises

   j. Explore the meaning of food and eating for the parents

   k. If more parental information is needed: NCAST feeding scale may be used as a means to identify for parents what is working well and where improvement is needed

   l. Nutritional interventions to be used if the immaturity of the infant/medical condition result in feeding relationship limitations (such as concentration of formula, tube feeding, etc)

   m. Provide support to parents, acknowledging and validating feelings of rejection, anxiety and depression from not being able to have a more carefree relationship with their child to nurture and feed them

n. Parental guidance is offered to address any concerns associated with food intake, selection/variety of appropriate foods, expanding food choices, and behavioral management techniques to improve the quality and outcome of mealtime

o. Referral for further evaluation and treatment. Referrals are made when indicated by significant growth problems, significant negative interactions associated with feeding, parent feels unable to feed child, parent is unable to pick up on and respond appropriately to infant cues (for example, overriding infant cues during feeding)

    i. public health nurse

    ii. early intervention center/Birth to Three

    iii. mental health referral

    iv. feeding intervention team

Attachment and Reactive Attachment Disorder

CASE EXAMPLE

Danny was 4 years old when his parents (Mr and Mrs Smith) sought intervention following a referral from their preschool teacher. Apparently, Danny was late almost daily to preschool and all efforts of encouragement from the preschool teacher did not yield the desired result. The therapist experienced difficulty obtaining the information she needed from Danny's parents to clarify what the problem was. Therefore, she met with Danny, Danny and each parent and the parents. Apparently, Danny was fussy and cried a lot as an infant so they soothed him by bringing him to bed with them, though there had been efforts to get Danny into his own bed to sleep, he was still sleeping with his parents. It was also discovered that Danny's mother had lost her twin sister at the age of 8 to cancer. She had been at ballet lessons when her sister died. She had never been able to let go of the feelings of guilt for leaving her sister and she feared that something might happen to Danny if she left him alone. She struggled every morning in sending him to school and Danny did everything he could on a daily basis to prolong breakfast, getting dressed, wanting to be held, etc. which resulted in being late. Additionally, when each parent and Danny were observed it was obvious that he demanded their constant attention and entertaining.

Treatment

1. Educating the parents about the importance of the developmental task of separation, social and emotional development
2. Educating, role modeling and reinforcing appropriate boundaries, limit setting, and behavioral management
3. Increasing and reinforcing autonomy, problem solving, resilience and age-appropriate social skills.
4. Establishing new night-time rituals to prepare and reinforce Danny sleeping in his own bed (review section on Sleep)
5. Refer Mrs Smith to therapy so that she can resolve her own attachment and loss issues associated with the childhood death of her twin sister. It was recommended that Mr Smith adjunctively participate with the focus on strengthening their parental alliance and dating (which meant getting a babysitter for Danny)
6. Establishing play dates for Danny with several peers from his preschool, which also reinforces Mrs Smith socializing with another adult instead of entertaining Danny

The phenomenon of attachment is rich with developmental concepts (Mahler et al, 1975; DeGangi, 2000; Schore, 2002, 2005; Thompson et al, 2008). Attachment refers to that deep and lasting connection established between a child and their caregivers during the first few years of life. Early experiences with caregivers shape a child's self-concept, belief about others, and life in general. These emotional experiences are encoded in the limbic system of the brain (the emotional center). These repeated encoded experiences become the child's internal working model or their lens from which they view themselves and others now and later in life. This is particularly true of their view of attachment figures and authority figures. These beliefs play a significant role in their interpretation of the present and the future. Attachment significantly affects a child's development along with their ability to develop relationships and effectively to express themselves. The parent or caregivers of a child experiencing attachment disorders feels helpless, physically and emotionally exhausted by their efforts to connect with the child. The responses they are often confronted with in this circumstance are opposition, defiance and indifference. This is because the child lacks the skills necessary to develop a meaningful relationship. The child's internal experience is indicative of low self-worth, a lack of interpersonal trust, fear of getting close, anger, and a need to be in control. They feel unsafe and alone. A fundamental contributor to attachment disorders is the consequence of negative experiences in primary relationships whereby they repeatedly feel abandoned, isolated, powerless, or uncared for. As a result, their experience is interpreted as they can't depend on others and the world is a dangerous and overwhelming place. Attachment problems develop when a child is unable to connect with primary caregivers due to poor nurturing skills, neglect and abuse:

- a baby cries and it does not elicit a response from caregivers or no comfort is offered
- a baby is hungry or needs to be changed and no one responds for a long period of time, maybe hours
- no one looks at or talks to the baby, resulting in feeling lonely and disconnected
- a young child only receives attention by acting out or exhibiting extreme behaviors
- a baby/young child is mistreated or abused
- there is inconsistency in needs being met, therefore, the child is unable to predict or depend on caregiver responsiveness and acts of love and care
- due to hospitalization the baby/young child is separated from primary caregivers -the baby/young child is moved from one caretaker to another as a consequence of the loss of a parent, adoption, foster care
- the primary caregiver is emotionally unavailable due to depression, substance abuse or another form of mental illness

FACTORS CONTRIBUTING TO INCREASED RISK FOR DEVELOPING ATTACHMENT DISORDERS

Caregiver Factors
- Care is insensitive/ineffective
- Teenage parent
- Mental illness
- Abuse/neglect
- Substance abuse
- Extensive absence (hospital, abandonment, incarceration)
- Intergenerational attachment difficulties (separation, loss, mistreatment)

Child Factors
- Genetic factors
- Congenital/biological problems/neurological impairment, in-utero exposure to drug/alcohol
- Premature birth
- Medical conditions/hospitalizations
- Failure to thrive (FTT)
- Lack of parent–child fit/difficult temperament

Environmental Factors
- Low SES/poverty
- Lack of support (absent parent, isolation, lack of services)

163

- Violence (domestic violence, victim, witness)
- Multiple out of home placements
- Significant stress (environment that is chaotic and disorganized, marital conflict, home instability/moves a lot/violent neighborhood)

The DSM IV-TR defines Reactive Attachment Disorder as a condition of "marked disturbed and developmentally inappropriate social relatedness in most contexts; symptoms begin before age 5 years and are associated with grossly pathological care". Furthermore, two subtypes are described: (1) a "pattern of excessively inhibited, hypervigilant, or highly ambivalent and contradictory responses; and (2) indiscriminate sociability with marked inability to exhibit appropriate selective attachments". The DSM also states that the diagnosis cannot be given in the presence of a pervasive developmental disorder which is also associated with social abnormalities. A more useful description is offered by the DC:0–3 which describes Deprivation/Maltreatment Disorder of Infancy as a disorder that manifests in some children who have been severely neglected or have a documented history of physical or psychological maltreatment, or have not had the opportunity to form selective attachments due to abandonment, frequent changes in caretakers or unavailability. The DC:0–3 suggests that children with this disorder have "markedly disturbed and developmentally inappropriate attachment behaviors in which the child rarely or minimally demonstrates preference to a particular attachment figure for comfort, support, protection and nurturance". Three patterns are described: (1) emotionally withdrawn or inhibited; (2) indiscriminant or disinhibited; and (3) mixed. This information is distilled down to the fact that when a child 0–3 years of age is responded to in a consistently caring and sensitive manner and receives comfort when required by an emotionally and physically available consistent caretaker they learn that they are worthy of love and care which results in the development of positive expectations about relationships in general. Likewise, when this is not their experience the outcome is opposite. Attachment therapy is a rich diversity of approaches designed to promote, develop or enhance a reciprocal attachment relationship.

SOME SYMPTOMS OF INSECURE ATTACHMENT VERSUS REACTIVE ATTACHMENT DISORDER

Insecure attachment	Reactive attachment
Avoids eye contact	Aversion to touch
Doesn't smile	Aversion to physical affection
Rejects efforts to be calmed	Control issue/disobedient/defiant
Cries inconsolably	Anger problems/acting out
Doesn't visually track caregiver(s)	Difficulty showing affection
Disinterest in interactive games/toys	Inappropriate affection
Rocks/self-soothes	Underdeveloped conscience

Goals

1. Rule out medical problems and Pervasive Developmental Disorder
2. Improve parenting skill
3. Improve infant/child feelings of trust, security and bonding with caregivers
4. Facilitate parental attachment to child
5. Individualized interventions
6. Improve self-awareness and social intelligence
7. Changing the impact of mother's attachment history

Treatment Focus and Objectives

1. Rule out medical problems and Pervasive Developmental Disorder
   a. Consult with pediatrician to rule out medical problems and thoroughly assess to assure correct diagnosis. Thorough assessment including history of treatment,

psychological history, educational history, medical history, attachment and social history (including breaks/disruptions in attachment), developmental history (including prenatal and birth), family system functioning, intellectual and cognitive skills and deficits, and differential diagnosis. The family's emotional response to therapy needs to be monitored, as well as the child's

2. Parenting. Positive effective parenting results in improving the parent–child relationship. If the attachment bond is insecure (i.e., the caregiver responds to the infant/child's distress in ways that are rejecting, inconsistent, or frightening/frightened/disassociated/ atypical) then intervention is focused on changing the quality of caregiver response to their child's distress. Such intervention is directed at training the caregiver accurately to read the child's cues and signals of distress and respond sensitively and in a manner that promotes health attachment and development. Parent–child interactions that are key to establishing a healthy attachment are central to their interactions in therapy, i.e., eye contact, physical contact, tone of voice, smiles, additional non-verbal communication and gestures, etc. For example:

   a. Employ a positive psychological perspective. While exploring unresolved issues, therapy takes into account past and present family dynamics. A central therapeutic activity, to benefit the child, is for the family members to express their emotional responses to past and present situations that are interfering with attachment

   b. Be patient. The process of change may not proceed as quickly as one feels it is needed, but it is a slow process and other bumps in the road can complicate and slow things along the way

   c. Maintain a sense of humor and joy. Repairing attachment problems is hard work. Humor and joy refuel energy, thus, spend time with people who make this easy. It is necessary for maintaining a positive perspective and being patient with the child

   d. Keep a realistic expectation. It takes a long time. Focus on small steps and rejoice over small accomplishments. The small steps are the sure steps and easiest to reinforce and build upon

   e. Remain positive and hopeful, the sensitivity of the child will pick up on this which has a contagious effect. Likewise, if a caregiver is feeling discouraged, a child picks up on that too. It is not an emotional response that any age person can feel secure and close to

   f. Self-care and stress management are imperative. Be sure to allocate time for a break and self-soothing (soak in the tub, reading for pleasure, coffee break with a friend, etc.). If a caregiver doesn't take care of themselves, they are going to lack the resilience necessary for the patience of working with the child

   g. Identify and seek support. This is a long haul. Rely on friends, family and community resources for support and necessary respite care. Learn to ask for help before it is necessary to avoid getting to a breaking point. It may also be beneficial to join a parent support group

   h. Parenting classes are a good way to get parenting education and learning about attachment along with other parenting skills

   i. Assist parents in developing healthy parenting strategies, such as:

      i. support the parents' authority and need to maintain control over the family environment, while assisting the child to feel safe enough to let go of their compulsive need to be in control

      ii. increase the child's readiness to rely on the parent for safety, help comforting, nurturing

      iii. encourage a positive, supportive family atmosphere

      iv. encourage a high level of nurturance

      v. encourage structure and limits

      vi. increase reciprocal, positive interactions between parent and child

      vii. help the child make choices that are in their own best interest, in the best interest of their family, and to accept the consequences of those choices

165

      viii. help parents become emotionally available for their child as healthy and safe caregivers (this could include exploring their own issues, marital relationship, infertility, grief/loss, early life traumas, etc.)

      ix. help family and child develop reasonable expectations of success

  j. Parents may have problems, which must be understood and addressed if they are to help their child resolve attachment problems (and/or other problems)

*For the adoptive/foster parent. All of the above parenting recommendations are to be utilized with the validation that the child's anger and unresponsiveness may be very emotionally difficult to take. Remember that child in this situation, while the gift of loving parents and a home are being offered, their young lives have already been confronted with loss and instability. Their life experience has not prepared them to bond, and they are not able to recognize their new caregivers as a foundation/source of love, comfort and stability. Be patient, it takes time, consistency, being firm, but always a lot of love.

3. Helping a child to feel safe and secure

  a. Set limits and boundaries. Children need structure and to know the parameters of what is okay and what's not. Consistent boundaries and consistent love make the world predictable for a child with attachment problems. A child needs to know what is expected of them, what is not acceptable, and what the consequences are for the choices they make. A child feels more secure when they come to understand that life is about choices and every choice has a consequence. In the same manner, behaviors have two outcomes; they bring people closer together or push them apart. They need to learn that they have more control over what their experiences are than they think

  b. Remain calm and in charge. When a child engages in problem behavior it is often due to their lack of management skills for the situation they find themselves in, they need the firm, but calm support of the caregiver. Staying calm demonstrates to the child that whatever they are feeling is tolerable and manageable. If they are purposefully being defiant, just be consistent with them receiving the established consequence for the behavior, but do it in a cool, matter of fact, in charge manner. If a caregiver disciplines a child in an emotionally charged state it may reinforce the bad behavior as well as reinforcing feeling unsafe and insecure

  c. Remain emotionally available. Be immediately available to reconnect with a child following an episode of negative behavior and ensuing consequence/discipline. This reinforces love, consistency, safety and develops trust that the parent is a constant no matter what happens

  d. If the parent makes a mistake they need to take responsibility for it. When low frustration tolerance results in parental out of control (yelling and intense, etc.) behavior they need to be willing to take responsibility, make amends and strengthen the parent–child bond

  e. Maintain predictable routines and schedules to provide comfort during times of change. A child with attachment issues lacks the instinct to rely on caregivers, resulting in feeling threatened and overwhelmed with transition and inconsistency

  f. Coach parents/caregivers to be sensitive to the child's signals but, at the same time, be able gently to challenge the child's miscues and misperceptions that nurturance is not needed when in fact it is. The goal is to help the child understand and communicate their needs more directly and effectively

4. Facilitate feelings of love for a child with attachment issues. When a child has developed attachment issues they have a hard time accepting love, in particular physical demonstrations of love. A child learns to accept love over time with consistency and repetition in a predictable environment. Trust and security develop from seeing loving actions, hearing reassuring and calming words, and feeling soothed/comforted over and over again

  a. Identify the nurturing things that feel good to the child such as rocking, holding, cuddling, stoking/rubbing their back. This is the fertile ground of attachment missed earlier. Always be respectful of the child and touch, it needs to be what feels good and comfortable to them. If they are resistant to touch (earlier trauma?) go slowly

b. Be astute to a child's emotional age and respond accordingly. A child with attachment issues acts younger emotionally and socially. Thus, they need to be treated as a younger child, using more non-verbal methods of comforting/soothing

c. Emotions can be overwhelming; help the child to identify what they are feeling and help them to identify what they need. Be consistent in reinforcing the idea that all feelings are okay and help them to learn healthy and appropriate ways to express them

d. Communicate and interact with the child. Listen, talk, and play offering full, focused attention in a manner that is comforting. Quality time together, without other distractions, provides the child with the necessary opportunity to practice trusting and opening up

e. Basic habits of sleep, eating and exercise are even more important with children experiencing attachment issues. Healthy lifestyle habits decrease stress levels as well as level out mood swings. When the child with attachment issues is relaxed, eating well, well rested and feeling good, daily life challenges are so much easier for them to manage

    i. nutrition. Offer easy to understand literature about good healthy food. If there are allergies, a consultation with the dietician about good, basic healthy foods is a good choice

    ii. sleep. Children need a sleep schedule so that they can be well rested. Being rested supports them to make better choices and more focused on tasks

    iii. exercise. Physical activity is important for dealing with stress and frustration – especially anger. It also triggers endorphins, which feels good

f. Consistency. Strive to develop a system within which the child seeks out the parent in times of distress or when pleased with achievements, as well as parental sensitivity to, acceptance of, and timely response to the child's needs

5. Individualized considerations

a. Family therapy which involves fun and rewarding activities designed to enhance and reinforce the attachment bond. It is also an opportunity for other children in the family to understand their sibling's experience and effective ways to deal with them

b. Individual psychological therapy/counseling for the child, while the parent is able to observe. This offers practice and skill building for both child and caregivers. The goals in this environment encompass direct intervening with the child with monitoring emotions and behavior

c. Play therapy helps a child to learn appropriate social skills for peers and other social situations

d. Special education services offers specifically designed programs in the school setting to facilitate and reinforce the learning of skills necessary for academic and social success, while at the same time addressing behavioral and emotional difficulties

6. Enhance the child's understanding of emotions, social cues, and interpersonal situations. A common theme in these interventions involves an emphasis on the nurturing, empathy building and affective attunement by the caregiver coinciding with consistent behavioral consequences (Figure 3.7). Consistency is extremely important for the child to develop predictive dyadic reliance

a. Play games that reinforce social understanding and knowledge as well as offering an opportunity to practice social rules in a fun way. One way to do this would be to modify a 5-point scale to identify emotional intensity

b. Using pictures telling a story in a sequence – allow the child to practice putting them in the right order

167

FIGURE 3.7
Family river rafting together.

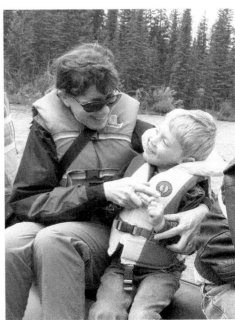

    c. Address issues of interacting appropriately and safely with strangers, as well as checking in and seeking out primary caregivers in times of need

    d. Affect regulation skills and impulse control are addressed by a therapist working with parent and to
        i. problem solve issues of daily living
        ii. assist parents in learning to recognize when their child is frightened and when to offer reassurance
        iii. translate the meaning of a child's behaviors to their parents

    e. Intervention strategies include the use of play, physical contact and language to promote healthy exploration, contain overwhelming affect, clarify feelings, and correct misperceptions

7. Changing the impact of mother's attachment history. The influence of a parent's own history and how it impacts their parenting style must be addressed as a significant factor in the course of treatment for young children. The impaired responsiveness (lack of involvement and non-reciprocal interactions) is indicative of the parenting style of a depressed mother and is associated with difficulties with infant/child emotion and regulation

    ○ Decreased ability to cope with frustration
    ○ Increased negative affect and emotional lability
    ○ Decreased level of soothability and positive affect
    ○ Increased risk for insecure attachment

The ripple effect for the child is significant. Not only is the child at risk for developing insecure attachment to the parent, but their resulting relationship skills may create difficulties in establishing positive relationships with other caregivers who could ameliorate the attachment consequences created by the depressed mother. Considerations for the effective intervention with the depressed mother

    a. Referral to a psychiatrist or primary treating physician for a medication evaluation
    b. Routine follow up with physician to monitor, reinforce and offer support
    c. Therapy
        i. non-directive counseling allowing the mother the opportunity to express fears or concerns associated with parenting or other aspects of life (such as marital relationship issues, etc.)
        ii. CBT focusing on parent–child interaction and matching of guidance in identifying infant/child cues to respond to and management of infant/child emotional and developmental needs
        iii. dynamic psychotherapy focused on understanding the mother's representational/interpretation of her infant/child and her relationship with them by exploring her own attachment history

The goal of these interventions is to:
    ○ Provide a validating and safe environment
    ○ Increase competency in meeting the child's needs
    ○ To model and reinforce positive, interactive, and developmentally appropriate mother–child dyad
    ○ Decrease isolation by activating the mother and mobilizing resources

Anxiety Disorder

Anxiety is a common emotion. It is often associated with fear when an individual is confronted with danger or a difficult situation. As a general response it may be exaggerated or out of proportion to environmental threats. Anxiety tends to be related to worrying about what will happen or what has happened in the past. Anxiety becomes a problem when it interferes with a child being able to enjoy normal life experiences. With regards to young children, anxiety is a normal part of development. For example, infants may show anxiety or fearfulness to loud noises or a sudden loss of physical support, and the 9 month to 2 year old commonly experiences separation anxiety which is an indication of the development of a healthy attachment to caregivers. Most children experience anxiety directly in relation to psychological, social and environmental influences (Figure 3.8). In other words, anxiety disorders are not necessarily inherited, although some appear to inherit a risk or vulnerability from an anxiety disorder from their family. Types of anxiety disorders include:

- Generalized anxiety disorder
  Characterized by excessive worry about future and past events and is usually accompanied by physical symptoms such as stomach ache, headache, sleep disturbance etc.
- Separation anxiety disorder
  The fear of separating from primary caregivers or familiar surroundings
- Specific phobia
  The fear associated with a specific object or situation such as the dark, heights, animals, etc.
- Post-traumatic stress disorder
  Characterized by the presence of severe anxiety reactions/feelings following a traumatic event (being involved in a tragic/frightening experience, near death, witnessing death, being sexually abused, etc.)
- Social phobia
  The fear of being embarrassed/humiliated in front of others, stressed about being the center of attention, fear of meeting new people, etc.
- Obsessive compulsive disorder
  Characterized by intrusive, obsessive thoughts which are usually alleviated by compulsive behaviors (excessive hand-washing, checking behaviors, etc.). Not seen often in children
- Panic attack
  Characterized by a discrete period in which there is a sudden onset of intense apprehension, fearfulness, or terror often associated with feelings that something terrible is going to happen (impending doom) and accompanied by physical symptoms (chest pain or pressure, difficulty breathing, etc.)

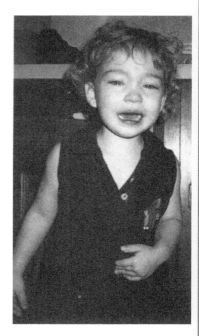

FIGURE 3.8
An irritable child cries inconsolably.

169

Factors that reinforce anxiety symptoms:

- Self-talk (automatic thoughts) refers to what the child believes can/will cause an emotional reaction. This catastrophizing contributes to a lot of anxiety with the associated belief that "I can't deal with it", "I am going to get hurt", etc.
- Avoidance (escape behavior) reinforces or gives power to a fear. It is not uncommon for this type of response to expand and potentiate what is to be feared
- The responses of adults interfacing with the child (caregivers, childcare, teacher, etc.) that contribute to feelings of shame, guilt, and inadequacy contributing to self-defeating thoughts and avoidance (for example, a parent ridicules a child for feeling fearful instead of reinforcing, encouraging and rewarding a child's effort, approximation of change and courage).

SEPARATION PROBLEMS

It is normal for a child to feel anxious when a caregiver says goodbye. In early childhood, crying, tantrums or clinging are natural reactions to separation. However, there is a difference between normal separation fear and separation anxiety disorder (SAD). SAD is an emotional problem not a developmental issue or stage. Separation anxiety can begin before a child has their first birthday and/or any other time before the child is 4 years old. However, some children experience a higher level of intensity of separation anxiety that does not subside. There is no predictable pattern of time frame and intensity from child to child. A cue that there is a more significant problem is when separation anxiety either continues or recurs as a child enters kindergarten. Children may inherit a tendency to develop anxiety disorders from their parents and these temperamental factors may be triggered by severely stressful events such as child abuse, the loss of a parent or parents, institutionalization, or a seemingly less stressful but difficult life event like the death of a family member or moving.

Just as with adults, anxious and nervous children will try to avoid feeling bad. Eventually, this results in making choices based on feared situations and not realities. However, in most cases, the consequence is learning to avoid and escape the normal challenges of life through isolation, avoiding daycare/school, thrill seeking, etc. Over time, a child may even come to express anger instead of their fear because anger feels better than fear and is easier to blame on other people or situations when they cannot escape (problem solve or practicing the learning of new skills or resources). These circumstances lead to a lack of self-confidence that negatively impacts thriving at home and daycare/school. An added consequence to these losses in building functional skills is depression. The types of factors which may contribute to increased separation anxiety include:

- Change in a child's routine
- Changes in the family system (divorce, birth of a baby, parent hospitalized for health crisis, etc.)
- Child becoming ill
- Change in caregiver, daycare/preschool
- Child being tired (needing to be soothed, decreased coping ability, etc.)

CASE EXAMPLE

Ben, age 3½, and his family recently moved to a new city. His parents were excited about the move and had already found an enrichment program for his daycare. They were surprised when he started making comments about not wanting to go to "school". He began to have difficulties sleeping and on the day that he was to begin school he threw a tantrum, started crying and refused to go to school. His parents finally calmed him down and took him to school. There he kept clinging to his mother begging her to not leave him and complained of a stomach ache every day. They thought that as he became familiar with the school, his teacher and started making friends that all of this would subside. After several months little had changed and he was now having nightmares. They consulted with Ben's pediatrician who referred them to a child psychologist.

Treatment

The psychologist identified the numerous symptoms of separation anxiety disorder that Ben was experiencing. It appeared that the relocation, loss of other frequent caregiver contacts (his grandparents and three cousins that he often played with) and general stress associated with change had triggered the separation anxiety disorder. Numerous efforts were put in motion to increase his feeling of security. Arrangements were made for his grandparents to visit on several occasions. They demonstrated their normal interest in what he was doing and asked him to take them to his school so that they could meet his teacher and new friends. His parents made play dates that helped to extend the continuity of his new friendships. Much orchestrating of consistency in his schedule and who he was with took place. Every Monday and Wednesday he went to school 15 minutes early (before the other classmates arrived) to spend time alone with the teacher which calmed his fears and distracted him from being left by his mother. The parents remained calm through all of this distress, being sure to offer their son choices, but also setting appropriate limits. The therapist employed play therapy where Ben revealed his fear and worries associated with his refusal symptoms, nightmares and stomach aches. Directly and symbolically he was presented with validation and choices for appropriately dealing with his fears and developing some basic skills for mood management. All of his efforts were praised and reinforced and before long he was looking forward to school and demonstrating age-appropriate adjustment.

Common Symptoms of Separation Anxiety Disorder

1. Worries and fears (nightmares about separation, getting lost, etc.)
2. Refusal and sickness (refusal to go to childcare, reluctance to go to sleep, headache/stomach ache, clinging)

Common causes of Separation Anxiety Disorder

1. Changes in environment
2. Stress
3. Over-protective parent

Goals

1. Decrease or eliminate separation anxiety
2. Increase confidence
3. Routines and structure
4. Identify feelings
5. Comfort and encouragement
6. Behavioral activation and exposure

Treatment Focus and Objectives

1. Improve and stabilize feelings of safety and security associated with separation. Educate and instruct caregivers.
   a. Practice separation for desensitizing. Leave the child with a trusted and caring adult for brief periods and short distances, and increase the time frames accordingly. Keep the child calm during separation. Participating in activities may be useful as a positive distraction which helps time to pass and decreases recurring anxiety provoking thoughts
   b. Schedule separations after naps or feeding. Babies are more susceptible to separation anxiety when they are tired or hungry
   c. Develop a good-bye ritual. Rituals are predictable and reassuring and can be as simple as a special wave goodbye
   d. Maintain familiar surroundings when possible and make new surroundings familiar. For example, have the sitter come to the house or, if the child is leaving the house, have them take a familiar object with them. Don't prolong departure
   e. Have a consistent primary caregiver. If a child-care provider is hired, keep them, changing this role on a child is distressing to them
   f. Leave without making a big deal out of it. The parent should inform the child that they are leaving and will be back. After that don't stall
   g. Minimize scary media. For example, some things on television may be scary and provoke fearfulness. Be sensitive to their experience
   h. Be consistent. Don't give in; reassure the child that they are going to be fine. Setting limits will benefit adjustment to separation
   i. Praise the child's efforts, reinforcing approximations of change/adjustment toward the goal of alleviation and elimination of separation anxiety. Focus on the positive things that will happen when the caregiver is gone, and/or plan something special for when they return/pick them up
   j. Educate the caregiver(s) regarding the importance of their own efforts to be calm and centered and how it benefits their child, possibly by:
      i. talking about their own feelings. Expressing what they are going through may be cathartic, even if they are unable to change the stressful circumstances

     ii. exercising regularly. Physical activity plays a key role in reducing and preventing the effects of stress

     iii. good nutrition. Nutrition is important to physical coping of stress

     iv. practicing relaxation. Stress levels can be managed with relaxation techniques such as yoga, deep breathing, and meditation

     v. getting adequate sleep. Feeling tired decreases resilience to stress and negatively impacts rational thinking

     vi. maintaining patience and a sense of humor

  k. Empathic listening is the active process of accepting and confirming the child's fear and involves:

     i. give undivided attention

     ii. always acknowledge the problem

     iii. be non-judgmental and sensitive

     iv. listen for feelings behind the behavior

     v. allow silence for reflection

     vi. restate to clarify their message in order to help them more effectively to communicate their feelings

     vii. an empathic/understanding acknowledgement can be helpful to validate their experience and initiate problem solving

  Parents are in the best position to teach their children about anxiety because a parent's reaction in a situation either demonstrates how to confront a situation and problem solve it or how to react with fear. When parents react with fear they are reinforcing their children's fear

2. Increase confidence

  a. Practice approximating change. This offers the opportunity to

     i. challenge irrational self-talk

     ii. develop new and accurate information about what can really take place by learning to participate instead of avoid

     iii. positive reinforcement, "it feels good" and "I want to do that, it is fun"

  b. Modeling by caregivers and other significant adults

     i. a child observes another person interacting effectively with the feared object/situation

     ii. adaptive responding demonstrated with guided instruction, encouragement. This offers productive and positive practice of thinking and behavior change which improves perception and creates the opportunity for constructive feedback and positive reinforcement

  c. Contingency management refers to the manner in which external events that follow a child's fear/anxiety reactions are manipulated using rewards for successful interaction and bolder steps of appropriate risk taking

     i. rewards are withheld for refusing to interact

     ii. children are reinforced (made to feel better) for facing their fears

  d. Self-management. Subjective and physiological reactions are altered/modified by teaching the child adaptive ways to appraise and interpret an upcoming event/situation

     i. challenging irrational self-talk with accurate self-statements

     ii. being taught to break tasks down into manageable steps to avoid feeling anxious and overwhelmed

     iii. identifying choices for adaptive responding

     iv. being taught relaxation techniques (deep breathing, visualizing a positive outcome, etc.)

3. Routines and structure. Routines reduce anxiety and regular daily patterns emphasize predictability

  a. Establish consistent daily routines and structure. Anxious children do not cope well with a disorganized spontaneous family lifestyle

  b. A regular routine develops a sense of control

  c. Take care of basic child needs, especially paying attention to prevent states of hunger (low blood sugar) fatigue

  d. Provide opportunities for exercise. It relieves stress and helps a child's body to relax

  e. Set limits and provide natural/appropriate consequences for breaking the limits/ boundaries. Children feel secure when there are limits setting restrictions on inappropriate behaviors

4. Identifying feelings

  a. Help the child identify different feelings by naming various feelings they experience

  b. Explain how people show their feelings (facial expressions, body language, words), thus demonstrating that showing your feelings is an important way for others to understand how you are feeling

  c. Help the child make the connection of the physical response to various emotions. To notice the different feelings of their body, for example, anxiety may bring with it a stomach ache/butterflies, headache, tight muscles/tight hands

  d. It is helpful for children to speak about their feelings, even though it may not be easy. Caregivers need to pay attention for appropriate times to facilitate such sharing and, if initiated by the child, listen carefully with genuine interest and care

5. Comfort and encouragement

  a. Provide soothing and comforting strategies to relieve anxiety

    i. verbal assurance of security and love, rocking, cuddling, holding, massage, singing, telling stories, etc.

    ii. respect the child's fears (just telling them to not be afraid is discounting). Let them know that (whoever the adult is) they can be helped to overcome the fear

  b. Model brave behavior. Children look to others for guidance on how to respond to unfamiliar situations

    i. demonstrate the cues that are used to help determine if a situation is safe or not

    ii. caregivers need to acknowledge and understand their own anxieties and make an effort to contain them when appropriate in the presence of children. If adults around a child are overly anxious and overprotective, this anxiety is communicated to a child with the accompanying message that the world is a dangerous place. Sometimes adults need to act brave when they don't feel that way

  c. Encourage brave behavior and appropriate risk taking. It is not generally helpful to demand that a child face their fears all at once

    i. gently encourage a child to approach the feared situation. Exposure to feared situations leads to desensitization and reduction of the fear and anxiety

    ii. break down the goal into approximations or small steps so that each step is achievable and gradually becomes more difficult (the first steps are easiest to program success of effort and to reinforce effort – it feels good!)

    iii. reward the child for trying to approach a feared situation

    iv. remind the child that the fear will get smaller over time. Reinforce this by reminding the child of fears and difficult situations that they have overcome in the past

  d. Teach relaxation skills. It will help them to learn that they have some control over their own bodies rather than being controlled by the anxiety

    i. encourage slow deep breathing. This can be practiced in conjunction with developing the skill of visualization. Have the child imagine they are slowly blowing bubbles

    ii. have them practice tensing and relaxing their muscles. It teaches the difference of feeling stressed vs relaxed

    iii. teach how imagination can be used to relax

      - have the child imagine a safe and relaxing place and to notice the coinciding good relaxing feelings in their body.

- imagine a container (like a big box) to put their worries in so that they are not letting their mind run wild with negative/fearful thoughts when they need to be directing their energy toward more positive endeavors
- imagine the "fearful thermometer" to visualize just how fearful they are of a specific situation. This could also be done by coloring a picture of a thermometer to match the intensity of their fear or using a 5-point scale modified to the concept of fear (1 = not afraid, 5 = very afraid). *These types of techniques can be used as a before and after measure for a calming technique.

e. Encourage "feeling good" activities
   i. playing with a favorite toy, playing a game, doing a fun art or craft activity, playing outside, reading a book, playing with friends
   ii. assist and attend to a child to engage in these activities when they are exhibiting stress and anxiety – it will distract them

f. Storytelling. Find some books that specifically deal with anxiety, they can show helpful ways of coping with fear and anxiety. Incorporating puppets, where the adult identifies specific worries, triggers, and obsessive/intrusive thoughts and beliefs through the puppet, encouraging the child to join in

g. Teach problem solving strategies
   i. basic problem solving; identifying the problem, brainstorming all of the possible solutions and their consequences, and choosing the best solution
   ii. give the child ample time to express their negative feelings where the adult is just listening, acknowledging, and validating their feelings before jumping in to help them find a solution. *Take the time to create a "coping menu" which lists soothing strategies in a fun and visual manner

h. Challenge unhelpful thoughts
   i. help the child understand that negative/pessimistic thinking is not helpful and can influence how they feel and behave
   ii. help them identify more positive and accurate ways of thinking, "if I keep practicing…", "I will get better…", "Even if I make a mistake….", etc.

6. Behavioral activation and exposure. These two techniques for dealing avoidant behavior are coupled in a framework to encourage a young child to seek out (vs avoiding) rewarding experiences

a. Parent involvement is imperative. They need to be trained in the basics of exposure therapy and graded anxiety experiences (hierarchy)
   i. psychoeducation and treatment rationale – educating parents about how a child's behavior is associated to the reinforcing of their feelings of anxiety
   ii. give examples to parents to show how what may appear to be a common experience is interpreted in such a manner that it results in anxiety and avoidance
   iii. educate about the fight or flight response and normal reactions to withdraw and avoid from what is interpreted as a threat (young children may be unable to describe their somatic and emotional experience)
   iv. active practice of relaxation and coping with negative affect. This entails interrupting the anxiety response with active coping. This could include a reassuring caregiver slowly proceeding through an experience (guided) demonstrating it is not fearful and offering choices of response to counter avoidance and reinforce coping. Coping could include asking an adult for help, having the steps broken down, coupling the approach with taking a deep breath to relax the body
   v. transition is now made to approach instead of avoid (able to do as a result of the guided practice previously provided). Graded engagement is developed and utilized
   - select a practical attainable goal
   - the goal is one the child is highly motivated to complete
   - the goal chosen is one that will alleviate the degree of distress and make strides in decreasing anxiety with every effort they make (self-reinforcing)

174

- increasing engagement and activation is accomplished by providing in vivo
practice experiences with guidance provided to the parents on how to craft
graded hierarchies with associated plans. By design, these experiences are
not highly structured and more interactive (but the skills practiced in these
experiences can be transferred to the central goal), building in preparation to
challenging the most feared experience/situation
- with the increased skill, the child is ready to challenge the central goal with the
guided approximations provided by the guiding of the parents and successfully
accomplished with the positive reinforcement experienced at every step
- relapse prevention. The child is too young for this review, other than the
reinforcement of everything/skill they have been demonstrating. For the
parents, it is an opportunity for being prepared for monitoring, problem
solving what kinds of situations may pop up as a problem (so that they can
plan ahead how to help their child deal effectively with it). *The most common
issues, daycare/school, night-time, small animals, separation, social phobias
b. Psychoeducation and treatment rationale-educating parents about how a child's
behavior is associated to the reinforcing of their feelings of anxiety

Depression
DEPRESSION AND THE LINK BETWEEN ANXIETY AND DEPRESSION

There is a strong relationship between depression and anxiety. Children with both anxiety and
depression tend to be older versus the younger child. However, since there is a high prevalence of
anxiety disorders in childhood, it is important to acknowledge and be aware of its association to
depression. Just as important is that children who experience anxiety are more likely to experience
anxiety as adolescents and adults where the existence of co-morbid depression is increased.

Toddlers and young children can suffer from depression that is not recognized because they
are not able to understand or communicate their negative feelings. Additionally, while they
may display classic depressive symptoms (sad, withdrawn, lack of pleasure in activities, etc.),
symptoms may also be less detectable in the form of behavioral problems and acting out.
Therefore, diagnosing young children with depression can be difficult.

CASE EXAMPLE

Sunny, age 2½, is evaluated by her pediatrician during an appointment made by her mother
associated with concerns expressed by the mother's observed changes in her daughter.
Apparently, the parents had separated about 2 months ago following a period of escalated
conflict (domestic violence denied). Sunny has been withdrawn, not enjoying her normal
activities, more tearful than usual and acting out. The acrimony between her parents
continues and Sunny is not seeing her father on a regular basis, in fact, several visits were
cancelled because her parents got into a fight. Sunny has now started to cry when it is time to
go to her daycare-enrichment program.

Treatment
1. Sunny's pediatrician identifies that she is experiencing both anxiety and depression and
makes two referrals: a conjoint therapist and a pediatric mental health specialist
2. Sunny's therapist consults with the conjoint therapist regarding the impact of acrimony
in the marital relationship and Sunny's experience of feeling abandoned with her father
moving out. The following decisions are made to improve Sunny's feelings of security that
are determined to be the source of her depression and anxiety
   a. Daily routines to increase comfort and security. The parents have both been nurturing
   parents who engaged in activities with their daughter and as a family. They have
   been instructed, following problem solving with Sunny's therapist, how to maximize
   positive interaction approximating their normal routines with Sunny as much as
   possible while residing apart

175

    b. Predictable time with both parents. Parents were educated about childhood depression and anxiety. While their family patterns have changed, Sunny needs to feel secure about mommy time and daddy time

    c. Helping Sunny to deal with her feelings of fear, frustration and anger

    d. The therapist used art and puppets as a means for Sunny to express her emotions and help her to adjust

---

Goals

1. Evaluation by the pediatrician to rule out associated medical problems

2. Improve interpretation of experiences

3. Increase pleasant activities

4. Improve social skills

5. Improve self-control

6. Interpersonal development

7. Working through grief

Treatment Focus and Objectives

Some of the objectives may seem challenging to carry out in an age-appropriate manner. Be creative, patient, a good guide and, most of all, reinforce feeling good about learning and developing new ways of thinking and doing.

1. A referral is made to the pediatrician to rule out any medical influences and/or initiate their participation on the treatment team with identified intervention of medical management

    a. Recommend a brief assessment of parental depression and refer for intervention if necessary

2. Improve assessment and interpretation (negative thinking)

    a. Challenge irrational thinking with accurate and rational thinking

    b. Challenge helpless thinking by modeling and guiding the child through the options that they don't consider

    c. Identify how they view themselves and challenge it with positive reinforcement for efforts and accomplishment

    d. Help children to learn that every experience, regardless of how it turns out, offers the opportunity for learning, new information, choices for future experiences and skill development

3. Increase pleasant activities

    a. Increase positive reinforcement from the environment by increasing activity. Everyone feels better when they have things to look forward to that they enjoy. Increased participation is the way to increase skills and contributes to positive feelings

        i. make play dates

        ii. outdoor play with family and friends

        iii. making simple forts for creative play

        iv. participate in organized activities (could be school, church or community based)

        v. parent–child-based activities where a father–child or mother–child meet with other dyads for a specific activity or social routine

        vi. positive daily structure

    b. Monitor effort to elicit resources and guidance when necessary

4. Improve social skills using role modeling, role-play, books that focus on specific skills, and practice

    a. Increase rewarding interactions

    b. Increase and improve social skills

        i. initiating conversation

        ii. responding to others

      iii. appropriately refusing requests of others
      iv. making requests
      v. waiting their turn to talk
  c. Provide experiences for skill development. For example, a day at an amusement park with a friend offers a concentrated experience of waiting for a turn and taking turn, but it is fun and cooperativity and other positive social behaviors make it work successfully. The concept is similar to being a good family member or class member, everyone has a role
  d. Be sure to provide adequate feedback reinforcement
      i. if they are having a difficult time offer a reminder to facilitate calming or the use of another skill
  e. Requires patience and repetition
5. Improve self-control (emphasizes cognitive processes)
  a. Self-monitoring
      i. be clear about the goal and what it takes to reach the goal. When the basics are identified it makes it easy to see what is working and where help is needed. For the younger child, criteria could be identified during play therapy and symbolically self-monitored by using the object/figure that represents the child and monitoring how the object/figure feels and deals with situation. This helps the child increase self-awareness
      ii. learn to take responsibility for choices and associated consequences. Ask questions of what could be done next time or differently, etc. Using the symbolic object/figure, the child may initially be able to offer responses of good choices and process through to associated consequences
  b. Self-evaluation
      i. this skill allows a child to participate in setting a goal, determine what needs to be done to accomplish the goal and to "self-monitor" and evaluate their progress and skill level (what is working and what are they learning)
      ii. there may be times they need help or guidance and part of improving self-control is recognizing when additional resources are needed. Being helpless is not an option. Again, some aspects of self-evaluation can be accomplished directly (age appropriate) and/or from the use of a symbolic representation of the child that the child evaluates and role models meeting goals
      iii. a 5-point scale also has utility for rating skill acquisition and can be used to determine what the criteria are at each level, making it clear what they need help with or need to do differently to advance their goals
  c. Self-reinforcement
      i. a positive feedback loop associated with skill development is self-reinforcing. It feels good to be productive, to apply oneself and to do a good job. It is important to be able to evaluate accurately what one does and how they do it and feeling good about it. *Children internalize the responses of their caretakers. For example, picking up toys at the end of the day with a caregiver and being praised→getting older and being praised for picking up their toys→older child resisting picking up their room but it still feels good when it is done. *Good parenting is planned obsolescence
6. Improve interpersonal skills
  a. Interpersonal relationship skills
      i. learning to live the golden rule even when one doesn't get it in return. It is a difficult lesson learning that it feels good to do the right thing even when the right thing isn't done to you
      ii. learning when it is one's turn to talk or when it is important to be a listener
      iii. learning to share
        - asking to take a turn and sharing when someone else asks for a turn

- preparing a child for a social experience where they need to be prepared to share their possessions or other objects
- use a felt board/story board or other similar media which allows a child to see visually what will be happening so that they can prepare themselves
- reinforce their efforts and accomplishments

iv. learning to demonstrate caring and kindness
- role modeling and role playing caring behavior
- reading books about caring and sharing behaviors
- storyboard with examples of caring and sharing behaviors
- use a token economy for an hour. A child can be given a token for every caring and sharing behavior they demonstrate. This is a fun way to clarify skill level and reinforce efforts. At the end of the hour they can redeem their tokens

v. learning what it means to be interpersonally respectful

b. Social adjustment
  i. validating normal feelings associated with the experience of a variety of events
   - using a book or story board address a variety of challenging emotions associated with making adjustment or experiencing different events to demonstrate how the characters deal with challenging emotions. It will give a child additional coping choices
  ii. preparing for change can circumvent potential negative emotions. Change is a normal part of life. Young children watch to see how the adults in their life respond to change (they rely on those adults to give them guidance/modeling in how to deal with such changes)
   - use a story board/white board to demonstrate scheduling as an aid for adjustment. Pictures of the child involved in the activity schedule for the day is another fun way to prepare a young child for transitions
   - role play how to join in play with other children (walking up and asking "can I play too", "can I have a turn", etc.
   - offer a lot of practice
  iii. reinforce efforts and successes

c. Mastery of social roles
  i. young children demonstrate surprising flexibility in learning to respond differently in different environments. For example, some rules are different at school/day care than at home (one reason is that there are a lot more people), etc.
   - a fun activity is to create a story book of the child with pictures of them in their different roles. Identify what they do well (got it!), what they need to work on (getting there!), and how to go about mastering it (do they need reminders, a daily activity picture with the steps of each activity made clear)
   - a 5-point scale to rate behaviors in their different roles to signify 5=mastery, 1=needs help
  ii. reinforce their efforts and accomplishments. It helps the teacher when everyone follows the rules just like it helps mom when rules are followed. Children need to know that caregivers/adults are proud of their behavior and contributions. Always reinforce what works.

7. Processing grief and loss
   This is a particularly difficult issue. Talking to children about death/loss must be at their level. The range of reactions displayed by a young child could be emotional withdrawal, regressive behavior, acting out behaviors, repeatedly asking the same question

a. Helping young children to cope with grief
  i. caregivers need to allow young children to teach them about their grief experiences. Give children the opportunity to tell their story – be a good listener and a good observer

ii. don't assume that every child the same age understands death/loss in the same manner or with the same feelings. Children are individuals with their unique view of the world which is shaped by personal experiences

iii. allow adequate time for each child to grieve in the manner that works for them. Grieving is a process not an event. Expecting a child to resume their normal/regular activities without the opportunity to deal with their emotional confusion or pain may actually result in additional problems or negative reactions

iv. tell children the truth about what happens – using language and concepts that are age appropriate. Lies or half-truths deprive them of the real-life experiences that we all have to learn to cope with the normal challenges associated with skill development

v. encourage children to ask questions about death/loss. Caregivers don't need to be concerned about knowing all of the answers. Treat all questions and concerns with respect

vi. everyone grieves in their own way. Grieving is not an orderly and predictable process of the "correct" way. They may seem uncaring at times and exhibit grieving at times

vii. sometimes children are upset because they don't know the words to express what they are feeling and thinking. Let them know that the adults in their life want to understand
  - using books and movies (carefully selected) which deal with issues of loss can be a useful approach to opening dialogue and processing grief
  - if the loss is a family member or a pet, honoring them and time spent with them can be helpful for processing grief. Making a picture book, photo album or story about them can all be useful approaches for dealing with grief in a positive way

viii. grief is hard and children need long lasting and dependable support. The more losses a child suffers, the more difficult, complicated and protracted recovery can be. *Consistency is the key of so many issues when it comes to helping children
  - remain emotionally available and be a good listener
  - caregivers need to be authentic "some days I am sad too"

ix. caregivers need to be aware of their own need to grieve. Therefore, while it is important to focus on the needs of children, adults may need to get help for themselves. The caregiver that lacks effective self-care is likely not emotionally available to a child
  - there may be times when a child would benefit from a grief group for children. Generally, the foundation is processing grief through art and offers a normalizing of the grief experience in association with processing the loss

Attentional Problems ADD/ADHD

There appears to be a strong genetic predisposition to ADHD. Therefore, when a child is presented for treatment of an attentional disorder, the evaluation and, if necessary, the treatment of other family members should also take place. A comprehensive plan of intervention is required to address the functioning of the child in the family system along with the parent–child interactions. Additionally, ADHD seems to have a high rate of co-morbidity with other psychiatric disorders that may have different etiologies, which also highlights the importance of a thorough assessment.

CASE EXAMPLE

Tommy was referred at the age of 4 by his preschool teacher due to attentional difficulties. Developmental history revealed that as a baby he often cried for long periods of time, was not able to self-soothe, and needed to be held constantly. As he grew, his parents noticed that his activity level seemed much higher than that of his older brother and children his age. Aside from a delay in language development, all other developmental milestones were met appropriately. Tommy had a positive disposition, but his parents and his teacher were concerned about his ability to maintain attention, his high activity level, and impulsivity in "touching everything". He was clumsy and experienced numerous accidents, often engaging in unsafe behaviors. Tommy struggled a lot with transitions, moving from one task to another, such as transitioning from play to dinner. Regarding peer relationships, he had friends, but sometimes experienced difficulty interacting with them and playing what they wanted to play. His play behavior was better when he was doing what he wanted.

Treatment

1. Support the parents to encourage Tommy to figure things out for himself, being available for guidance and reinforcement of his efforts. Allow him to take pleasure in his accomplishments in the presence of his parents/teacher. His parents used a star chart at home to reinforce his completion of tasks and compliance. He was also instructed in problem solving: (1) ask himself "what is my problem?"; (2) think, think, think of some solutions: (3) what would happen? and (4) give it a try

2. Parents to engage him on a verbal level and back off on their physical proximity. Positive ways to highlight their connection could be through calling him on the play phone, using binoculars or a long cardboard tube to watch/check on him. When he feels the need he can respond in kind, thus allowing for healthy attachment–separation

3. Create a calming get away. His parents got a pop-up tent and filled it with soft pillows. This allowed Tommy to calm and regroup when the stimulation of interaction became overwhelming. He was reinforced for appropriately choosing quiet time for himself

4. To reinforce engagement and attention during play he was given materials that were highly visual and provided proprioceptive input

5. He was encouraged to express his difficulty with impulse control through play instead of becoming disruptive or impulsive in the course of daily routines. He increasingly became more self-directed and able to get back on focus when he became impulsive or accepting the redirection of his parents/teacher. His attention span and behaviors were improving

6. His interactive play with peers was improved by his mother scheduling brief and structured play dates with careful attention to preparing him for the transition and giving him a few choices of what he could take to the play date. While there she was clear regarding the relationship skills he needed to refine and created opportunities for him to practice. His mother always made sure to reinforce his positive behaviors and good choices

---

SIGNS AND SYMPTOMS OF ATTENTION DEFICIT OR NORMAL CHILD BEHAVIOR?

Likewise, as a result of similar symptoms observed in RSPD and attentional problems, a clear and correct diagnosis can at times be challenging. Some children have both RDSP and ADHD. However, if a child does soothing or stimulating activities that should be calming, and regardless, they are not able to calm down (such as providing deep pressure and heavy muscle movement and they can't calm down), and if they present with difficulties in ability to focus and pay attention (with the exception of hyperfocus as well as being situational) it is likely ADHD. The three primary characteristics of ADD/ADHD are inattention, hyperactivity, and impulsivity. The conundrum is that just because a child has symptoms of inattention, impulsivity, or hyperactivity does not mean that they have ADD or ADHD. Children with ADD/ADHD may be:

- Inattentive, but not hyperactive or impulsive
- Hyperactive and impulsive, but not able to pay attention
- Inattentive, hyperactive, and impulsive (*most common form of ADD/ADHD)

180

Additionally, observable symptoms which reinforce the attention deficit diagnosis:

- Cannot stop impulsive behavior regardless of sensory input
- Craves novelty and activity which is not necessarily related to specific sensations
- Does not become more organized after receiving intense sensory input
- Has difficulty waiting and taking turns
- Waits and takes turns better with cognitive input rather than sensory input
- Tends to talk all the time, impulsive interrupting, has trouble waiting for their turn in conversation

Before a diagnosis of ADD/ADHD diagnosis can be made, a mental health professional will explore and rule out the following possibilities:

- Learning disabilities (problems with reading, writing, motor skills, or language)
- Major life events or traumatic experiences (recent move, death of a loved one, divorce, bullying, any major change)
- Psychological disorders including anxiety, depression, and bipolar disorder
- Behavioral disorders (oppositional defiant disorder, explosive anger, etc.)
- Medical conditions (thyroid dysfunction, neurological conditions, epilepsy, sleep disorders, etc.)

DeGangi (2000; Barkley, 2000) espouses the complexity of attentional problems (whether associated with ADD/ADHD or RSPD) requires a comprehensive multifaceted treatment approach not only being multidisciplinary, but utilizing the integration of cognitive-behavioral, sensory integration, and dynamic interactional approaches. She further states that additional approaches that have been used include:

- Special education and tutoring to address learning needs
- Language therapy to improve auditory processing
- Sensory integration to address sensory problems that affect attention and activity level
- Sensory diet
- Visual training and eye desensitization to improve eye focus
- Auditory training to decrease hypersensitivities and improve auditory discrimination
- EMG biofeedback to inhibit excessive body movement
- Relaxation techniques for self-calming and body inhibition
- Homeopathic medicine
- Dietary supplements and dietary control of sugar intake

181

This creative individualized treatment approach is necessary to address and improve the negative impact to the challenging manifestations of inattention, hyperactivity, and impulsivity as well as other possible challenges, such as poor motor planning, low motivation, poor emotional regulation, and problems with sensory integration, language processing, and perceptual organization. Another point made clear by DeGangi is that children with an attention deficit diagnosis don't always present consistently or uniformly within diagnostic criteria. *Drawing upon DeGangi's conceptual framework, the presentation of sensory processing dysfunction is initiated, due to the interweaving of symptoms and challenges of children with ADD/ADHD, the information in this section is to be extrapolated into the RDSP section which follows (instead of duplicating it).*

Impaired sensory registration is a common difficulty impacting attentional abilities. Dr. DeGangi explains this in the following manner: "a pattern of overarousal is seen when there is difficulty filtering extraneous information. Accompanying this are orienting to irrelevant stimuli, distractibility, excessive motor activity, and a decreased attention span. In contrast, a pattern of underarousal may be manifested by (1) a high activity level associated with stimulus gathering behaviors, or (2) a low activity level with difficulty orienting and acting on novel stimuli. (2000, p. 242)". DeGangi (2000; Mulligan, 1996; Parush et al,

1997) reports that research indicates that it is not uncommon that children with ADHD demonstrate evidence of somatosensory dysfunction such as tactile defensiveness and developmental dyspraxia along with difficulties processing vestibular input. The following symptoms of sensory registration impairment that negatively effect attention are provided by DeGangi (2000), with minimal changes to wording in an effort to maintain the degree and specificity of information given in the outline:

1. Sensory overload in active environments (classrooms, playgrounds, shopping centers). The central nervous system integrates and processes information from the environment which is to be translated into a meaningful response. The child that does not struggle with sensory overload responds effectively.
   a. Sensory avoiders shun experiences and sensory seekers tend to go for the intense dare-devil experiences. Both children need their responses to be rechanneled. The avoidant child has trouble getting started and needs tools that allow them to get in sync by facilitating timing, body awareness and motor planning. They need simple choices that facilitate entry into interaction. The sensory seeking child's behavior may be unsafe/inappropriate. This child needs help to stop and interpret what is about to happen before jumping in, thus being guided into more appropriate behaviors. Various members of the treatment team provide the child with suitable alternatives. Guiding and redirecting a child into appropriate activities promotes sensory processing. A child is as old as they act, therefore, "developmental ability" is a central consideration in providing the aforementioned opportunities for growth and change. When observing a child (whether at home, school, or play), watch to see what it is that they like to do, build on their interests and instill a sense of control. When the child is facilitated toward behavior modification that is fun and satisfying behavior becomes self-reinforcing

2. Auditory hypersensitivities to particular sounds:
   a. High-pitched sounds such as a whistle or children squealing/laughing
   b. Low-frequency background noises (heater, appliance, etc.)
   c. Loud noises (vacuum, garbage disposal, toilet flushing, doorbell, etc.)
      i. The ability to understand sounds or the skill of auditory comprehension is acquired as vestibular sensations are processed. Gradually, as the child interacts purposefully with their environment, a child learns to interpret what they hear and to develop the complexity of sophisticated auditory processing skills. When interpreting sounds is the problem, the child benefits from speech and language therapy, occupational therapy-sensory integration, or other sensory integration based intervention. The goals of auditory integration therapy of sound stimulation is to improve listening and communication skills, learning capabilities, motor coordination, body awareness and self-esteem

3. Visual distractibility with difficulty screening out relevant from non-relevant visual stimuli and poor coordination of the eyes for focused work:
   a. Problems converging eyes in midline for near-point work
   b. Overwhelmed by competing visual stimuli
   c. Need for clear special cues such as encasing blocks of information on the blackboard with a boundary
      i. Vision is a highly complex process integrating information in combination with other senses (especially the vestibular sense) and prepares the child to make an appropriate and effective response. As the child matures and integrates information from other senses, visual-spatial skills evolve and are refined. When visual dysfunction is not identified, it can result in problems with reading, learning, physical, emotional, and social skills development. Visual training/visual therapy, occupational therapy-sensory integration may benefit basic eye movement or complex visual processing skills. Simple, but purposeful vision games with a

progression in complexity can be designed to aid the child in a reassuring manner as well as they may present with difficulties with transitions and separation. An example of an activity would be a daily calendar or schedule board which is a visual demonstration of daily events allowing them to see (visualize) the structure and progression of their day. Much like a class schedule which is broken down hour by hour, each block signifies a specific activity for the child (eating breakfast, brushing teeth, washing face, getting dressed, riding to school, playing with peers, class instruction, etc.). Daily activities must also build into the structure time for challenging transitions as well as predictable pleasurable moments

4. Tactile hypersensitivities to particular types of touch:
   a. Bumps/pushes other children when in close proximity and bothered by random touch of others (standing in line, sitting in cafeteria, sitting on bus)
   b. Complains about tags in clothing, can't tolerate some fabrics, only wants to wear certain types of clothing
   c. May dislike and complain about face washing and being hugged or patted/touched by unfamiliar persons
   d. May become upset with normal tactile input from the environment such as the feel of the chair when sitting on it
      i. The tactile sensory system is a key factor in determining mental, emotional, and physical behavior. Starting at birth, tactile stimulation is necessary to be organized, functioning, and to develop healthy relationships. The ability to process tactile stimulation is important to visual discrimination, motor planning, and body awareness, as well as for emotional security, social skills and academic learning. If a child suffers from tactile dysfunction, they will have problems with their ability to modulate, discriminate, coordinate, and/or organize tactile sensations in a meaningful, adaptive and effective manner

5. High/elevated need for proprioceptive input (weight, pressure, traction):
   a. Likes to pull/push on heavy objects (crash play trucks together)
   b. Likes to hang from jungle gym bars/banister, dangling off of furniture
   c. Likes to butt head into things
   d. Roughhousing activities (pillow fights, wrestling)
   e. Likes deep massage on their back
   f. *Take note: when a child is seeking these things, they tend to be more organizing
      i. Body position or the sensory messages about position, force/pressure, direction and movement of body parts is referred to as the proprioceptive sense. It aids in integrating vestibular and tactile sensory information. Proprioception functions to increase body awareness and plays a role in motor control and motor planning, thus being able to move body parts effectively and efficiently. Proprioceptive dysfunction results in a child being out of sync in the positioning and movement of the body, thus influencing a smooth gait, sprinting, climbing stairs, carrying objects, etc. Ultimately contributing awareness, alertness, and countering overresponsivity of other systems

6. High/elevated need for vestibular movement activities:
   a. Likes swinging high and fast for long periods of time
   b. Likes to move about, run, or to find opportunities to move on playground equipment
   c. Often gets up and leaves their desk at school on the premise to get something
   d. When seeking vestibular activities, it is important to evaluate whether the child is benefitting from the movement or energizing activity by doing it
      i. Balance and movement are referred to as the vestibular sense and is a unifying system. In other words, the vestibular sense is what imparts the sense of where one stands or the ability to orient themselves in their environment. Special receptors for movement and gravity reside in the inner ear. As a unifying system, it gathers messages associated with balance and movement from the positioning and

movement of the neck and body, and eyes telling the child where their head and body is in relation to the surface of the earth. Consider the significance. It informs the child if they are upright, upside down, not standing straight (bent over or tilted sideways), moving or static, the movement or motionless state of objects in relation to one's body. Additionally, it relays where one is going, how fast or slow, whether it is a relaxing place or if there is danger

7. Motor planning difficulties:
   a. Problems initiating and planning new movement activities
   b. Prefers repetition in movement games
   c. Needs physical assistance and verbal prompts to learn a new motor activity such as tying shoes, putting on a jacket or skipping
      i. while learning new skills, allow a child enough time to practice on their own, but don't allow them to get stuck and overwhelmed. Observe without hovering. If they are not making progress, simply state "would you like me to help you with that?" Also, during the course of observation, some recommendations may be made and practiced for the benefit of skill development.

Attentional deficits may be related to impaired information processing. Problems associated with accurately distinguishing stimuli or detecting sensory information may be the outcome of an inability to maintain attention. When a child lacks the ability to screen novel stimuli, effectively comprehend, and/or organize effective efficient responses, it is seen in their performance and impact to overall functioning. They don't finish activities, follow directions, pay adequate attention to detail, or give adequate attention when someone is speaking to them. In addition, there may be problems with executive functioning. This is particularly true of the child with ADHD and their behavioral inhibition, poor self-control.

In the treatment section, though there is separation of goals for interventions associated with parenting and for the school setting, much of the information in either section can be modified for either environment. Therefore, a duplication of information was not made.

Goals

1. Consultation and medication evaluation
2. Improve arousal and alerting for focused attention
3. Improve behavioral management
4. Improve social skills
5. Improve cognitive skills
6. Developing parenting skills
7. Enhancing school strategies

Treatment Focus and Objectives

1. Medication evaluation is determined by pediatrician, psychiatrist, or a consulting psychologist specializing in evaluating and making such a recommendation
2. Improved focus attention
   a. Environmental modifications: it is important to make sure that children understand what the expectations are. Doing so indicates "we are a team" and everyone on the team is expected to help reach the goals whether it is a classroom task or family system (Figure 3.9). Respect and responsibility are key to positive and effective systems functioning
      i. organize all material and toys into bins or cubbies
      ii. limit the number of toys or objects to manipulate per setting
      iii. routine of putting toys, objects away at close of playtime
      iv. recycle toys every couple of weeks to retain novel experience and, therefore, maintain focus

   v. utilize enclosed spaces such as a pop-up
   tent or large cardboard box filled with soft
   blankets and pillows (take allergies into
   consideration when choosing materials)

   vi. create and encourage seating along the wall
   or in the corner of the room (home and
   classroom)

   vii. decrease distraction at a desk by constructing a
   cubicle of cardboard

   viii. make available a bean bag chair for reading

   ix. seat the disorganized, distracted child by an
   organized child who role models positive and
   effective cues

b. Productive playtime

   i. a variety of activities meets physical needs,
   provide rules, interaction and repetition for skills development (soccer, karate, wall
   climbing, wrestling, horseback riding, tactile games, etc.). Shop at an educational
   store where a wide variety of resources are available and find additional creative
   ideas

   ii. encourage movement on swings and other playground equipment in the
   afternoon

   iii. schedule play dates with specific activities such as bowling, miniature golf, treasure
   hunts, etc.

   iv. evening is a cue to decrease activity level and provide calming activities such as
   reading, being held and rocked, self-rocking, etc.

c. Auditory stimuli

   i. soothing music (chants, Mozart, female vocalist, etc.)

   ii. nature sounds (rainfall, waterfall, bird sounds, etc.)

   iii. use of ear buds, or headsets to buffer from environmental sounds

   iv. the use of carpeting is a consideration for decreasing environmental noise

d. Visual stimuli

   i. increase attention to visual information by highlighting with bright/bold colors
   and outline the perimeter with an outline

   ii. maintain organization for objects

   iii. at school, it is recommended that homework assignments and other important
   pieces of information be printed or listed in a box on the blackboard

e. Arousal versus calming states

   i. observe the child to determine at what time during the day that they demonstrate
   their highest alert state. During this time, plan tasks that involve quiet
   concentration to support academic development

   ii. for children who are always on the move, harness their arousal level by giving
   them a task to help or a "job" to provide goal directed movement activity as well
   as providing social and emotional reinforcement

   iii. prior to the onset of a focused cognitive activity, engage in activity highlighting
   body organization for a period of 5 minutes

   - interesting squeeze toys where squeezing creates interesting patterns or
     eye pop out, therapy putty, etc. *Often, the child with ADHD can do this
     simultaneously while completing academic tasks
   - bury hands or feet in a bin of dried beans
   - snack of crunchy hard foods (apple slices, carrot sticks, pretzels, rice-cakes, etc)

   iv. evening wind-down cues/routine

   - warm bath or shower
   - back massage and pressure to palms (particularly the web space of thumb)

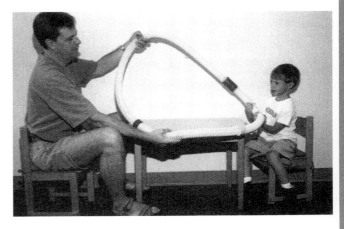

FIGURE 3.9
This father is helping
organize his child's
attention in a game
where they try to move
the steel ball inside the
large tubing.

185

- rocking (linear, forward–back) while participating in a visual focusing task like reading, looking at pictures or listening to soothing repetitious music
- it may feel safe and calming for a child to lie under a heavy quilt or snuggle up in a sleeping bag

 v. create a cozy corner in a room for a child to seek out for calming. It could be a small pop-up tent, a sheet over a small card table, or a large cardboard box. Whatever it is, line with soft blankets and pillows (consider allergies when choosing materials)

 vi. for increasing the child's awareness of his internal drive state associated with activity level, ask them to identify what level their engine is running at "high, medium, low". Given the child's response, direct their activity to get their engine running at the desired running level (this is a good barometer to use for any desired activity level, i.e. work, play, homework and how to best guide the structure to help program the child's success)

 vii. to facilitate and reinforce the child's objectivity in identifying their own states, label for them when they are intense or calm and focused. For example, "your engine is running at the right speed for….". Also a 5-point rating scale can be creatively adapted

*The occupational therapy use of sensory integration therapy approaches work quite well for some children in dealing with the arousal associated needs of attention

 f. Interactive metronome (IM). Computer-generated programming (i.e., beats through a set of headphones) guides the child (or adult) to perform different repetitive exercises that are measured through the hand and foot sensors. After each movement is completed, the computer attached to the sensor assesses the accuracy with which the user performs each exercise. The accuracy is essentially the difference between the metronome beat and the individual's response. The goal is to lower the amount of time of this difference. IM improves motor planning and sequencing so that a child can carry out a multistep process. As timing improves sequencing improves. Additionally, IM improves coordination, motor skills and attention span. Therefore, IM would appear to be beneficial for any attentional problem, distractibility and motor coordination

3. Improve self-control, sustained attention, and self-monitoring. It is important to ensure that the behavioral intervention plan be based upon a careful functional assessment of behavior. Antecedents and consequences of both the problem and replacement behaviors need to be studied. Antecedents indicate environmental changes that set the child up for success or failure. Consequences will identify the environmental contingencies that reinforce both desired and undesired behavior. The goal of the intervention is to shape, change and reinforce desired behavior.

 a. Floor-time activities

  i. to facilitate self-organization (versus free time play where they may be lost), it is recommended that caregivers structure 20–30 minutes/day to engage in play with the child. During this "special time" the child is encouraged to choose something they would like to do and the caregiver joins in with them

  ii. play should be both fun and interactive. Caregivers are not to structure or direct unless it is necessary to initiate the activity or at any point in the activity to maintain the activity. *Pleasure is an important motivating factor

  iii. steer away from the structure of board games. If the child likes board games create other times, such as a family night to play board games

  iv. maintain the caregiver–child connection. This means that if the child gets up and leaves, the caregiver can ask them to come back as soon as they disengage and inquire as to what they are doing, and if necessary gently redirect. The caregiver needs to keep the caregiver–child connection and, if necessary, keep the activity and the interest engaging. If the child is confused or lost about how to participate in the activity, the caregiver may role model or take turns to facilitate the child's skill development or repertoire of responses

b. Behavioral intervention

    i. identify triggers and use prevention strategies to soften them

- anticipate and cue
- use visuals. Photograph schedules give a child a clear sense of time and routine. Mini schedules allow for predictability with individual activities within the daily schedule. Activity task sequences represents steps within an activity
- prompt/cue children
- state clear and simple expectations. When redirecting, let a child know what you want to see. Say "quiet voice" instead of "no yelling". Visual cues can be used to communicate clear expectations
- signal and warn
- use "first-then" statements. Combine statements with visual if child needs visual support. "First clean up, then go outside to play"
- use proximity
- offer choices. Ask the child what they want to do. Choice is a powerful learning tool
- encourage/praise
- embed preference
- adjust length of activity. Extend activities that the child is actively engaged in when possible. Move on to a new activity when it isn't working. Follow the child's lead
- modify materials
- use timers
- model
- allow for flexibility

    ii. positive reinforcement: focusing on what is right. It is important to give much encouragement, praise and affection as these children are easily discouraged. It is important to keep in mind that rewards used with these children lose their reinforcing power quickly and must be changed or rotated frequently

    iii. time out: removing the student from positive reinforcement, or time out, generally involves removing a child from a classroom. Time out can be effective in decreasing aggression and disruptive actions in the classroom (especially when the behaviors are reinforced by peer attention). Time out should not be over used and the time frame should be brief, ended based upon the child's attitude. When it is over, there needs to be a discussion on what went wrong and how to prevent a repeat of the problem. It is recommended that time out be used only with the most disruptive classroom behaviors

    iv. response cost: this is a behavioral tool which provides mild punishment when problem behavior is displayed. A child may lose earned points or privileges when previously specified rules are broken. A response cost program may decrease impulsivity. A specific response cost program involves giving a specific number of points at the start of each day. When a rule is broken (problem behavior), points are taken away. Therefore, to maintain their points the child must avoid breaking the rule. At the end of the day, the child is generally allowed to exchange the points they have earned for a tangible reward or privilege

    v. token economy systems: these systems generally involve giving a child tokens (like poker chips) when they display appropriate behavior. These tokens are then exchanged for tangible rewards or privileges at specified times. *It is critical that a token economy be set up with the individual goals in mind. An economy based on a reward at the end of the day may be too delayed for a child with ADHD

   vi. daily report cards/star charts etc.
   vii. natural consequences are an alternative to discipline. They are the actions or responses following a child's inappropriate behavior that serve to discourage the child from engaging in that behavior again
   - implementing logical consequences
   - discuss logical consequences with the child before implementation
   - only select options you are willing to enforce
   - presented to the child as a choice
   - be sure the child understands the options and can choose (i.e., clean up or no outdoor play)
   - don't help the child by intervening before the consequence takes place
   - behavioral options logically link current activity to resulting action. They should not be threatening

c. Task duration: in order to accommodate short attention span, classroom assignments should be brief with feedback being given as quickly as possible. If a project is longer, it is recommended that it be broken down into manageable parts. Be specific about short time limits for task completion, this can be reinforced with a timer

d. Direct instruction: attention to task is improved when the child is engaged in teacher-directed activities versus independent seat work. As a child gets older they can be taught skills such as note taking to increase the benefit of direct instruction. Comprehension and on-task behavior improve with the development of these skills

e. Tutoring: tutoring provides many of the instructional factors that program the child for learning/academic success. It offers frequent and immediate feedback. When combined with a token economy, tutoring can offer significant learning/academic gains

f. Scheduling: on-task behaviors for the child with ADHD generally worsens as the day wears on. Therefore, it is suggested that the academic block take place early in the day/morning. Plan that the afternoon be structured with more active, non-academic activities

g. Novelty: presentation of novel/interesting material will be motivating, thus improving attention. Increase novelty and level of interest in tasks by increasing stimulation through color, shapes, textures, etc. This also decreases the undesired activity level, enhances attention and improves overall performance

h. Structure and organization: lessons are structured and important points clearly identified (and when possible reinforced). Performance and memory/retention are improved when material is meaningfully structured

i. Rule reminders and visual cues: rules are to be clear, well defined, specific and frequently reinforced. Well-defined rules and clear consequences are fundamental. Visual reminders/cues should be placed throughout the classroom. There is also benefit in reviewing the rules before making the transition to a new activity and following breaks/recess. A token economy system is an effective tool when the rules for programming are reviewed daily

j. Auditory cues: it is beneficial to offer auditory cues that prompt appropriate/desired classroom behavior

k. Pacing of work/task: it can be beneficial at times to allow a child to set their own pace for task completion. Sometimes, the intensity of problematic behaviors is decreased when work is self-paced versus work being paced by others

l. Productive physical movement: the child with ADHD has difficulty staying in their seat. Therefore, productive physical movement should be planned. There should be time allowed for controlled movement and to develop a classroom routine of physical activities such as intervals where everyone stretches. Other examples include such tasks as watering class plants, sharpening a pencil, feeding classroom pets, taking a note to the principal's office or to another teacher, even standing at their desk while they complete their work. It is also a benefit to alter seat-work activity with other activities to break it up and allow for movement. The educator needs to be flexible to make modifications because some days will be more difficult than others to stay in their seats

m. Active versus passive involvement: it is essential to be creative in providing productive physical movement, i.e. tasks requiring active responses to channel disruptive behavior into constructive responses

n. Distractions: when a child has difficulty paying attention, it is important to minimize desirable alternatives to the desired task. For example, distractions like mobiles, aquarium and an activity center should not be in the child's field of vision

o. Anticipation: it is important to prepare for anticipated challenges of the ADHD child. This allows for appropriate accommodations to be made. When an educator is presenting a task that they think might exceed the child's capacity to attend, it is appropriate to decrease assignment length and focus on quality versus quantity

p. External reinforcement: a cornerstone of understanding the child with ADHD is that contingencies and consequences need to be delivered immediately and frequently. It is also likely that the magnitude of consequences will be higher than for the child without ADHD in the class. These children benefit from external criteria for success and need reinforcement for increased performance. Intangible rewards are not enough. It is important generously to offer praise, encouragement and affection as incentives to reinforce desired behavior. Additionally, when negative consequences are given, it should be done in a manner as not to embarrass or humiliate a child. *For the ADHD child rewards lose their effectiveness or reinforcing power fairly quickly and must be changed or rotated regularly

q. Problem solving: instruct the child
   i. ask yourself, "what's my problem?"
   ii. think, think, think of some solutions (choices for dealing with the situation)
   iii. ask, "what would happen?"
   iv. give it a try

4. Social skills development
   a. Scheduling regular play dates with peers to develop organizing attention and appropriate play in a child-centered setting. No competitive games at play dates
      i. teach skills that lead to friendships. Sharing, giving compliments, taking turns, helping others, organizing play ("let's build...", "let's play tag")
         - provide toys/activities that promote cooperation
         - give attention and time to children who engage in friendship
         - model and role-play friendship skills
      ii. play dates should at first be brief and structured. The types of behaviors to be promoted and reinforced that are important for successful peer interaction include the following:
         - getting a friend's attention: "Gage let's go play on the swings"
         - sharing objects/toys: "Armondo, here is one of the cars"
         - asking a peer to share an object/toy: "Kelly, can I have a crayon?"
         - providing a play idea to a peer: "Justine, let's build a sandcastle"
         - saying something nice to a friend-giving a compliment: "thanks for the gluestick", "I like your new shoes"
      iii. prepare, with the child, ahead of time what they will take to the play date that they are willing to share with a friend
      iv. hands-on play requiring materials should offer plenty of materials for each child
      v. provide simple foods that the children can prepare together (prepared cookie dough, microwave popcorn, etc.) so that they can have a snack while listening to a story being read, etc.
      vi. be the safe base – introducing the child to others while in the safety of the parents' arm or holding their hand (and keeping them close). The child will observe positive non-verbal cues

     vii. pair a slow to warm up child with a more outgoing child (but who will not over stimulate them). This will facilitate an increased feeling of comfort with the one child and is likely to generalize to a larger group of children

     viii. provide numerous opportunities for social interaction like going to a park with a lot of other children, or to the library, community events for children, etc. Each environment provides an opportunity to practice skills (some repetitious and some unique to the specific environment)

     ix. be prepared to intervene when help is needed to resolve conflict, prevent escalation of an argument, or soothe emotional distress. If they get too excitable, direct and encourage them to express it in socially-appropriate ways – keeping in mind the freedom of one ends where another begins
- if a child needs to be pulled away for calming, use the concept of the anger thermometer or 5-point scale to have them identify the level of their challenging emotion so that they can decide on what self-calming skills to use, if they need support calming and if there are other problems to solve (like taking turns or waiting)
- these challenging situations are a great opportunity for learning about the golden rule (treating others as one would like to be treated themselves) or "thinking about you thinking about me"

b. Social skills group

  i. teach problem-resolution skills such as appropriate play behaviors and developing repertoires of appropriate play outside of group

  ii. talk about the golden rule and solicit examples of it from the child. This is an important step in facilitating the understanding that other people have different perspectives from their own. The concept behind "thinking about you thinking about me" helps a child to understand the validity of their own experience has to be worked out (resolved) in the context including the experience of another

  iii. read stories which reinforce empathy and social awareness

c. Problem-solving family meetings

  i. a family member can address something that happened to them and what they did

  ii. they can request feedback from other family members about whether what they did was right or if there are other suggestions

  iii. the goal is to highlight to the child with ADD/ADHD that everyone has things to work on (a self-responsibility concept)

d. Dealing with specific behaviors

  i. wanting what someone else has. Prevent the problem: (1) provide multiples of the same object/activities that have a high child preference; (2) use a timer to indicate turns; (3) anticipate the child's preference and cue them to ask/gesture to join in play (can I play? my turn); (4) use first-then cue "first ask, then play"; (5) use a "my turn" visual cue chart for highly preferred objects/activities. Intervening: (1) remind the child to ask/gesture to play; (2) remind the child to ask/gesture for a turn; (3) offer an alternative object/activity; (4) remind a child when their turn is on or off

  ii. difficulty waiting for their turn. Prevent the problem: (1) use a timer to indicate turns (better if it is one that indicates time passing in a visual manner); (2) use a "my turn" visual cue chart where a child puts a photo with their name on the chart when it's the child's turn; (3) provide alternative choices that are of high interest, create and play outside choice board available; (4) use the turtle technique with visuals and puppet to discuss and model "anger control" when waiting for their turn throughout the day. The turtle technique: recognize feelings of anger, think "stop", go inside "shell", and take 3 deep breaths, think calm, think of a solution; (5) encourage when uses/attempts to use new skill in place of challenging behavior. Intervening: (1) remind the child to wait by showing "my turn" visual cue and offer alternative choices; (2) remind the child that when the timer goes off then it is their turn and cue to watch the timer

    iii. child doesn't want to leave the activity and get in line to go outside. Prevent the problem: (1) give the child transition signal (2 more times, 5 more minutes, 3 more turns then it is time to get in line); (2) cue class to line up by removing class visual of "line up" off of the visual schedule, then go over directly to cue child using the picture; (3) say to the child "let's look at the schedule to see when we will play _____ again." Then ask the child "do you want to put _____ away by yourself, or do you want help?" Help the child if needed and say, "I know this is fun, you can play it again_____"; (4) use visual schedule showing the child what activity is coming next; (5) give the child a special job to do during the transition or in the next activity (holding the door, line leader etc.). Intervene: (1) verbally/visually re-cue with "first-then" statements (first line-up, then outside); (2) state "all done play" while repeating class cue, "do you need help, or can you line up on your own?" Help child if needed, and immediately praise; (3) validate feelings ("I see you are mad") and remind with visual schedule when the child can do the activity they were doing again; (4) teach the child how to line up/imitate peers

    iv. child doesn't want to clean up after an activity. Prevent the problem: (1) give the transition signal (2 more times, 5 more minutes, 3 more turns then it is time to clean-up); (2) cue class to clean up (clean up song, bells, light off) then go directly to the child to cue; (3) turn-take cleaning up with the child (first I put these blocks away and then you put those blocks away…), add the visual cue by pointing where to put the blocks away; (4) praise children that are cleaning up; (5) use verbal and visual, "first clean up, then (choice of preferred object/activity)". Intervene: teach skills of the clean-up process

    v. child doesn't know what to do with the items at the activity center. Prevent the problem: (1) pair the child with a peer who knows what to do at the activity center to serve as a model; (2) provide a visual choice board, and limit the number of toys to teach play schemes (new toys and activities can be overwhelming); (3) join the child at the center and, in a brief, fun way, teach play using features that the child prefers (music, light, favorite color, textures, favorite character, etc.); (4) choose a preferred item to teach new play schemes; (5) cue the child to look at how their peer (they were paired with) is playing; (6) praise for playing and using the new scheme/skill "you're doing it!"; (7) help the child finish play by putting each toy/object away in its space. Intervene: (1) provide a visual choice board of a limited number of toys/objects to play with; (2) help the child learn to play by using least-to-most prompting (verbal, gesture, physical assist) to teach play scheme/skill; (3) prompt the child to ask/gesture for help; (4) if beginning to fidget, say "one more, then all done"

*Choice charts/boards allow for children to have opportunities for socially appropriate power and control. Give choices at every possible opportunity. When making a choice chart start with one item at a time. Examples of choice charts:

- songs
- activity choices
- toy choices
- food/drinks
- places
- clothing/shoes

e. Self-control (self-discipline). Self-control means being able to express and cope with challenging emotions in appropriate ways. For example, being able to say "I am mad at you" instead of biting or hitting. Using a 5-point scale to identify intensity of emotion is a good starting place for defining the right choice(s) for managing the challenging emotional state versus acting out. It should also be made clear to a child if they are starting to get overwhelmed and struggling to cope to engage in calming strategies or seek the help and support of a caring adult

    i. facilitate self-soothing. The calmer the child can respond the higher the degree of self-control. There is quite a range of soothing techniques/skills. Sometimes physical (rocking, hugging) contact and soothing are necessary, or removing themselves from overstimulation. Give them adequate time to calm down. Afterwards, they can use the experience not only to reinforce the benefit of their effort but to identify if there are other methods of self-calming that would be helpful

    ii. empathize with the child. Let them know you understand what they are experiencing. They may be being offered choices they don't want (an activity they don't like, visiting a place they don't want to go, etc.). Ask them if they can do it themselves or they need help to do it

    iii. Teach acceptable behavior. Give the child option "what they can do". This helps them to learn right from wrong and to channel energy and interests in acceptable ways

    iv. provide opportunity for choices. Giving children the opportunity to choose lets them know you trust them to make good choices. It also helps them to feel in control. If necessary offer gentle guidance, reinforcing their choice or building upon it or redirecting

    v. help them to develop a "feelings" vocabulary. Learning to identify and label feelings helps them to calm down and be in control. This doesn't mean giving in to demands. Instead offer choices, "we can read a book, or put a puzzle together…"

    vi. help the child learn to wait. This teaches them self-control and that others have needs too. Much of what we do is a cooperative effort, therefore, there are times we have to wait

    vii. play time. Playing with friends offers many opportunities to help a child practice many skills such as sharing, waiting your turn and having to wait

    viii. dealing with anger. Teach the turtle technique: recognize feelings of anger, "stop", go inside "shell" and take 3 deep breaths, think calm, think of a solution, try it. There is also the anger thermometer or the 5-point scale to slow things down, identify intensity of emotion and problem solve

    ix. provide opportunities for practice. There are numerous daily moments for teaching new skills. Be thoughtful in creating the opportunities to practice waiting, taking a turn, dealing with making an undesirable choice. Praise and reinforce their efforts

5. Cognitive activities

  a. Teach self-talk skills, "your inside voice" or "voice in your head". This is initiated by offering a narration what the child is doing, and then asking the child to reflect or talk through the steps of the task

  b. Observe and determine the child's learning style and try to magnify their best way of learning (multisensory, visual, auditory). Be creative

  c. Teach visualization skills

    i. use this with motor skills, i.e., picture the ball flying over and hitting the basket. Then have the child do it

    ii. show a child the finished product of an activity and then say, "now I will show you how to make it"

  d. Give instructions in an attention getting manner

  e. Teach focusing and organizational skills

    i. use pictures or photographs to depict the sequence or steps to take place

    ii. actually draw out what should take place as instructions are given

    iii. use "check-ins" either with parent or teacher at specific junctures to reinforce completion of each step. One way of doing this is to chart explicitly the steps from beginning to end

f. Provide immediate feedback to reinforce what is right. These children get so many negative responses from their environment be sure to seize the moment to reinforce positives

g. Teach sequences in everyday activities

  i. give simple chores to complete and reinforce. (This can be done with verbal praise, stars on a chart, etc.)

  ii. utilize a picture board of activities for the day. This additionally offers a form of self-monitoring whereby the child can check off the activities as they happen or use the board as a reference

  iii. provide the child with toys that have a concrete beginning and end

h. Use consistent rules, routines, and transitions to insure frame of organization and predictability. Parents can work on flexibility and spontaneity in interactional play, or making subtle changes when carrying out routines

6. Developing parenting skills

  a. Educate caregivers about ADD/ADHD. The symptoms and impairment may change throughout the child's life and development. Discuss the effect of ADD/ADHD on learning, behavior, social skills, family function, and effects on daily life. Discuss treatment options and side effects (if medication is chosen). Periodically review the child's and family's functioning, problem solving and/or offering new child/family system skills as needed. Offer to connect child/family to pertinent community resources and national organizations

  b. Teach parents how to help their child improve function instead of pointing out dissatisfying behaviors

  c. Attention deficit runs in families, and many parents of affected children had difficult school experiences themselves. Explore with them how they dealt with their experiences as a child, in their family, and at school. This process may shed important light on their interpretation of their child's behavior

  d. Provide updated information to the parents as these developmental stages approach to provide information and associated tools to help them face new challenges and anticipate and prepare for the future developmentally related issues

  e. Self-control strategies

  i. exercise can help burn off excess energy. Steer the child toward organized sports (soccer, t-ball when old enough), martial arts, tumbling class, running games, etc. Consider the child's need to be in constant motion, and then the added benefit of sports which require mental discipline

  ii. nature time such as playing in the park, going for nature walks and exploring plants and bugs. It is interesting and relaxing

  iii. nutrition is so important. Educate their palate to enjoy good food. This will help them to make the connection between eating well and doing well

  iv. social and emotional intelligence. Teach the child to read the cues other people are trying to give them. How to read faces, listen to words, what behavior means, etc. Role playing is reinforcing for skill development. Teach them how to listen and speak less

  v. teach self-management of anger. Teach the turtle technique: recognize feelings of anger, think "stop", go inside "shell" and take 3 deep breaths, think calm, think of a solution

  vi. support groups may be available for parents and children to address their issues and skill development

  f. Ideas for parent management of challenging behavior

  i. keep expectations realistic. It is only fair to a child that the parents know and understand their abilities and limitations. If expectations are too high or too low it can result in problems and frustrations for both parent(s) and child

  ii. plan ahead in an effort to anticipate what a child may need in a variety of situations. It is the programming of successes. It is key always to have a back-up plan and be flexible

193

iii. clearly state expectations in advance. As challenging as it is, some undesirable behaviors are the result of the child just not wanting to act differently, but other times they simply can't act differently (lack of ability and limitations). Be clear and consistent in communicating instructions to the child

iv. offer limited, reasonable choices. This helps the child to learn how to make decisions and develop the internal compass of what is okay and what is not. It is an important step in learning to take personal responsibility. They will need not only a lot of support, but a lot of practice and reinforcement as well. It is important to offer an abundance of support, practice and reinforcement

v. use "first…then…" statements. This is a simple and direct instruction to a child that clearly tells them what they must do to earn a desired outcome. This is also known as a contingency statement. A contingency statement should
  - give a positive frame and focus
  - be stated only once
  - set a reasonable time limit
  - follow through for reinforcement
  - be flexible and prepared for the child's response – even their refusal to comply

vi. catch the child being good. Instead of focusing so much on correcting what the child doesn't do right. Instead give specific, positive attention to the desired behavior and effort. This teaches the child what a parent wants them to do and increases the possibility that the desired behavior will occur repeatedly

vii. stay calm. When the child's behavior is unacceptable, a parent can respond to it or ignore it. *The least response necessary is best. Responding in a calm manner with a minimum of attention will decrease the risk of strengthening the undesired behavior (i.e., they don't get environmental reinforcement for it). A parent remaining calm affords the child time to think about what has happened and what is desired of them. The calmer the parent the more in control the child. A parent's calm response is also good role modeling for learning appropriate ways to respond to difficult situations

viii. use neutral time. Neutral time exists when everyone in the family system is calm enough to think, talk and listen. Neutral time can occur either before or after undesirable behavior occurs. That is the time to talk about what has happened and positive ways that the problem can be managed in the future. Parents should practice identifying neutral time so that these opportunities can be created

g. Promoting social-emotional development. It is the development of the capacity to experience and regulate emotions, form secure relationships, and explore them in the context of family

i. provide responsive care. This requires observing what the child is doing. Observing involves looking at what the child is doing, listening to what they are saying, and learning about their individual way of approaching the world. Taking time to sit with the child and observing these factors can teach a parent a lot. These clues allow parents to make better hypotheses about why a child does what he does, and to respond in a manner that is productive and supports their development

ii. be affectionate and nurturing. There are so many sweet moments to be shared with a child. Whether it is a fun bath time, snuggling, telling them how special they are and seeing them filled with joy – it can fill one's heart for a lifetime. The limitless array of similar interactions provides the kind of stimulation a developing child needs. Loving touches and encouraging words send messages to a child that they are someone special

iii. help the child learn to resolve conflicts in a healthy, appropriate way. Think of the classic 2 year old and all of the struggles they have with sharing, management of emotion, wanting to do it themselves, etc. This is the time when they are beginning to develop a sense of self, and have a hard time keeping themselves from acting on their impulses. The ability of self-control comes with time, brain maturation, practice, and the encouragement and support of caring and loving adults. By helping young children identify/name their feelings, and letting them see and practice ways to control their impulses, they learn over time how to do it themselves. This helps them learn how to resolve conflicts on their own. Let them explore what they are capable of doing and that a loving parent is there to give them support

h. Help the child to learn the joy and pleasure found in the "give and take" of relationships. Again, think of all of those sweet moments shared between a parent and young child. They are in love. Gazing into one another's eyes and the sharing of loving touch and loving words. This results in a child learning that others care about them, and what they need. This results in the beginning of the child understanding that their actions affect other people's feelings and actions. When a parent enjoys play with a child they learn that satisfying relationships feel good, building healthy relationships, and feeling good when they make other people happy. This is the fertile ground of the sharing and the concept of "give and take" that prepares them to go out into the world and recognize their own feelings and to care about the feelings of others too

i. Facilitating feelings of being safe. When a child has a reaction to a negative experience and the parent is there to protect, validate and offer solutions for dealing with a situation the child feels safe because a caring parent is there to support and protect them

j. Facilitating the development of frustration tolerance
   i. help children learn to wait by engaging with them about what you are doing. In other words, while they wait the parent talks to them about what they are doing and when they will be available to focus on them. "I am dressing the baby right now, and when I am done I will help you, I am almost finished, thank you for helping me"
   ii. help children cope with frustration. When they have a melt down, validate them for the difficult time they are having. "I know it is hard". Coach them through reinforcing what they were doing right and to keep persisting because they were almost there, etc. When coaching, it is fine to offer a suggestion or to offer a demonstration. Thus, help them think through a problem to the solution without taking over and doing it for them
   iii. join them in their activities/play and use humor. Humor is a good tension reducer – it can be not only appropriate but useful to be silly at times. Just because a child is persistent and occupies themselves in an activity does not mean that they do not benefit from a parent's time and attention. A parent should demonstrate their interest
   iv. be emotionally available and willing to help. This actually goes hand in hand with the positive feedback a child is given for working independently. Make sure they understand that it is okay to ask for help when they have persisted and need support and guidance – we all do from time to time. Knowing when to seek a resource is an important skill. Of course, asking for help/support should only take place after a child has made an earnest effort
   v. be creative, seizing the moment for fun and challenging activities. Making life interesting supports and encourages children to build and expand their skills. Give a young child different sizes of blocks and ask them to build a skyscraper/tall building

k. Helping a child deal with emotional intensity and reactivity
   i. be creative by conjuring up interactive games such as rolling a ball back and forth, playing with a Velcro ball and matching mitt, etc. Interactive play is about taking turns which keeps a child engaged
   ii. keep and maintain their attention. Sharing the stage as entertainers is a lot of fun for young children, singing together, dancing together, playing with puppets, rough housing

195

      iii. utilize soothing music and modify lighting to set the stage for a fun activity, but to keep it from being too stimulating. A dimmer switch is a useful tool. Offer several sensory choices as well like finger painting or playing with play dough

      iv. be emotionally available and nurturing. When a child is distressed offer them physical comfort such as holding close, massaging their back, rocking them. Verbally validate their experience of stress, "I know it is hard for you...". This is also an opportunity to help them see the different ways they can express their difficult emotions

      v. teach the turtle technique: recognize feeling of anger, think "stop", go inside "shell" and take 3 deep breaths, think calm, think of a solution, try it

      vi. use a 5-point scale or emotion intensity thermometer to identify emotional intensity. There could be pre-established choices for management at each level of intensity

l. Dealing with a low or high level of activity

      i. accept their pace of activity and interests and make available to them numerous choices of activities to choose from that they enjoy and promotes dexterity, interest, and skill development

      ii. incorporate movement in activities that they already enjoy. For example, children singing/dancing CDs, take turns singing or watching the other in creative dance or do it together, etc.

      iii. offer numerous opportunities for safe and active exploring of their world. Make an obstacle course, use an expanding tunnel to crawl through, play hide and seek, freeze tag, Simon says, etc. Expand this as a tool for increasing skills as a helpful family member. For instance, helping pack for the picnic (as instructed), setting or cleaning the table, etc.

      iv. don't expect a child to lay down/incline or sit for too long. Just because it seems easier to the parent to position the child, there are times when being sensitive to their need versus stretching their tolerance is beneficial to them

      v. free time. While appropriate structure is important, it is also important for children to not be overscheduled. What almost every child wants is for their parents to spend more time with them playing what they want to do

m. Facilitate skill development of learning to deal with change

      i. ease the anxiety of transitions by using familiar objects to maintain a feeling of security. It can also be helpful to allow them some control over how a transition is made, "would you like to play for 5 more minutes before we go?"

      ii. aid adjustment to transitioning into new activities. One way to do this is to talk about the steps of change that we are going to be engaging in, thus allowing a child to become comfortable about change or an activity coming to an end

      iii. offer a variety of experiences. The variety maintains interest and practice that feel fun and positive for developing the desire of new activities, talking about them and looking forward to them

      iv. just because a child adapts and adjusts easily doesn't mean it should be taken for granted. Be emotionally available to offer support when they experience stress in making a transition or doing something new for the first time

      v. carefully observe to prevent overstimulation. Help and support as needed

n. Dealing with defiance (after validating your child's feeling, if appropriate)

      i. set appropriate limits, be brief, clear, and direct, "It is time for dinner now, come to the table and sit down"

      ii. offer a few acceptable choice when appropriate: "We laid out two outfits last night choose which one want to wear today and get dressed"; "Do you want to put your pajamas on before or after daddy reads you a story?"

     iii. be creative to engage them. "Your books are saying that if you don't put them away they want to stay on the shelf tomorrow"; "You can get into the car seat yourself or I can put you in it"

     iv. when necessary enforce the limit. This takes place after allowing the child to make the right decision and they continue to resist. For example, the child has refused to get into the car, without emotion the child is picked up and placed in the car seat and buckled in. If a tantrum ensues then initiate a conversation designed to distract from the situation. It is important to not acknowledge the tantrum. In this case, ignoring the negative behavior will help eliminate it

     v. be consistent. We do not want the child to learn that if they don't give in you will. Therefore, parents cannot allow themselves to be worn down. If they are not consistent, the non-compliance will sustain and it will impede the child learning that with every choice there is a consequence. Some consequences are positive and some are negative.

o. Discipline: the goal of discipline is to facilitate learning to think and behave in appropriate and positive ways. Another way to understand it is that discipline helps a child develop self-control. *Understanding the factors that may be maintaining the function of the challenging behaviors are also critical (for example, is the challenging behavior attention maintained? Escape maintained? etc.)

     i. separation. When asked to keep their hands to themselves or they can't stop arguing, being apart allows a child to calm down. Once calmed down a child is encouraged to make better choices of behavior (thinking about their choices and the associated consequences)

     ii. behavior management means talking calmly with a struggling child so that they can learn from what happened, why, and what they can do differently for a desired outcome. A child gets to learn to control their behavior and take responsibility for it. Use the turtle technique: recognize feelings of anger, think "stop", go inside "shell", take 3 deep breaths, think calm, think of a solution

     iii. redirection is used to stop the child when they are in trouble, explain what the problem is, and suggest or redirect the child to another activity

     iv. taking responsibility – fixing it or getting help. If they spill a drink, give them a cloth or a paper towel so they can clean it up (fix it)

     v. ignoring undesired behavior when the goal is attention. But don't forget to give attention for desired behavior

     vi. be firm and respectful. Make statements that are brief, clear and firm instead of being weak and sounding like one is asking or pleading for change instead of making it clear

     vii. remain in control and intervene in a situation before it escalates and gets out of control. Remember you can't be rational with someone who isn't. So if things have escalated where children are angry and frustrated create a calm down time. An escalated situation may be the result of parents not intervening early enough

     viii. don't become emotionally involved – be detached when undesirable behavior takes place. Try understanding from the child's perspective, why it happened, so that intervening and redirecting offers a learning moment as well

p. Focus on the positives

     i. emphasize and reinforce the positive desirable behaviors and choices. Tell the child what to do instead of what not to do. Speaking to a child respectfully while giving guidance creates a respectful authoritative frame for the parent–child or adult–child relationship

     ii. be positive and reinforcing instead of using negative words and negative expectations (I don't expect you to do well). There should be a lot more "dos" than "don'ts"

iii. set positive limits to help a child deal with difficult emotions. Encourage them to use their words instead of acting out their emotions. This facilitates identification of emotions, self-control and recognizing choices for dealing with difficult emotions

- Grieving
  Grief is a normal emotional experience associated with death and loss. When a child experiences grief they need to be comforted, supported and guided through dealing with their loss. Death is a part of life and young children may not understand that it is permanent and all that lives at some point dies. Generally, when a child grieves it is brief and intermittent, thus, needing to be addressed at different times as they grow. It is not uncommon that a grieving child demonstrates regression requiring a parental response of patience, nurturance and understanding. If someone close to the child dies they might feel unsafe and fearful, leaving them with concerns about uncertainties and what is going to happen. If it is another child/sibling they could fear that they might die next. If a parent(s) is consumed with their own grief and not emotionally available to the child, this may result in the child not feeling safe and secure. Consequently, potentially leading to numerous possibilities associated with the child's interpretation of their experience and the loss of an important for understanding emotions and learning how to deal with them
- What to tell a child when someone close to them dies
- First of all the parent(s) need to be in the right state of mind themselves. Be thoughtful and if necessary ask someone else close who is in a better state of mind to be there and be supportive. Even if a child seems unaffected by the loss keep in mind that they process grief differently
- Be brief and honest. Death is a reality, but be caring and developmentally appropriate in the sharing of information and giving details
- Allow the child to express their emotions and validate them. If asked questions only give as much information as needed to answer the question, but in general don't go into details
- If the death was the result of some terrible violent act that the child has some awareness for, be reassuring of the child's safety
- Offer the child choices in dealing with their grief. They may feel comforted by their normal daily routine and have moments of sadness. Meet the child where they are at
- Be reassuring to the child, and offer support in simple statements, "I'm sorry…" "tell me about how you feel", etc.
- Feelings of loss associated with change.
- What do they miss. This needs to be identified so that there can be a facilitation of problem solving to adjust to changes and appropriately meet their needs which are currently destabilized
- For example, making new friends by structuring play dates, consistently participating in activities to increase proximity to new people, places and situation until it becomes a routine and feels secure
- What are the different ways to resolve the loss by creating new or different resources "an appropriate replacement" that also reinforces resilience. This is an important opportunity because life brings with it continuous challenging change
- Dealing with feelings of guilt. Sometimes young children think they caused something that happens resulting in feelings of guilt. It is important to make sure that the child understands that nothing that they said or did caused the death of someone they loved

q. Reinforce for parents: while ADD/ADHD is not caused by ineffective or bad parenting there are helpful strategies. Fundamentally:
- provide structure

- be consistent
- communicate clearly
- help them to understand and learn from the consequences of their actions
- give them lots of love, support and encouragement

The very basic issues these children struggle with such as difficulty sitting still, listening quietly, and paying attention does not mean that they cannot be successful at school. It starts with evaluating a child's individual strengths and weaknesses, then coming up with creative strategies for helping the child focus, staying on task, and learning to their full capacity

7. School plan/strategies (a number of these techniques can be used in other professional environments as well)

Don't forget to utilize information from the above section when applicable. The manifestations in the classroom are often similar to those experienced in the home environment. However, there are times when a hyperactive child may not demonstrate the same difficulties in the classroom. Most commonly, the hyperactive child is engaged in out-of-seat activities, difficulty completing assignments, frequently noisy and disruptive, poor social skill, poor awareness for consequences, and aggressiveness toward peers. This can be further complicated by learning disabilities which can play a role in oppositional defiant disorder and conduct problems. As with the interventions above, treatment is not meant as a cure but as efforts to decrease inappropriate behavior and to improve the occurrence of more appropriate behavior through development of skills with replacement behaviors. Educators must strive to maintain their awareness with regards to how they interact with the chronically frustrating and challenging hyperactive child. There is the likelihood of responding to a hyperactive child with commands, limits, and consequences (overall general negativity), versus praise and positive tone of interaction with children who do not present with these problems. It is important to interact with this child in a manner which does not draw unnecessary attention to their behavior. The three most targeted behaviors of change are inattention, off-task, and disruptive behaviors

Instruction of desired behavior is most effective when it is embedded in the child's daily routines and in meaningful activities. Katz & McClellan (1997) offer the following suggestions and examples for teaching social skills as part of classroom activities

- ○ Modeling: demonstrate (model) the skill while explaining what you are doing. A puppet could also be used (to increase focus and attention) to model the skill while interacting with the child. A puppet can explain to the teacher (like a child would explain their thoughts/feelings to an adult caregiver) so that the child learns vicariously. For instance, telling the teacher how they became angry and hit a peer because they wanted the toy that the peer had. The teacher could then talk to the puppet about considering other options for dealing with such a situation
- ○ Preparing peer partners: enlisting the help of a child who has mastered a skill to show another child how to do it, "Bobby, Cindy is learning how to wait and take turns, can you help her?" This could be reinforced by using a photo showing how the children line up at the drinking fountain and wait their turn
- ○ Singing: introduce a new skill through a song. Using the tune of a familiar song create simple lyrics that guide the thinking of a child to practice a new skill in a fun way.
- ○ Doing fingerplays: introduce the skill with finger play. As with singing, create a rhyme that coincides with adding one finger at a time (each finger representing the addition of a child/friend who is complying or cooperating with an skill/activity
- ○ Using a flannel board or white board: flannel boards/white boards are fun for introducing new skills through activities and stories
- ○ Using prompts: multisensory prompts. Give a child verbal, visual and/or physical prompts to use a skill during interactions and activities. If a child has difficulty initiating playing with others, recommend, "remember to use your words and ask to

play", show a series of pictures with the dialogue of initiating play with others, walk a child up to peers and tell them you will walk over with them so that they can ask

○ Giving encouragement: provide specific feedback when a child has been instructed in the use of the skill and they do it. "You did great, good job!" A child can be encouraged verbally or with a smile and a thumbs-up

○ Supplemental or incidental teaching: during the course of interactions/activities guide the child to use the skill. "Benton, I can see that you are angry that all the balls are being used. Let's go over the choices you have to deal with feeling angry". Included in this example would be the skills of asking if they can join in play with others or asking for a turn

○ Playing games: games are a great vehicle for teaching a number of skills such as identifying and expressing feelings, taking turns, friendship skills/social skills. Children can take turns pulling a photo out of a bowl or bag and be asked to offer a compliment to the child in the photo or a photo might show a social challenge and each child could share an idea of how to deal with it

○ Reading books with a message: it is not difficult to find a book that offers almost any message one would want. With desktop publishing it is also easy to create a personalized book for a topic or a child (so that they have a picture reference).
*Children need repeated opportunities to practice a new skill in familiar and new situations for maintenance and generalization. They need occasional encouragement to reinforce the use of the skill and feedback when using it in new situations

The classroom offers a unique environment for developmentally appropriate practices. A well-organized, effective and engaging classroom will start with structuring the physical arrangement of the space to increase appropriate behaviors and decreasing the probability of engaging in challenging behaviors. In general, classroom practices include a developmentally appropriate and child-centered environment crafted to promote successful interactions, engagement in learning, social competence and the development of independence

○ Arrange the classroom for a good visual overview for monitoring all of the children

○ Attend to details such as wall color, lighting, temperature, noise level, and number of children in the space to decrease the probability of engaging in challenging behaviors in association with sensitivity to environmental factors

○ Arrange activity centers to structure and support appropriate behaviors (staging the sequence of an activity and limiting the number of children at any given time)

○ Being prepared to provide assistance to children as they need help and support them to remain focused and attending to the task at hand

○ Daily scheduling of activities embeds predictability and communicates to children (you know what you need to do) the organization of daily events. Once the routine is mastered, choices can be slowly interjected. Also, place the most difficult activity at a time when children are the most alert and attentive

○ Rules/rituals/routines provide beneficial structure. They foster a sense of community, convey values and remind children of what is expected of them. Teaching these requires patience as they are taught in small steps with repetition, positive feedback and embedding to assure practice leads to generalization

○ Facilitating smooth and easy transition from one activity to another (locating the activity centers as a progression for ease of change, organization of materials, etc.)

○ Being thoughtful as to the arrangement and organization of materials in the room to facilitate and promote engagement, mastery and independence

Educators have a lot of responsibility coinciding with multiple roles:

a. Range from teacher/classroom to multidisciplinary team

b. Informal classroom modifications

c. IFSP and IEP meeting (IDEA)

d. Section 504 plan

e. Positive reinforcement methods

   i. employ a high rate of intrinsically rewarding activities (privileges) such as access to games, free play at recess, permission to be the "teacher helper"

   ii. token or points program (tokens, poker chips, or other symbolic reinforcers). Tokens are intermittently exchanged for earned choices – tangible, intrinsic rewards – that the child desires. The educator will prepare a list of 10 activities that the child may exchange their tokens for. *The token system can successfully modify classroom and academic achievement. In other words, improvement in deviant behavior in the classroom can be accomplished by reinforcing correct academic performance (what they do right) without even focusing directly on the deviant behavior as a target of intervention. Choose a time frame for utilizing a token economy that is manageable and reinforcing for the child (waiting until the end of the day may be too long)

   iii. the application of tangible rewards or edible substances as a reward for appropriate/desired behavior. *Generally outruns its usefulness after preschool

   iv. contingency contracting. This technique is not an actual reinforcer of behavior, but this contract can target a disruptive/inappropriate classroom behavior/poor academic performance, or both by allowing the child to earn desired reinforcers by completing the agreement set forth by the contract

f. Punishment methods (careful negative attention can be reinforcing too!)

   i. withdrawal of positive activities. When withdrawal of attention is combined with positive attention and other rewards it can improve the rate of change. Especially, withdrawal such as ignoring unacceptable behavior alone may escalate the behavior. Be sure of the outcome that the tool of choice will result in

   ii. time out for reinforcement. This tool needs to be explored for amount of time, location and level of compliance. There is likely a school policy which provides the answer of specifically how to employ this intervention

   iii. response cost. Taking away tokens or some other intrinsically motivating activity upon occurrence of the undesired behavior

g. Improving self-control. The tendency to act without thinking. Child's role in self-control training. This techniques requires self-monitoring, self-evaluation, self-instruction, and recognizing associated consequences. As can be seen, this age group presents obvious developmental issues associated with being able to employ the factors comprising the technique of self-control. However, aspects of it may be used with some children at the older end of the 0–5 age range. A realistic expectation is necessary. When reviewing what consists of training self-control, the limitations for utilizing this technique with little guys will be evident. However, the concept still has merit for increasing awareness, using the decision chair to take a moment to think about making the best choice and reinforcing approximation of change/shaping and change:

   i. children are taught to watch, note/record their behavior in specific situations. Young children could create a record of sorts by choosing a picture that represents their behavior, thus giving them a cognitive (thinking) and a visual cue of what the behavior looks like

   ii. children are taught to identify situations in which they have problems

   iii. children are taught active responding vs responding impulsively in specific problematic situations

   iv. children are taught to express verbally what their struggle is (factors describing why they have the problem) in a situation/environment where they have problems. Part of this is teaching them "feeling vocabulary". Help children understand and label their own feelings and the feelings of others. Add to this a 5-point scale for identifying emotion intensity. "This is what I feel and this is how strongly I am feeling it" can be an important aspect of a verbal expression of their challenge

    v. children are helped to create a list of possible responses or solutions to the problem situation/environment. This includes the evaluation of the short- and long-term consequences associated with each choice

    vi. children are helped to identify and use which response will work best for them to achieve the desired outcome in each situation. This effort is continued as an evaluation of results of change, i.e., what works, teach/model what to do with a feeling before it leads to a challenging behavior. "Boy am I mad. I need to take 3 deep breaths and calm down"

    vii. children need to be encouraged to use self-reward or clarification for reinforcing success of behavior change

    viii. for improving insight, a child can be asked a question, but they are not to respond for 15–20 seconds, long enough to think about it first and not just respond impulsively

    ix. to improve out of classroom behavior, allow the child to earn a reward based on the compliments they receive on their behavior from other teachers, lunchroom staff, playground aids, and the principal, etc.

  h. Educator's role in self-control training

    i. programming success. Provide success experiences. This can be accomplished by
- break tasks into parts to make more manageable
- give tasks in an increasing level of difficulty
- modify material to a child's ability
- provide reinforcing reviews

    ii. organize experiences of success both at school and home for reinforcement and generalization
- educator and parents structure demands on children that match their capability successfully to accomplish the task(s)
- reward effort, approximation and completion of tasks
- praise specific behaviors

    iii. teach basic steps for accomplishing tasks (this can be done in a fun practice manner with a lot of reinforcement)
- identify what is needed to accomplish the task
- assess what they are capable of doing on their own and/or where they may need help (encouraging them to make every effort on their own and avoiding the building of frustration)
- identify all of the different choices
- identify what is the best solution
- teach them how to check the accuracy of their work
- role play the problems, and possible solutions ahead of time. Have the child practice these responses during the school day. Have them and others give feedback on the success they are experiencing

    iv. encourage independence and self-efficacy
- encourage their effort and appropriate risk taking in directed situations
- discourage dependence – they need to develop confidence in their efforts and abilities
- encourage children to think through their own solutions
- teach them the difference between making a careless mistake (not paying enough attention to what they are doing) versus making mistakes due to a lack of resource, knowledge or capability
- frequently move about the room. When you catch a child working on task, reward them with a simple smile or wink, followed by a reinforcing statement about how hard they are working

    v. increase awareness: it is also critical for educators to understand that children often attribute success and failure to internal/external factors differently
- discourage excessive and inappropriate talking
- draw awareness to diminished attention or hyper behavior
- encourage them to increase their effort beyond a superficial approach to a task

i. Teaching problem-solving skills
  i. actively teach and model strategies that increase attention and concentration
- focusing strategies
- how to check for what is important (critical factors)
- careful listening for important information

  ii. teach strategies/plan and offer suggestions that increase inhibitory control and develop organizational skills
- sit on hands until they have thought through all of the possible solutions
- model how to arrange things such as assembling materials for a project, clothes to be laid out to wear the next day, etc.

  iii. teach strategies/plan and offer suggestions to improve alertness and arousal
- label states of arousal/naming feelings
- teach self-calming techniques
- create interesting breaks between time frame of demand for concentration
- be sensitive to their struggle to fight boredom as well as their need for stimulation

  iv. when there is a failure to learn a skill
- model, practice and reinforce task steps
- teach strategies for specific academic activities
- practice

  v. problem-solving process
- ask yourself, "what is my problem?"
- think, think, think of some solutions
- what would happen?
- give it a try

j. Decreasing classroom distractions/stimulation
  i. identify the type of stimuli that are of high appeal to the child
  ii. identify the pattern of when the child does best and utilize the information for developing the structure which will offer the most benefit to maximize academic performance and behavioral compliance

8. Cognitive exercises
a. The coin game. To improve memory, sequencing, attention and concentration. An added benefit is that it is fun, fast paced and kids enjoy it. Put together a small pile of coins, a small piece of cardboard to cover them and a stopwatch. Choose five coins from the pile (e.g., "choose 2 pennies and 3 nickels") and put them in sequence. The child is told to look closely at the coin arrangement. Then the coins are covered with the cardboard. The stop watch is started and they are asked to make the same arrangement from memory. When they are finished write down the time it took to complete the pattern (whether it is correct or not). Keep doing it until they get it right, practice it a few times and then increase the complexity by adding a different coin (e.g., 2 pennies, 3 nickels, 1 dime) and continue to be creative in increasing complexity in tune mastery

b. Relaxation and positive imagery. Combining simple relaxation techniques such as deep breathing with positive visual imagery helps the brain to improve or learn new skills. Similar to what is done in sports psychology, instruct the child to see themselves paying attention in school, etc.

c. Mind–body integration. Encourage the child to sit in their chair without moving. Either the educator or parent can then time them to have a baseline. Repeat the activity and find how the practice yields improvement in self-control

    d. Crossword puzzles and picture puzzles. These games improve attention for words and sequencing ability. Picture puzzles have the added benefit of identifying what is wrong with a sequence as well putting the pictures in the right sequence (social and emotional intelligence play a role here too). Another fun picture game of these skills is looking for the hard to find objects in the picture

    e. Memory and concentration games. There are a lot of board game options and card games as well as the techie ones like Simon. Simon is fun because it stimulates a child visually and auditorily. Encourage and reinforce their efforts

As always, it is important to highlight strengths when challenged by deficits. Those with ADD/ADHD also exhibit the following positive characteristics:

- Energy and drive. When children with ADD/ADHD are motivated they work and play hard – striving to accomplish and succeed. In fact, it may be difficult to distract them from the task that is motivating them. This is especially the case when the task is hands on or interactive
- Enthusiasm and spontaneity. These children are anything but boring. They are lively and have numerous interests. When you aren't exhausted and frustrated by them, they exude energy and are a lot of fun
- Creativity. These children can be highly creative and imaginative. It is not uncommon to find them daydreaming with numerous thoughts colliding. Another benefit of this characteristic is that they may at times see what others don't
- Flexibility. This is one of the flip-side benefits. Because the child with ADD/ADHD may consider a lot of options at once, they don't rigidly focus on one option early on and are more open to different ideas

Regulatory Disorders of Sensory Processing (RDSP)

This diagnosis will be presented somewhat differently than other diagnoses in this chapter. It is a highly challenging treatment arena that demands creative individualized interventions. Therefore, the treatment team must be vigilant in finding ways to achieve freedom of choice. This is accomplished by shaping the choices available to the child (providing equipment, objects, pictures, etc. that meets the needs of the intervention and still allows them to choose from what is presented). It is believed that inner-directed choices are more ego syntonic and result in increased investment by the child.

Children presenting with difficulty regulating and processing sensory input typically demonstrate sensory processing difficulties, motor difficulties, and specific behavioral patterns. A child with RDSP will be sensitive (either hyper/over or hypo/under) to touch, sights, sounds, smells, and sensations of movement in space.

The therapist must take into consideration the child's arousal level, attention, motivation, motor planning, and problem solving. The therapist is assigned the role to understand the child's deficit, allowing the child to assume control over actions during the treatment session (by purposeful design), and modify the environment in order to achieve the desired adaptive response. The treatment team creates the necessary "sensory diet" of a variety of sensory experiences designed to help a child with RSPD properly and correctly interpret their environment.

Basically five interconnected elements comprise the sensory integration mechanism (Williamson & Anzalone, 2001).

THE ELEMENTS OF SENSORY INTEGRATION

- *Sensory registration* takes place when a person first becomes aware of a sensory event. There is an individualized level of sensory awareness or "sensory threshold". In other words, a person may not be aware of a certain sensory input or message until it reaches a certain level of intensity or threshold and this threshold varies from person to person. Additionally, this threshold is dynamic, meaning that it changes during the course of a day depending on numerous factors such as prior emotional experiences, prior sensory experiences, fatigue, stress, level of alertness

- *Sensory orientation* allows a person to pay attention to new sensory input – determining what can be ignored and what needs to be attended to. This functional mechanism of inhibition vs facilitation is referred to as *modulation*. This mechanism is important because it would be impossible to attend to all incoming sensory input. Modulation is necessary for the ability to select relevant stimuli for a specific situation/experience. Sensory modulation describes changes in the state of the nervous system regarding the continuum of sensory registration and responsivity with orientation at one end of the continuum and failure to orient at the other end. As a child matures, he develops regulation allowing for the ability to maintain a calm alert state. This regulation skill equates to the ability to achieve, monitor and change one's state to match environmental demands. Overall, the goal of the nervous system is to achieve and maintain homeostasis. Children with regulatory disorders tend to work against their threshold for stimulation as a way to reach their homeostasis

- *Integration* or interpretation of sensory information allows a person to determine not only what to respond to but what is threatening. New sensory experiences are compared to old ones via numerous related processes such as memory, emotion, language, etc. A well-known role of the nervous system in the interpretation process is the fight or flight reaction to protect/escape from harm

- *Organization of a response/adaptive response* can be physical, emotional or cognitive and it is the brain that determines if a response to sensory input is necessary or if it is responded to at all

- *Execution of a response* whether it be cognitive, emotional or motor to the sensory input or message is the final step of the sensory integration mechanism. And then it starts all over again. Thus, the circular process or feedback loop of sensory integration

*Neuroplasticity is what underlies interventions for sensory problems. By providing carefully designed sensory experiences, positive neural connections are enhanced and reinforced, thus providing the template of change.

Sensory intake>sensory integration>planning and organizing behavior>adaptive behavior and learning>feedback

SENSORY SYSTEM AND SENSORY-RELATED INTERVENTIONS

Sensory integration therapy strives for an outcome of helping a child to put it all together: where they begin and end, relationship functioning, functioning well in their environment and being flexible. Therefore, when developing a treatment plan for a child with RDSP, the treatment should be thinking backwards from the goal in selecting the "best fit" intervention which translates to:

- Improve attention/focus to task
- Increase independence in self-care tasks
- Decrease fear and anxiety (avoidance)
- Improve communication
- Improve flexibility
- Increase socialization
- Increase self-confidence/self-esteem
- Improve ability to explore choices and take appropriate risk

Therefore, when choosing objectives to meet a goal, consider the different aspects of a child's needs that will be met. This requires an understanding of how each task will address several areas of deficit. It may look like a game, but it could entail listening, personal space, relationships, and taking turns. Regarding intervention choices being the "best fit" for the child, establish realistic expectations and adhere to consistent guidelines.

CASE EXAMPLE

Noah is 4 years old. He has difficulty adjusting to new activities and when it is time for recess he wants to play but experiences difficulty joining in. Additionally, especially during recess, he tends to get to frustrated while engaging in play with his peers. He screams, pushes other children and grabs toys. His teacher, Ms Cooper, has introduced several interventions. To facilitate self-soothing, Ms Cooper has worked with Noah to identify his feelings and have a 'tool box" of self-soothing activities and a quiet, safe place where he can find refuge. To help him with transition he is reminded of the daily schedule with a picture board and she has made a special laminated sheet with progressive pictures of him successfully engaging in activities. She has also introduced a 4-step problem-solving process as a class learning activity along with picture cards portraying the problem-solving process: (1) ask yourself, what is my problem?; (2) think, think, think of some solution (what are my choices?); (3) what would happen?; (4) give it a try.

Noah has been doing pretty well using the problem-solving process during play, but Ms Cooper recognizes that Noah needs prompting and reinforcement in new situations. Today, the class is on a field trip to a children's science exhibition (hands on). While at school and preparing to assemble for leaving on the field trip, Ms Cooper gave Noah a picture card depicting Noah getting on a bus, smiling and talking with a friend on the bus, unloading the bus, and standing in a group with the other children preparing to go in. She also gives him a stress ball to keep in his pocket that he can squeeze when he starts feeling frustrated or overwhelmed. Before entering, Ms Cooper respectfully takes Noah aside and reviews the problem-solving skill.

Once inside, there is a gravity experiment with several launching tubes, but they are all in use. Ms Cooper sees Noah squeezing the ball in his pocket and moves to close proximity with Noah offering him support and reminds him about using the problem-solving steps and to stop and think, think, think, about what to do. Noah turns to one of the children engaged in the activity and asks, "can I play too?" The child hands him the object to place in the tube and when it completes the journey Noah hands it to the other child. They are taking turns. Ms Cooper catches Noah's eye, winks, smiles and gives him a thumb's up.

When engaging in "sensory-play" it can be messy. Make sure clothing and surfaces are protected as needed. All of these activities require a knowledgeable adult providing guidance and supervising the activity to assure safety and benefit of the activity. What follows is a minimal demonstration of the type of creativity to work with these little guys!

1. Tactile sense
   a. Using a flat surface (counter top, baking sheet, tray) apply unscented shaving cream or bath foam. This is like finger painting without the paint. Encourage the child to put both hands into and draw figure 8s/swirls, write letters or words, make shapes
   b. Make play-dough (or purchase it). There are numerous recipes on-line. It can be made different colors and the child can take a marbled piece of it and work the color through to consistency. Making shapes, rolling, using objects to create shapes. This is a great tool for visual sensation and teaching how 2 colors are combined to make another (yellow + blue = green, blue + red = purple, etc.). To increase the tactile experience, sand can be added or other pieces of plastic like plastic beads or cubes. Fragrance can also be added (vanilla, because some fragrance bases like mint or cinnamon can be hot or hurt eyes – be sure to test first). *Dust hands with flour so dough won't stick to them if necessary

c. Theraputty (therapeutic exercise putty). For small children, "soft-resistance" is the best choice

    i. to decrease over-responsivity. Instruct the child to hide their hand in the putty. Then with that hand have them slowly make an arc of going up (ascending) and then slowly coming down (descending). When done, ask the child if they can show you their hand and encourage them working to get the putty off)

    ii. take small objects such as buttons, beads, pebbles, coins, small plastic figures, etc. Bury a few objects in the putty and have the child search the putty to find them

d. Sand tray. Have available all kinds of small plastic people and toys (including beach type object, i.e., small paper umbrella, palm trees, turtles, etc) to engage in imaginary play for the sand tray. A child can make roads, or give them a spray bottle with water to wet the sand and they will be able to make structures with it – make sure they have some small molds to use on wet sand

e. Cook spaghetti and once cooled give a child a couple of strands to touch and manipulate into shapes, numbers and/or letters. They can let the shapes dry on a cookie sheet. Once dry they can be glued to paper/cardboard and painted if desired

f. The over-responsive child will benefit from sifting food through their hands or playing with their feet. Take dry goods such as beans, rice macaroni, etc. Using empty coffee cans (or other containers) fill the can about half full

    i. encourage the child to sift their fingers through the dry foods or stir it with a spoon

    ii. using small plaster figures (animals or people) pretend that they are engaging in activities like diving, swimming, eating

    iii. walk barefoot in material, pick up the objects with their toes

    iv. if there are a lot of objects have the child sort them

g. The tactile path. This activity requires different textures to walk on that are laid out in a circle or wandering path. The different textures could includes such things as a carpet square, fake fur, velvet, satin, terry, sandpaper, egg crate-bedding, etc. The child can be instructed to walk or jump from one texture to the next and can go forward and backwards

    i. child cannot tolerate getting messy

       - adapt materials (glue stick instead of paste, finger paint with plastic spoons, allow to wear gloves, use play dough instead of clay, etc.

       - cue verbally to remind the child of the expectation (glue on paper, hands on finger paint paper, etc.)

       - have wet wipes available on table for the child to use clean hands

       - use first-then statements ("first glue and then I will help you clean up")

       - have a scripted story about "being messy" to shape tactile adjustment and reinforcement

       - send the child to an activity with a peer who can model the steps

h. Character dress up. It is a great idea to have a variety of "costumes" and accessories for children to play in (go excessive versus limited)

    i. it is an opportunity to handle a variety of textures and help with tactile discrimination

    ii. orienting the body for getting dressed, motor planning, and awareness of body position

    iii. encourages imaginative play using different roles and different personalities

i. The Mummy Wrap (provides uniform deep pressure to calm the oversensitive nervous system). A 50-yard length of latex free stretchy exercise band is recommended. Wrap the child up like a mummy from shoulders to ankles. It should be taught but not too tight. The pressure needs to be applied as evenly as possible. The taut binding organizes the tactile system

    j. The human roll. The deep pressure of this activity feels good. Because the oversensitive child seeks deep pressure, this activity is calming and relaxing. The activity can be done in a few different ways

        i. have the child lie down on a beach towel and then taking a beach ball roll and press the ball (consistently firm) all over their body. This can also be done with flat hands

        ii. roll them up in a mat and with open hand press consistently and firmly

2. Vestibular sense (balance and movement)

    a. The T-stool (easy to build or buy from Theraplay) compels a child to find balance and stay in the center. It also improves body awareness and posture stability. If the child struggles with balancing have them sit on it with their back against the wall for support

    b. Teeter totter. Easy to construct using a railroad tie or other thick piece of lumber like a beam remnant (using it as a fulcrum) and then take another flat and wide board to place evenly over it. Have the child stand on the board over the fulcrum in the balanced position. Next have them practice applying pressure on either side to tip the balance

    c. Therapy ball. Allow a child to sit on a therapy ball for sensory input

    d. Mini trampoline. Jumping is beneficial for improving rhythm and regulating the nervous system. Place pillows all around the trampoline so that if the child bounces off in any direction there is ample (several layers) cushioning protection. While the child is jumping read or sing to them. Get them to jump to the beat

    e. Gentle roughhousing. Children love physical play with caregivers. There are numerous ways to go about it and kids love them all. Such play with an adult builds trust, security, self-esteem and social skills. They also benefit balance, flexing and extending muscles, deep pressure, and strengthening body awareness

        i. rowboat. Sitting on the floor facing each other, take each other's hands and press the soles of your feet together. As you sing row, row, row your boat pull the oars (hands) back and forth

        ii. airplane. Lie on your back, knees bent and toes pointing forward. Take the child's hands, place your feet on their lower abdomen, and then lift up for a smooth take-off. It is up to you and the child how adventurous this play will be

        iii. horsey. Kneel down and have the child come up behind you and put their arms around your neck. Slowly lower your hands to the ground so that they can stabilize. A long scarf can be put around the girth and used as reins

        iv. wheelbarrow walk. Have the child lie down on their tummy, then take their ankles in your hands and gently draw them up like the handles of the wheelbarrow

        v. piggyback ride. Load them up in whatever means easy for you (kneeling down, or standing up with them on a chair, etc.)

        vi. hokey pokey. Take a piece of rope to create a circle. "You put your left hand in.., you take you left hand out you put your left hand in and you shake it all about, you do the hokey pokey and you turn your self around – that's what it's all about…" duplicating the verses with the other arm the legs, head, belly button, bottom, whole self

3. Proprioceptive sense (sensory messages about position, force, direction and movement of one's body parts.) These activities provide pressure, body awareness, motor planning, problem-solving skills, and self-esteem

    a. Crash pad (mattress, several layers of egg-crate material or large dog bed). The child leaps from their bed onto the crash pad and rolling around on it

    b. Bottle babies. Depending on the size of the child, use a water bottle or a one liter bottle. They can be filled with different types of liquid, different color, sparkles, shells or other objects in the fluid

        i. carry it in their hands

        ii. cradle and rock it like a baby

      iii. shake it

      iv. push it with a stick

  c. A box fort provides a quite place to go. Have the child help make and decorate the box. You can get a big box from an appliance store, either cut a hole in it for a door or place it open side up with a sheet over it so that the child can climb into it. It needs to be decorated with numerous soft pillows and a blanket (all hypoallergenic). One can also purchase a small pop-up tent for the same purpose

  d. Simon says: touch your toes, bend over and place your hands on the ground, choose any position or take turns imitating each other

  e. Stretchy bands. Have a collection of them varying in resistance. It gives joints and muscles a work out. Use them in every way imaginable

  f. The tunnel. One can be purchased or made using hula hoops and knit jersey tubing fabric. Kids can crawl, creep, go through on knees and elbows, they can push a ball through

  g. Shopping game. This game requires a laundry basket or large plastic bucket to use as a shopping cart. Now set up the store. Have all kinds of interesting things from the pantry (sizes, shapes and weights)

  h. Jiggling on the dryer. Sitting on top of the dryer while on. Depending on a child's needs, this can stimulate or calm

  i. Helping mom. Basic household chores can provide benefit in a daily routine. For example, sweep, dust, push chairs in after dinner, etc.

  j. Physical activities/sports such as pillow fights, play wrestling, roller skating, gymnastics, karate, running, soccer, etc.

4. Visual sense is a complex process used to identify different aspects of one's environment and to anticipate what is coming so that one can prepare for a response. "Listening with your eyes"

  a. Schedule board offers a visual line up of the day's activities, allowing a child to prepare for transitions from one activity to another. Actually, a single activity could be used with the same concept, but breaking down all of the steps from beginning to completions

  b. Citrus ball. Gather several types of citrus. Take a paper bag, open it and face the opening toward the child. Have them roll the citrus into the bag. But they can also name and count the fruit, identify the color, smell it to see the variation in fragrance, put the fruit in order of size, they could also peel the fruit

  c. Bean bag catch. Take empty plastic bottles with a handle (like small bleach bottles). Wash thoroughly and cut a section out of the bottom. Make several small bean bags. Toss the bean bag back and forth with the scoops

  d. Peanut hunt. When a child isn't watching, take the peanuts in a shell outside and hide them. Later give them a bag and have them hunt for the peanuts

  e. Hose 'em. Kids love playing with a hose. Identify a place in the yard that they can be a "helper" to water plants. It is also fun to line up objects and let a child hose them over. Good target practice

  f. Flashlight tag. Have the child lie back down on their bed. Give them a flashlight and turn off the light. Shine your flashlight on the ceiling and have them follow your path. It can be done drawing different shapes, or a different point pattern. You can also play tag (tag my light)

5. Auditory sense. The ability to hear does not guarantee that one will have an understanding of the sounds heard. Comprehension is acquired while processing vestibular sensations

  a. Using a recorder is fun. A kazoo is just as fun. A child can copy your tune or make up their own tune

  b. Tapping tunes by clapping or tapping hands or beating a drum. Tap, clap or drum the rhythm of a song, or singing along

    c. Matching sounds. Shake a container and guess what is inside (buttons, paper clips, pennies, etc.)

    d. Identify animal sounds, environmental sounds (siren, hourly chimes, recess bell)

    e. Use songs that also have a message or can be used for learning. There are some fun tunes for learning

6. Olfactory sense/gustatory sense. Smell plays an important role in establishing and eliciting/reviving memories. Taste provides essential information about a variety of flavors which, with experience, provides information, i.e., did it make us sick, did we like, etc.

    a. Smell and tell. Put together a good collection of different smells. It could be stimulating or calming scents. Scents could also be transferred to cotton balls and placed in sequence for identification

    b. Make a pomander ball using an orange and press whole cloves into as much of the surface as possible tie a ribbon to it and hang it in a closet

    c. Smash and smell. Take things with a fragrance, flowers and herbs. In a tray and using a rubber mallet, let the child smash one at a time, finding if the aroma is intensified

    d. Scented flashcards can be made by taking plain index cards and putting different fragrances on them. They can be further distinguished by punching holes or applying patterns to separate them for another form of identification

    e. Taste and tell is a game with a variety of food bits (goldfish cracker, jelly bean, citrus fruit section, popcorn with different seasonings, different slices of fruits or vegetables, etc.). Make the game more challenging by guessing with eyes closed

    f. Lettuce samplings. Using pieces of lettuce and a variety of salad dressing, have the child smell the dressing to identify different herbs and then taste them. This promotes olfactory/gustatory discrimination. The activity is enhanced if the lettuce was grown in a home garden where the child could water and weed the garden area and see the lettuce grow

GENERAL SKILL BUILDING

1. Relationships

    a. Clarifying the concept of family

        i. make a poster of a family tree

        ii. use opportunities such as phone calls or social gatherings/holidays to clarify the meaning of family relationships (i.e., Uncle Bob is mom's brother)

        iii. make a collage – let the child cut out and glue or just glue pictures of family on a poster board and label them

    b. Understanding the perspective of others

        i. help a child to understand that relationships are bidirectional (2-way street, the golden rule, thinking about you, thinking about me)

           - observe children taking turns at a game and discuss why it is important/ respectful, cooperative team work, how/why it makes an activity work better

           - observe friends talking to another at the park – they are listening to each other. Discuss the value of that and why it is important (everyone wants to be heard)

        ii. have the child list why listening is important

    c. Identifying friends

        i. work with the child to make a list of friends. What do they like about their friends? What do they do to make their friends feel good?

        ii. what are the characteristics of a good friend? (make a list)

2. Learning to listen

    a. Using eye contact "I look at the person I am listening to with my eyes"

        i. the winking game; take turns winking

        ii. a version of hide and seek where the child has to make eye contact with you when you find them (they are listening, therefore quiet and communicating with their eyes)

   b. Don't interrupt
      i. when the child is talking to you interrupt them. Ask them how it felt for you to interrupt them. Then explain to them when someone interrupts the other person feels ignored and possibly angry. *Practice talking without interrupting
      ii. practice being a statue. Statues don't move. So when someone is talking to you "be a statue, make eye contact and listen"
      iii. practice appropriate responding. Take turns talking about a specific topic (such as a field trip that everyone shared or when there was play day at the park)
3. Personal space
   a. Identify personal space. Have a child take a hula hoop and stand in the middle of it. This is a great demonstration of personal space
   b. A squeeze is not a hug. For the child who is always squeezing arms and being too physical, give them a stress ball to keep in their pocket. When they want to squeeze someone they can squeeze the stress ball instead
   c. Make a "how close can I get poster". It depends on who it is and what kind of relationship that it is that defines how close one can get (issues of intimacy and safety). Clarify levels of closeness and discuss all the different types of relationships and make associated posters
      i. family relationships
      ii. friends, teacher, daycare provider, etc.
      iii. people seen regularly, but we are not close to. These are contextual relationships (gardener, housekeeper, waitress, etc.)
      iv. strangers
4. Waiting. Sometimes a child experiences difficulty waiting
   a. When to wait. Make a list of when they need to wait. Practice
   b. What is hard to wait for? Make a list of things that they have a hard time waiting for (e.g., taking turns in class, waiting for their turn at play). This is also an opportunity to learn about the golden rule (treating others and one wishes to be treated)
5. Dealing with anger
   a. The anger thermometer. Draw a thermometer and indicate the intensity of emotion by graded levels. For example, the lower level could be frustration and at the top is furious. Another option is to adapt a 5-point rating scale. Additionally, there is the turtle technique: recognize feeling of anger, think "stop", go inside "shell" and take 3 deep breaths, think calm, think of a solution
   b. Management tools
      i. take a deep breath
      ii. count to 10
      iii. walk away/go to a safe spot
      iv. talk to a caring adult (identify the caring adults in a child's life)
      v. make a list of triggers that cause the child to lose their temper
      vi. make a list of replacement behaviors to substitute for the behaviors they engage in when they lose their temper
      vii. practice. "Let's pretend you are angry because Kenny wouldn't play the game you wanted to play at recess. What could you do instead?" Use real life examples
      viii. catch them being good. "I saw you playing with Kenny, you did a great job!" Shape and reinforce the behavior change
      ix. teach the turtle technique: recognize feeling of anger, think "stop", go inside "shell" and take 3 deep breaths, think calm, think of a solution, do it
6. Using your voice. Learning modulation. Learning to speak more quietly and with appropriate emotion
   a. Using musical instruments. Use musical instruments (like a drum) to illustrate loud vs quiet. One could also use the volume control on the radio for a similar demonstration
   b. Practice volume being low, medium and high

    c. Sound examples. Give examples of the tones associated with different emotions (anger, sadness, happy, etc.)

    d. Environment and tone. Make a list of all the environments the child is exposed to. Then identify the tone of voice that is appropriate for a specific environment (e.g., the tone of voice to use in the class, at the dinner table, on the playground)

7. Cooperation

    a. Cooperative tasks. Make an activity chart demonstrating the tasks that require cooperation. They should be typical requests (such as go to bed, sit at the table, brush your teeth)

    b. When to be a helper (it feels good to help and be appreciated). Identify how we help each other as family members, as a friend, at daycare, etc.

    c. Taking turns. Explain that taking turns provides the opportunity for everyone to do something they want to do when others are also doing it. Role model taking turns and create opportunities for practice

    d. Explain the reasons for limits and requests. Point out how rules help everyone, "when you help me pick up the toys and put them away they are easy to find next time"

    e. Take time to problem solve. Identify the problem, think of solutions, make a choice and redirect. Sometimes they need help in finding acceptable ways to channel their desires or goals

    f. Assign chores at an early age to learn the benefits of cooperation. "Together we can set the table, and then we will have time later to read a book together"

    g. Give specific praise for cooperative efforts to help them recognize their skills

    h. Offer suggestions, not commands. Suggestions elicit cooperation: "It's cold outside so you will need to wear a coat. Can you put it on yourself or do you need help?"

    i. Find a way to offer choices while maintaining the rules. "Your teeth need to be brushed before you go to bed. Do you want to brush your teeth before or after we read the book you chose?"

8. Behavioral management

    a. Help the child identify triggers for the problem behavior (could happen in a single situation or multiple situations)

    b. Determine if the triggers can be eliminated by environmental modifications

    c. Make a list of possible things that the child could do instead of the problem behaviors (replacement behaviors)

    d. Practice the replacement behaviors, using role playing or simulations

    e. Connect the use of the replacement behavior with a reward/reinforcement. Self-regulation works toward internalizing the problem solving process of a child asking themselves: "What is my problem?"; "What is my plan?"; "Am I following my plan?"; "How did I do?"

9. Impulse control

    a. Identify situations where impulsive behavior occurs (such as making the transition from one activity to another)

    b. Agree on a rule for the situations. The rule should focus on what the child can do to control impulses (i.e., use a quieter voice, wait their turn, keep their hands to themselves)

    c. Use a story board to tell the story of steps for how the child is "going to do it differently". For example, if they think they are going to lose control in a situation what are the agreed upon strategies for backing away

       i. removing themselves to a quiet/calming space that has been identified

       ii. removing themselves and asking an adult for help

       iii. counting to ten, going for a run, doing art (drawing), etc.

    d. Practice using the choices to see what works best in what situations. It will help the child understand themselves better, and improve their self-confidence

       i. make a "let's pretend" role play of various situations and choices. Make sure the list represents a range from a situation that presents minimal/no challenge to maximum challenging

10. Task management

    a. Identify the task and break it down into manageable steps. Reinforce the completion of each step

    b. When the child learns the principle to breaking a task down ask them how they would like to break it down. Offering to them the opportunity to practice this step of problem solving.

    c. A fun way to initiate this is to use a story board with sequencing to a variety of tasks provided. Initially, the cards of steps for each task are disorganized. Let the child practice putting them in order. Together talk through each step so that it reinforces the sequence from beginning to end.

    d. Reward their willingness, effort and accomplishment

11. Flexibility. Helping a child to accept changes without distress

    a. Using well rehearsed routines to decrease anxiety/distress. Predictable is comforting

    b. Informing a child ahead of time when changes are being made and prepare them for making the adjustment

    c. Use time ranges when possible to increase flexibility

    d. Use a schedule board showing the child the activities for the day or week. It can be done with pictures. Actually, the adult could make the activity list and ask the child to help create the activity schedule. The child could find the picture that corresponds to the activity on the list and place it on the schedule

    e. Review the schedule at the beginning of the day. If something changes during the day make the change on the schedule and talk the child through the change while they are looking at the visual and then problem solve with them how more effectively to adjust to the change

    f. Start to introduce graduated changes and reinforce the shaping of change

12. Routines. Daily patterns or routines which take place at approximately the same time everyday offer predictability, at a very basic level provide young children with a sense of safety, security, trust and emotional stability. The result is that children feel free to play, explore and learn from interacting with their environment. Additional positive consequences of routines are a decrease in power struggles, self-control, self-confidence, increased social skills, communication skills, and an increased ability to cope with transitions

13. Building self-confidence. Self-confidence is learned through the interactions and experiences with others (primarily caregivers). It is a belief in one's ability to master their own body, behavior and environmental demands. Caregivers reflect to children their strengths and encourage them to try new things – shaping and nurturing their abilities and self-confidence. Children with self-confidence have a positive expectation about how others will respond to them (they will be liked and supported) and are able to meet the challenges of their environment. Self-confidence is fundamental to all aspects of development, important for school success (eager to learn new skills), and social skills (cooperative, making friends). To nurture self-confidence:

    a. Establish routines (predictability) to reinforce feelings of safety, security and confidence in managing daily patterns

    b. Provide an abundance of time to play. Children learn about themselves and others during playtime. Playtime provides the opportunity to increase behavioral skills such as cooperativity, sharing, taking turns, and physical skills (how to use one's body manipulating creative toys, completing puzzles and getting the right shape into the right hole, etc.). Playtime also provides a vehicle for children to process their emotions. A child choosing the role of a superhero may be mastering fears, appropriately venting aggressive feelings or practicing assertiveness. A child pretending to be a mommy going to work may be demonstrating the complicated emotions of separation being processed. Playtime is also a rich opportunity for developing an understanding that others have different perspectives

213

c. Problem solving. It is important to encourage young children to find solutions to their problems to foster their feelings of being successful. Caregivers can offer validation for the frustration of their struggle ("I can see you are frustrated"), encourage the child to identify what the problem is, enquire about their thoughts for dealing with the problem and, if appropriate, offer suggestions. This is also a wonderful opportunity to try out the different solutions, without judgment, to learn about what works, what doesn't and why. They also learn that they can depend upon the caregivers in their life to encourage them. The key is to guide and support confidence, competence and mastery

d. Give responsibilities. Children need to feel useful and have purpose and one of the ways to accomplish this is to give age-appropriate chores. Examples for young children could be picking up toys, feeding pets, helping with laundry, putting old newspapers in the recycle bin, etc.

e. Encourage children to master struggles. Children learn by doing. If the task is overwhelming, break it down into manageable steps to foster and reinforce feeling safe, in control, and confident. Make sure they know you believe in them and there is no disappointment in making the effort and trying (that is how we all learn)

f. Acknowledge and celebrate successes. Take the time to reflect to a child recognition of their growing development and accomplishments

g. Be a role model. Children observe the behavior of their caregivers. There is no better source to learn how to deal with difficult emotions like hurt, disappointment, anger and frustration. Demonstrate persistence and self-confidence. Exhibit interest, love of learning and trying new things. When necessary, try and try again – we don't always get it right the first time around!

14. Communication and learning. Communication is associated with developmental progression. However, the numerous opportunities for simple interaction between a young child and a caregiver provide a rich source sharing pleasure, practicing language skills, and learning. Seize moments like spending time in the garden or buying produce at the grocery store/farmer's market. Through taking turns talking with an interested adult a child can be encouraged to explore all of their senses (smells, colors/shapes, sounds, touch/textures), counting/learning about numbers, learning new words, and practicing language skills.

15. Building communication skills

a. Be responsive. Whether a child is extending their arms for nurturance and comfort or they are in need of support, caregivers reinforce communication skills for expressing what they feel (verbal and non-verbal) leading to appropriately getting their needs met
   i. teach them about non-verbal communication such as different facial expressions, posturing, making eye contact, and being a respectful listener

b. Speaking and listening. When engaging in talking with a young child, be patient and allow them time to respond. Be at their level and make eye contact, thus conveying a desire to hear what they have to say. Ask them open-ended questions so that they have the opportunity to think about new ideas and share those ideas. This reinforces skill development and motivates them to be an active participant. When making a request be clear, simple and match the child's age-appropriate abilities

c. Narration. When spending time with a child they benefit from a caregiver talking through their activity, "I am going to take the clothes out of the dryer, and then take them to the sofa where I will fold them and then I will put the clean folded clothes away". Also talk to them when engaging in play activities and while doing basic routine behaviors like bathing (good opportunity for naming arms, tummy, belly button, etc.). Encourage children to ask questions and answer them without frustration

d. Acknowledge and respect a child's feelings. A child will be more inclined to share their feelings in a safe relationship that is not critical or judgmental. Also, be careful about teasing. There is an appropriate time to be playful and a child needs to understand the context

  e. Develop "feeling" words. Provide a child with the words that describe their emotional experience (sad, happy, frustrated, confused, lonely, excited, etc.)

  f. Encourage pretend play. It is an opportunity to change roles and safely to express difficult emotions such as fear. This also develops empathy

  g. Read to a child and read together. There are times when a story is read to a child. However, a child can also participate in reading time by choosing the book to read and turning pages. A caregiver can also ask a child how the characters in the story feel, what they think will happen next, or how it is going to turn out. Make reading a pleasurable experience

16. Discipline. The goal of discipline is to learn good behaviors and avoid bad behavior (choosing to engage in a good behavior over bad behavior)

  a. Avoid power struggles and do not overreact. Try to solve the problem as quickly as possible

  b. Be interested in a child. Give them plenty of attention and affection

  c. Accept a child's personality. While behaviors can be modified or changed a child cannot change their basic personality

  d. When intervening with a child, do not push them to the level of becoming fatigued and cranky. Also, it is a good routine to give them a head's up when a change is coming to support them making a positive transition

  e. Be consistent about rules, boundaries and consequences otherwise a child becomes confused. Consistency is also predictable which reinforces trust and security

    i. list rules and associated consequences (positive and negative). The list should be short and make sure that the child understands the rules and consequences

  f. Do not embarrass or criticize a child in front of others. That is not respectful and will not result in a positive outcome. Also do not tell a child that they are bad – it is the behavior that is the focus of attention during discipline

  g. Whenever possible, offer a child choices so that they can feel respected. However, limit the number of choices to prevent confusion. For example, do you want to wear the red dress or the blue one?

  h. Praise children for cooperation, a willingness to learn and being a good family member. A caregiver reinforces what works by letting a child know that their good choices are appreciated and helps the family

17. Helping young children manage the most difficult behaviors

  a. Tantrums/hair pulling/biting. All of these behaviors are indicative of losing control. Therefore, do not treat as a disciplinary issue. Instead, if a child is having a tantrum, get on the floor with the child to make sure there is nothing that will harm the child (such as sharp objects, furniture, etc.). These behaviors can happen when a child feels stressed/pushed and lacks the skill to manage it. Frustration builds, especially when a child's internal development does not match their ability to verbalize and manage what they are feeling. A young child's behavior has a purpose, but sometimes their feelings are so intense they act out. Nonetheless, the behavior is not acceptable and will not result in them appropriately getting their needs met. Some alternatives for management include:

    i. acknowledge the underlying emotion, look for the positive intent, and respond to the impulse ("I can see that you are angry...")

    ii. educate and provide a behavioral limit/boundary. Keep it simple ("We don't bite...pull hair...have tantrums"). Demonstrate gentle touch and then have them do it

    iii. encourage a child to find the words to express their feelings and use them

    iv. provide alternatives. If they need to sooth themselves provide options, if they are struggling with waiting to take a turn role model the right way to go about it or

215

how to make a different choice. For example, "if you are angry you can stomp you feet, go for a run, use your words, etc".

   v. if necessary, separate the child from the environment for calming, educating and redirecting. Use good judgment and do not emotionally overload the child

  vi. do not respond to the child with the behavior that they have demonstrated (biting, hitting or humiliating them by reflecting a tantrum)

b. Aggressive behavior – the bully child. It is not uncommon that aggressive behavior is an effort to control social dynamics by excluding other children. The child who acts aggressively has often been the victim of hurtful behavior by a peer. Children often exclude a peer because they have been excluded themselves. If bullying behavior is witnessed, immediately intervene:

    i. be clear and direct that the behavior is not acceptable

- don't touch. Direct: keep your hands down (model and say with eye contact). Reinforce: You are a good listener, you are looking with hands down!
- no yelling. Direct: use a calm voice/use your inside voice. Reinforce: (in a low voice) Now I can listen, you are using a calm (inside) voice
- don't hit. Direct: hands down. Hands are for playing, working, eating, and hugging. Use your words (give child appropriate words to use for expressing emotion). Reinforce: You are using your words. Good for you!
- no biting. Direct: we only bite food. Use your words if you are upset (give the child appropriate words to express their feelings). Reinforce: You're upset, thanks for telling me. What are some ways to deal with being upset?

   ii. redirect. Talk with them about appropriate ways to talk with and play with others. Offer choices, maybe they need to start a new activity that will help them discharge aggressive energy. Also, help them to use their words to express how they feel so that they can participate in problem solving

  iii. support a child's efforts to reach out to friends. This could be encouraged by structured play time, reinforcing positive behaviors, and then monitoring during free play to be assured that behaviors have generalized

  iv. it is easier to avoid bullying behavior when children play 1-1 such as on play dates or by arranged activities done in pairs. Monitoring is important

   v. *If a child is being chronically victimized (more than one setting), it could be the result of their difficulty being socially adept. This needs to be addressed. Help them to develop assertive behavior, how to deflect teasing, and how to demonstrate their strength. Victims sometimes remain the focus because they reward bully's by crying, looking fearful or withdrawing. Assertiveness stops bully/victimizing behavior from others

c. Disruptive behavior. Needing attention and approval is normal, and only becomes a problem when it happens all of the time, is excessive and is controlling. The most common reason for a young child to misbehave is to get attention. The goal is to eliminate the attention-seeking behaviors which are excessive and unacceptable while seeking to understand the underlying feelings and needs of the child so that those needs can be appropriately met

    i. strike a balance between attention seeking/need for attention versus demands for attention

   ii. give generous nurturance. Also give attention and approval for being well behaved – positive attention (negative attention is not a punishment it is a reward). When a caregiver ignores positive behavior and pays attention when a child misbehaves then the child is being taught to misbehave

  iii. make it a practice to catch a child being good and spend time with them playing and listening to them. Children want and need caring and nurturing relationships with caregivers

    iv. when to ignore misbehaviors associated with the demands for negative attention. Some misbehaviors should be disciplined. It takes timing and judgment:
- a caregiver cannot allow a child to push their buttons
- if misbehavior persists for more than a few minutes give a reminder, "I do not respond to whining (or whatever)". If the behavior persists for another few minutes beyond the reminder discipline, "stop now, or you will go to time-out"

  d. Defiance. The defiant child may seem rigid and inflexible. They may not want other children "messing up" their room or playing with their toys. They may not like going to the homes of other children where they do not have their favorite things

    i. a defiant child may be controlling and/or shy, stubborn or negative – dealing with their world in a bossy way. One view of the child asserting "no" is that it is an effort to define themselves

    ii. a common time frame for the display of defiance is around transitions. Therefore, make a practice out of preparing a child for the transition that is coming

    iii. many defiant children are very clever, deliberate, and purposeful – figuring out ways to defeat the most sophisticated arguments. They may even reject efforts to comfort them. Be respectful, offer choices (that means two choices for young children) and appropriately set limits, redirect, and reinforce positive desirable behaviors

    iv. basic rules
- set appropriate limits, "it's time to pick up the toys…"
- offer a few acceptable choices
- be creative to engage the child
- when necessary enforce limits (choices and associated consequences)
- be consistent. A lack of consistency is confusing and will interfere with learning

RSDP Hypersensitive/Over-responsive Type/Distractible

The characterizations include:

- Has a quick or intense response that results in
  - exaggerated responses (fight or flight)
  - or withdrawn (flight or freeze)
- Their behavior indicates that the child has
  - an intense and often scattered perception of sensory input from their body
  - a perception of their body in their sensorimotor cortex referred to as a "firecracker" perception which contributes to an exaggerated but scattered perception of themselves as they move and interact with their environment
- Responds to activities that provide a clear localized sense of their body
- Tends to be distractible and may display hyperactivity
- Patterns of directing their attention to the latest stimulus presented, which draws them away from what they are trying to accomplish
- They might be cautious about proceeding in some situations because they missed something
- Disjointed movement, wander from object to object (distractible vs focused)

TREATMENT

1. Providing very specific localized points of contact such as engaging in play on firm surfaces. This gives the child localized points of input with limited variability. Thus, providing the child with specific and intense sensory input. A sensory anchor, so to speak, to attend to in the morass of exaggerated responses
2. Avoid activities or handling that encompasses (wraps) the child's body as their body response indicates that this is an overwhelming experience. They usually get escalated in

soft surfaces (hammocks, lycra material, etc.). The sensory "firecracker" is overwhelmed by too much stimulation

3. Caregiver to position themselves in the child's line of vision so that they can anticipate what the caregiver is going to do by interpreting the caregiver's body language
4. A brushing program may help to address the sensitivity to touch. It is important to include compression after the brushing. It is the combination of brushing and compression that is an effective intervention for the sensory defensive child
5. Provide quiet, calm spaces when possible
6. Watch for cues from the child that the environment is overly stimulating (i.e., some children love loud noises, but the hypersensitive child may cover their ears)
7. Find out the best way to show comfort, and help the child's peers to show comfort in similar ways (i.e., let the child's peers know how close is too close)

RSDP Hyposensitive/Under-reactive Type/Withdrawn

The characterizations include:

- Slow to respond to sensory stimulus
- Requires a high intensity or increased duration to invoke an observed behavioral response
- Behavior suggests that this child has
  - a diminished perception of sensory input from their body
  - a cloudy or hazy perception of their body sometimes referred to as the "novacain sensorimotor cortex" which may contribute to a diminished perception of themselves as they move or interact with their environment
- Responds to activities that increase their sense of their body map
- Tend to appear uninterested
- Can have a flat or dull affect
- Low energy levels, act as if overly tired all of the time
- Self-absorbed, focused inward.

The brain is not getting what it needs to generate responses, and the child's inclination to respond in accordance with high thresholds results in an apathetic, self-absorbed appearance.

TREATMENT

1. Contouring of the caregiver body around the child's so that they have an increased sense of where their body begins and ends
2. Play in materials that wrap the child (lycra fabrics, hammocks, tunnels, etc.)
3. Lycra suits or similar fashion/fabric may be beneficial as it provides a second skin – each time the child moves the spandex of the suit provides another layer of feedback as the body moves
4. Following the child's cues if they are seeking out sensory input. The caregiver may be inclined to try to stop or inhibit sensory-seeking behavior. Unfortunately, that stops or takes away the stimulation which often makes the child more distressed and they will continue to seek input. Therefore, it is important to provide safe avenues for the child to fill and satiate this need fore sensory input
5. Slowly/gradually introduce any sensory stimuli such as lights, noise, or physical touch. A light dimmer switch is great, and starting the TV at a lower volume and slowing increasing the sound is helpful
6. Avoid loud crowded environments and overstimulating areas full of bright lights
7. Allow the child to wear ear plugs or head phones when they have to be in a noisy environment (such as a school bus)
8. Provide the child with sunglasses they can keep with them to help deal with bright lights
9. Encourage the child to experience new things, but do not force them to have contact with bothersome or aversive stimuli or environments which cause them to be fearful

10. Try slowly to introduce new textures into their diet with repeated exposure
11. Prepare the child ahead of time for places they are going. It also helps to illustrate the type of stimuli that they will be coming in contact with
12. Provide interactive input and exaggerated gestures
13. Reach out to the child: use animated expressions
14. Give robust responses to the child's cues (however slight the cue may be)

RSDP Sensory Stimulation Seeking/Impulsive/Sensation Seeking

The characterizations include:

- Active and continuously engaged in their environments
- Appear excitable or seem to lack consideration for safety while playing
- Add sensory input to every experience in the daily life,
  - they make noises while working
  - fidget, rub or explore objects with their skin, chew on things, and wrap body parts around furniture or other people as a means to increase input during tasks
- Breaking toys, things are always in their mouth.

TREATMENT

1. Provide a lot of opportunity for physical activities and movement experiences, such as jumping on trampolines, swinging, running, and sitting on a therapy ball for sensory input
2. Provide the child with constructive opportunities for sensory and affective involvement
3. Utilize weighted vests and blankets to help the child be more aware of their body
4. Have the child change positions frequently when doing activities, such as sitting, kneeling, laying down, etc.
5. Use a lot of hand gestures and animated tone of voice, possibly even sign language or a picture exchange communication system when speaking to the child to provide them with extra sensory input to illustrate the message
6. Encourage and teach the child to recognize their own limits, especially with regard to issues of safety
7. Encourage the use of imagination and support exploration of the external environment

219

The "sensory diet" is a personalized activity plan for children with RSPD to assure that their sensory input needs for the day are met. There is a basic rule of thumb associated to nervous system functioning. For example, some children need a more calming input (Figure 3.10) while others need more stimulating or arousing input. The sensory diet is viewed as resulting in meeting immediate needs and being cumulative as well. It is the structuring of activities that stimulate or calm a child effectively in the moment as well as aiding to restructure the child's nervous system over time. It is a challenge to identify the appropriate calibration of sensory input. The ingredients of a sensory diet can be found at http://www.sensorysmarts.com/diet.html

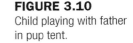

FIGURE 3.10
Child playing with father in pup tent.

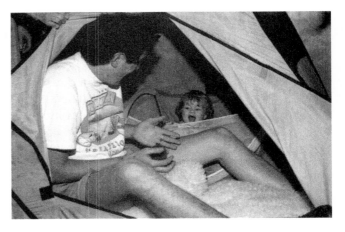

TREATMENT STRATEGIES FOR ALL CHILDREN

1. Show soothing and respectful support of the child's individual needs
2. Prepare the child for transitions. Announce transitions to the child who needs extra time to adjust; when significant changes are happening (such as moving to a new room), a slow and gradual change with plenty of emotional support to aid the child's adjustment

3. Show the child empathy and love. A caregiver who can manage a demonstration of caring in the face of negativism or rejection will support the child's development. It may take time, but persist with consistent demonstrations of empathy and care

4. Help the child engage, attend to, interact with, and explore their environment

CO-MORBIDITY AND STABILITY

Regulatory disorders of sensory processing can exist with other disorders, as with any condition. RSPD is often confused diagnostically with ADHD. Once diagnostic clarity is achieved, it may still be useful to pull from the treatment planning interventions from ADHD and integrate the objective into the treatment for the RSPD diagnosed child. The diagnostic issue of co-morbidity has an impact on the treatment frame. The hypersensitivity subtype who is fearful/cautious may also exhibit separation anxiety disorder, while the hypersensitive type who is negative/defiant may also demonstrate oppositional defiant disorder. The sensory, motor, and behavioral responses of the child with RDSP has characteristics that interact with and compound the problems presented by the symptoms of other diagnoses. Regardless of what diagnoses the child struggles with, the most important question to be answered by the treatment team is, "what can be done to prevent the progression of symptoms and improve their quality of life including maximizing learning capacity".

Dyspraxia and Developmental Coordination Disorder

Generally, children master developmental skills around the same ages which are referred to as developmental milestones. For children identified as having dyspraxia (difficulty in conceiving of, planning, and carrying out an unfamiliar motor action or series of motor actions) and developmental coordination disorder, there is difficulty learning new motor skills and, as a result, their motor development is delayed in comparison to their peers. While they are young this difference in motor functioning appears to be subtle. However, as they age, there is greater disparity in motor skills. Identification of delayed motor development is key to getting help and subsequently establishing a thorough understanding of what to expect from the child at various developmental stages.

1. Improve body awareness – as evidenced by appearance of being clumsy/awkward and frequently exhibiting difficulty with gross and fine motor skills/activities requiring subtle changes in posture, strength, force or dexterity. Body awareness is imperative for physical coordination and moving their bodies and objects regarding spatial orientation. A number of activities that can be presented as games make mastery of body awareness fun for a child:
   a. Play Simon says, instructing the child to copy or imitate movements or to respond to verbal instruction. For example:
      i. close your eyes, nod your head, turn your head, shrug your shoulders, wiggle your toes and fingers
      ii. touch body parts with body parts: nose to knee, chin to chest, ear to shoulder, hands to hips, wrist to ankle,wrist to ear, elbow to leg, chin to wrist, fingers to shoulders
      iii. touching body parts to objects, such as "touch your"….head to the wall, hands to the door, knees to the floor, nose/ears/mouth to the chair, elbows/finger/wrists to the …, feet/toes to the…, back/stomach/shoulders to the…
      iv. lateral physical action (do them on the right side and then instruct/model doing them on the left side). For example, stomp the right foot, wave the right hand, hop on the right foot, wiggle the toes on your right foot, slap the right thigh, wiggle the thumb on your right hand, point your tongue to the right, shake your right leg, bend the right elbow, slide to the right
   b. Have the child close their eyes and touch body parts as instructed

    c. Have the child get down on all fours on the floor and ask them to raise a right or left arm or leg. As their balance improves instruct them to raise an opposite arm and leg (e.g., right arm and left leg)

    d. Play hokey pokey including ears, chin, hands, arms, shoulder, legs, feet…

    e. Make a body puzzle. Instruct the child to lie down on a large sheet of paper and trace around their body. Then ask them to fill in the body parts, name them/color them. When this is completed, cut out the shape and then take the body parts (puzzle pieces) and have them arrange the pieces to look like their body. *We had fun doing this by using the cut body part pieces and using them as a template to make a life size cookie as a reward!

    f. Draw or show the child incomplete people/faces and ask then to identify the missing parts

2. The development of fine motor skills referring to the use of fingers, hands and arms. Such skills include reaching, grasping, manipulating objects, and using different tools like crayons and scissors. Supporting the development of fine motor skills is often overlooked until a child starts school. The following information is intended only as a guide. The professional working with the child and caregiver is responsible to ascertain if the child is capable of the tasks in that range. Additionally, individual differences influence rate of learning with some children acquiring skills more quickly than others

    a. 0–4 months: the baby will move their arms and hands together to bat at objects or visual stimuli. Bilateral control should be equal. The child will also develop the ability to move their eyes and head in a coordinated manner from side to side, which is required for further development of fine motor skills. For example, turning their head from left to right to track the sound of their caregiver's voice. Between 2 and 3 months the child begins to reach for objects and hold them in the middle of their body. At this age their grasp is reflexive, therefore, they will not be able to purposefully release objects in their grasp

    b. 4–12 months: at this stage the baby gains increased control over their arms and makes progress from reaching with both hands to reaching toward an object with one hand. Voluntary movement develops with demonstrated increased capability of grasping and holding onto objects. At about 4 months, they will not only grasp objects but squeeze and hold them in a closed fist. At about the age of 6 months, the baby will pick up small objects like a raisin. By 12 months they have achieved the dexterity to hold small objects between their thumb and index finger, as well as being able to transfer an object from one hand to the other and release the object voluntarily. To begin with they will learn to coordinate their eyes and head to move up and down in sync. This will progress to being able visually to find an object and purposefully reach for it. Also at the end of this stage of development (12 months) they will be able to mark with a crayon/marker, stack ring/blocks, turn pages and roll a ball

    c. 1–2 years: there will be a demonstrated improvement in the child's sitting balance and trunk control whereby they will no long need to use their arms for support. They will sit unsupported while using their hands for play. Hand and arm use is characterized by the whole arm moving together and both arms being used equally. As the child approaches the age of 2, hand preference begins to emerge, but is not solidly established, demonstrated by the use of one hand over the other to initiate activity, but there is still some alternate hand use. Hand use changes dramatically in other ways too. The child begins to move fingers. For example, pointing at bubbles, using whole arm movements to color and will hold the crayon in a closed fist with the thumb pointing up. Generally, by age 2 the child's coloring progresses from circular scribbles to either vertical or horizontal scribble

    d. 2–3 years: the child's balance and trunk stability allow them to maintain posture when they reach away from their body or shift their weight to one side. There is less shoulder movement during hand use and more movement from the elbow. Hand dominance continues, but still is not established. During such activities as opening a container, one hand will lead the other as one hand is used to hold the container and the other hand is used to remove the lid. The child continues to alternate use and assist roles between the right and left hand. When drawing, a crayon or pencil will be held with fingers pointing toward the paper (pronated pencil grasp). They now begin to follow drawing modeled by another, drawing vertical and horizontal lines and eventually circles, as well as imitating the drawing of a shape when shown how to do it by another (imitation). At about age 3, they should be able to draw horizontal and vertical lines and eventually a circle when shown a picture form of them (copying). They will always be able to imitate a shape or form before being able to copy it. At approximately 2 years of age, the child will use both hands to open and close scissors. By age 3, this has progressed to them being able to use one hand to snip a piece of paper in half. They will not yet be able to cut along a line at this age

  e. 3–4 years: finally, there is a demonstrated strong preference for a dominant hand, but switching continues. When drawing, the dominant hand will be holding the crayon while the other hand holds the paper in place. There is a progress from being able to draw lines and circles to drawing crosses (+) and tracing over diamond and triangles. They will not yet be able to accomplish keeping their coloring within the lines. By age 4, the child should be holding the crayon with 3 fingers, pinched between the thumb, index finger and middle finger (tripod grasp). This is the mature and efficient pencil grasp. During cutting, the child should be able to move the scissors in a forward direction and cut along a straight line, and when cutting a curve they begin to turn the paper cutting around the curve

  f. 4–5 years: at this age, hand use is characterized by refined wrist and finger movements as well as decreased elbow and shoulder movement. Drawing reveals a combination of finger and wrist movement and hand dominance is established or close to it (age 4–6). Therefore, hand preference is fairly consistent. As a result, the skill of the dominant hand begins to exceed that of the non-dominant hand. While coloring, the child has greatly improved the ability to stay within the lines. They are also able to copy crosses, diagonal lines and squares using a tripod pencil grasp. Scissors are held in a thumb up position pointing away from the body and should be positioned perpendicular to the floor

  g. 5–6 years: at this stage, both hands work together, and the roles of dominance between the left and right hand are easily identified. During pencil use, a tripod grasp should be strongly established and the child should be able to copy triangles and diamonds. Small precise finger movements are evident during coloring exercises, and the child is able to hold scissors in an adult manner

3. Fine motor activities for preschool children. The development of fine motor skills is imperative to a child's success throughout their educational experience. Fine motor skills are the ability to grasp and utilize an object with their hands. This skill, though taken for granted, is necessary for almost all our basic daily living skills (dressing, bathing, writing, cutting, etc.)

  a. Scissor ships. Draw broad, straight lines on a sheet of paper. Tell children that scissors are like big ships breaking through ice and they have to be opened wide before they can move through the ice

  b. Making pizza. Give a child a piece of clay about the size of their palm and instruct them to roll the clay into a ball using both hands. They are instructed to not roll it on the table. Once in a ball, they are to flatten it with their hands. Next they are to pinch off small pieces and roll them into tiny balls using the thumb and index finger of one hand (to represent sausage). They then place the "sausage" on the pizza

  c. Secret key. Get a box with a padlock and put snack goodies and prizes such as stickers or small super-balls, etc., into this box. Place several keys in front of the box. Only one key is the correct key and the child must manipulate the keys in order to get the prize they choose inside

   d. Rubber-band wrap. Give a child various sizes of rubber bands along with a couple of different size cans/jars. The child must stretch the rubber bands over these objects

   e. Scissor cutting activities. Using old magazines, greeting cards, and newspapers have the child look for specific letters or pictures, cut them out and make a collage out of them

   f. Jewelry making. Provide macaroni (could be dyed different colors), buttons and beds and have the child make jewelry

   g. Building block activities. The child uses blocks, Lincoln logs, legos, or tinker toys to build and/or copy designs

   h. Coloring. The child uses crayons, colored pencils or markers to color pre-drawn pictures

   i. Push pegs. Draw circles or other shapes on a piece of styrofoam. Give the child golf tees or small wood dowels to push through the Styrofoam. This reinforces tip-to-tip grasp with the thumb and index finger

   j. Sand writing. Place a layer of sand or flour in a baking pan. Ask the child to write or draw in the sand

   k. Chalk scraps. Give the child small pieces of colored scrap chalk. Instruct them to hold the chalk piece between their thumb and first two fingers (the last two fingers can remain next to the second finger, but not touching the chalk). Allow the child to draw on the chalkboard using this grasp. This grasp reinforces the proper way to hold a pencil for writing tasks

   l. Pick up objects. Have the child pick up small objects like pennies, paper clips, marbles or beans and place them in a box with a small opening

   m. Q-tip art. Have the child paint pictures with a q-tip

   n. Card bowl. Cut a small rectangular shape in the lid of a bowl (like a cool whip bowl). Have them put playing cards through the hole one card at a time

   o. Spoons. Have the child pick up beans with a spoon and transfer them from one container to another. Remind them to use the proper grasp such as holding a pencil

   p. American sign language. Teach the child basic letters and/or signs

4. Identify problem areas in a child's everyday life, and working out practical solutions. This is accomplished by observing the child at home, school and playing to see where problems are experienced. When a problem is identified the actions are broken down into small steps and practicing the individual movements. Examples:

   a. Dressing themselves

   b. Balance. Use of a balance board to develop balance, core strength and flexibility

   c. Use of crutches when walking/stair lift at home

   d. Using eating utensils

   e. Writing

   f. Reading and spelling

5. Perceptual motor training. These tasks include:

   a. Language skills (only able to make certain sounds, leave out parts of words, speak too slowly/quickly or too loudly/quietly)

      i. exercises to move the lips or tongue in a certain way

      ii. practicing producing a certain sound

      iii. learning to control their breathing

   b. Visual and auditory (hearing and listening) skills

   c. Movement skills

Intervention for Caregivers of Children with RSPD

1. Educate them regarding sensory processing. Identifying the problem early in life gives the child a better chance of decreasing the effects of that problem on their life

2. Educate them regarding the importance of engaging in activities that are appropriately sensory enriching for the child (based upon the specific needs of the child)
3. Provide activities or procedures that make engaging in life events pleasant and natural for the caregiver and child
4. Help the caregiver to feel all right about themselves and reinforce their efforts in using the tools provided to them
5. Help the caregivers create the correct type of control in the environment
6. Help the family system learn how to play to enhance and enrich positive family experiences

GREENSPAN'S FLOOR-TIME TECHNIQUES

Dr Greenspan's contribution to improving the lives of children is to be heralded. One of his contributions is the Floor-time techniques or strategies for helping a child tune into parent(s) and to their entire world so that they could build two-way communication. The quality of the parent–child relationship bears a significant influence upon the development of healthy social, emotional, and behavioral adjustment, as well as setting the framework for other settings such as school. So, for parents, a few gifts of ideas from Dr Greenspan:

- Follow your child's lead and join him. It doesn't matter what the activity is as long the child initiates the move
- Encourage and reinforce their persistence in their pursuit
- Treat everything your child does as intentional and purposeful. Give their apparent random actions new meaning and respond to them as if they were purposeful
- Help your child to do or accomplish what is important to them
- Position yourself in front of your child (1 to 1 and making eye contact)
- Invest in whatever your child initiates or imitates
- Join your child's perseverative play
- Do not treat avoidance or "no" as rejection
- Expand, expand, expand; play dumb, make the wrong move, do what your child tells you to do, interfere with what they are doing. Do whatever it takes to keep the interaction going
- Do not interrupt or change the subject as long as your child is interacting
- Insist on a response (stay engaged with your child and demonstrating interest)
- Use sensory-motor play-bouncing, tickling, swinging, etc. This is designed to elicit pleasure
- Use sensory toys in cause and effect ways: hide a toy, then make it magically reappear; drop a bell so that your child will hear the jingle; bring a "tickle feather" closer, closer and closer until you finally tickle your child with it
- Play infant games, such as peek-a-boo, "I'm going to get you", and patty cake
- Pursue pleasure over other behaviors and do not interrupt any pleasurable experience
- Use gestures, tone of voice, and body language to accentuate the emotion in what you say and do
- Try to be as accepting of your child's anger and protests as you are of their more positive emotions
- Help your child deal with anxiety (separation, getting hurt, aggression, loss, fear, etc.) by using gestures and problem solving

Specific Floor-time Strategies

While there are numerous Floor-time strategies to address processing difficulties, below are a few to offer an idea of how important it is to learn from masters, who earned their richness and depth of understanding by working for decades in the field such as Dr Greenspan and

224

Dr DeGangi. They collaborated often in their work. Dr Greenspan offered the following solutions to child actions:

Childa ctions	Therapist/parent solutions
Avoids, moves away	Persist in your pursuit, treat as intentional, provide visual cues, playfully obstruct, attract with "magic", insist on a response
Stays stuck, does not Know what to do next	Provide destination, return object of interest, use object in some way, expand, expand, expand, give new meanings, use ritualized cues to start, i.e., "ready, set, go"
Usesc ripts	Join in, offer alternative script, change
Protests	Act sorry, play dumb, restore, blame figure
Rejects,r efuses	Provide more things for him to say "no" to, expand, give other choices or time
Says something unrelated	Insist on a response, notice change, bring closure
Become anxious or fearful	Reassure, problem solve, use symbolic solutions
Acts out, pushes, hits	Provide affective cue ("uh, oh"; "no, no, no") to encourage self-regulation, set limits, reward for absence of negative behaviors

Additional Treatment Caveats

DETECTING VISUAL IMPAIRMENT

Some visual impairments are genetic and, as a result, are detected soon after birth. However, The American Academy of Pediatrics (AAP) recommends the following vision screening be performed at all well-child visits for children, starting in the newborn period to 3 years; ocular history, vision assessment, external inspection of the eyes and lids, ocular motility assessment, pupil examination, and red reflex examination. For children aged 3–5 years, the AAP recommends the aforementioned screening in addition to age-appropriate visual acuity measurements and ophthalmoscopy. The clinical practice guideline of the American Optometric Association can be accessed at http://www.aoa.org/eweb/Documents/CPG-2-pdf

225

DETECTING HEARING LOSS

Current technology allows for the accurate assessment of hearing in children starting within a few hours following birth. A child with an undiagnosed hearing loss may not be able to develop normal speech and language or acquire the cognitive abilities of knowing, thinking and judging which are needed for learning. Unfortunately, if a child's hearing loss is not identified until they are 2 or 3 years old they may suffer from permanent impairment of speech, language, and learning.

The initiation of treatment and rehabilitation that can be initiated by early identification increases the possibility of learning more normal speech skills. There are many subtle gradations between normal hearing and deafness. A child's hearing loss may not be apparent, therefore the early screening is imperative.

AUDITORY PROCESSING DISORDER (ADP)

Auditory processing is what happens when the brain recognizes and interprets the sounds that are heard. An APD means that something is adversely affecting the processing or interpretation of the information heard. Children with APD often do not recognize the subtle differences between sounds or words, even though the sounds or words are clear. Being in a noisy environment is an additional complicating factor for the child with APD.

LEARNING DISABILITIES

Learning disability is the common term used to describe specific kinds of learning problems. A learning disability can negatively impact the ability to learn as well as using certain skills. Learning disabilities vary from one individual to another, and the same type of learning disability may present different difficulties for two different children. The most common skills affected are:

- Reading
- Writing
- Listening (receptive language)
- Speaking (expressive language)
- Reasoning
- Math

Wolraich et al (2008) offer the following conclusion on how to enhance academic outcomes for children with learning disabilities:

1. Task analytic instruction is imperative. This refers to instruction being explicit and well organized. Thus, providing opportunity for cumulative reviews of prior mastered content
2. Strategy instruction. Teaching children strategic behaviors to maximize their performance by monitoring progress, setting goals, and transferring and maintaining skills
3. Peer mediation as an effective method for extending task-analytic instruction and strategy instruction. This is done by creating structured opportunities that enhance the gaining of knowledge and extend transfer of learned content into daily activities (inside the classroom and out)
4. It is recommended that teachers provide systematic instruction on academic performance to strengthen foundation skills while simultaneously working directly to improve comprehension
5. Gains are directly related to what is specifically taught. If interventions do not teach academic content, little academic learning will be achieved
6. A child's progress must be frequently monitored to allow for program re-evaluation and a child's individual response to programming in order to ensure adequate progress over time

Learning disabilities are life long without a cure. However, a child with learning disabilities can be a high achiever and taught ways to learn successfully. IDEA's definition of "Learning disability":

> "…a disorder in one or more basic psychological processes involved in understanding or in using language, spoken or written, that may manifest itself in imperfect ability to listen, think, speak, read, write, spell, or do mathematical calculations, including conditions such as perceptual disabilities, brain injury, minimal brain dysfunction, dyslexia, and other developmental aphasia"

> Learning disabilities do not include "…learning problems that are primarily the result of visual, hearing, or motor disabilities, of mental retardation, or emotional disturbance, or of environmental, cultural, or economic disadvantage." 34 Code of Federal Regulations ξ300.7(c)(10).

EXECUTIVE FUNCTION

Executive function describes a set of mental processes indicative of social and emotional intelligence. It connects past experience with present action. Executive function is known as the operational system which performs activities such as planning, organizing, strategizing, and paying attention to and remembering details. The executive functions are a set of processes associated with managing oneself and one's resources in order to achieve a goal. There are a related and overlapping set of skills. Daily functioning, regardless of environment is seen in abilities such as:

- Making plans
- Being able to track more than one thing

- Keeping track of time
- Being able to include knowledge from past experiences in a meaningful way
- Engage in group activities in a cooperative way and managing group dynamics
- Evaluating ideas
- Being able to reflect on work product
- Being flexible to change one's mind in the middle of a process and making corrections
- Staying on task to finish work/project on time
- Asking for help (resources)
- Waiting to speak until called upon or waiting to take their turn
- Knowing when to seek more information.

Another way of viewing these skills or using psychological terms would be the following list. *Remember, it is important to understand that children often attribute success and failure to internal/external factors differently:

- Delay of gratification
- Flexibility (shift from one situation to another)
- Emotional control
- Initiation (ability to begin a task)
- Working memory (being able to access the information needed to complete a task)
- Planning/organization (the challenge of managing the current and future demands of a task)
- Organization (imposing order on play, school, organizing personal space)
- Self-monitoring (monitoring one's own performance)

Obviously, children who experience problems with executive function have problems with planning, organizing, and managing time and space, in addition to impairment or weakness with a "working memory". This difficulty negatively impacts a child in finishing their work on time, asking for help when needed, and seeking more information. Strategies that may be helpful:

1. General strategies
   a. Take step-by-step approaches to work and use visual organizational aids
   b. Employ tools like time organizers, timers, computers or watches with alarms
   c. Prepare visual schedules and review them several times a day (i.e., schedule board)
   d. Plan and structure transition times and shifts in activities
2. Managing time
   a. Create checklist or to do lists, allocating adequate time for completion and be prepared to offer reminders and positive reinforcement
   b. Break long assignments or tasks into chunks and assign time frames for completing each chunk or approximation
   c. Use visual calendars to keep track of longer-term assignments, due dates, chores, activities
3. Managing space and material
   a. Organize work space
   b. Minimize clutter and distractions
   c. Consider having separate work areas with complete sets of supplies for different activities to decrease confusion and distractibility
   d. Schedule time to clear and organize
4. Managing work/assignments
   a. Make a checklist for task management. For example, get out pencil and paper, put name on paper, put date on paper
   b. Check with teacher when task is complete (or they think it is complete, thus allowing for redirection and reinforcement for what has been completed)

227

PERVASIVE DEVELOPMENTAL DISORDERS

Pervasive Developmental Disorders describe a child who demonstrates severe and persistent difficulties in several areas of development. Social interactions, language, communication, repetitive and stereotypical behavior (restricted range of behaviors, activities, and interests) may be affected by Pervasive Developmental Disorder (PDD). The diagnostic category of PDD serves as an umbrella for Austistic Disorder, Rett's Disorder, Childhood Disintegrative Disorder, Asperger's Syndrome, and PDD NOS. Autism is the most common diagnosis in this disorder spectrum and will be the focus of this section. Mental retardation may or may not be associated. There is no cure for PDD and treatment is a complex and time-consuming task. Treatment typically involves the framework of an individualized intervention program with multiple independent interventions, coordinated to meet the short- and long-term goals for the child while interfacing with family intervention.

This brief explanation is being added because of the political/legal role currently addressing mandated treatment.

According to Johnson et al (2007), there are three major diagnostic challenges for professionals making a comprehensive assessment of a child with suspected ASD:

1. Determining global level of functioning
2. Clarifying the diagnosis of an ASD
3. Determining to explore and identify associated etiology

To accomplish these three diagnostic tasks of the comprehensive evaluation should include the following

1. Health, developmental, and behavioral histories of at least 3 generations and a review of systems
2. Physical examination including an exploration of dysmorphic features and neurologic abnormalities
3. Diagnostic and psychometric evaluation (age/skill appropriate) to determine the child's overall level of functioning and if there is incongruence between motor-adaptive problem-solving and social communication skills is evident
4. Determination of the presence of a specific DSM IV-TR diagnosis (preferably identified with standardized tools that operationalize the DSM diagnostic criteria)
5. Assessment of the parent's knowledge of ASD's, coping skills, and associated available supports
6. Referral for further lab testing to explore etiology or coexisting conditions as guided by information elicited in steps 1–5

The treatment range is diverse. On one hand is Applied Behavioral Analysis (ABA) and on the other are the treatment interventions associated with sensory processing. ABA uses behavioral learning theory (based on Skinner) to modify behavior by focusing on the observable relationship of behavior to the environment. An assessment is made to determine the relationship between a targeted behavior and the environment (behavior transaction), and then selected ABA interventions are employed to change that behavior. ABA targets areas that are of social significance. Thus ABA signifies practical importance (social importance) as that being essential and not necessarily any underlying cause (Sprectley & Boyd, 2009).

Regarding sensory processing, if one were to be sitting in an audience of a presentation being given by those who recognize the influence of sensory processing (Greenspan, DeGangi, Trott to name a few) they would espouse the importance of gathering information associated to medical history, past and current family history, home environment, attachment, interactions between parents/caretakers and the child, the child's behavior and coping in the full range of their daily experiences (who, what, where, and when), and most meaningfully seeking to understand the display and patterns of challenging behaviors and emotions.

Therefore, interventions are based on *functional behavioral analysis* for the family and the child by utilizing sensory integration and behavior strategies. In order to develop an effective behavior change program it is essential to determine to the greatest extent what components of the behavior are primarily sensory and what components are conditioned.

Children with autism have differences in the development of their thinking, language, behavior and social skills. No single treatment was identified as being superior in the treatment of autism. What is key is to start treatment as early and intensively as possible in an effort to improve their behavior, communication and social skills. Treatment may include support and facilitation, behavior modification, educational therapy, and pharmacological intervention.

http://www.nidcd.nih.gov/health/voice/autism.asp

http://autismspeaks.org/science/programs/atn/

http://www.cdc.gov/actearly

INTELLECTUAL DISABILITY

Intellectual disability refers to limitations in intellectual functioning and associated skills of communication, self-care, and social skills. As a consequence of these limitations, a child will develop and learn at a slower rate than the typical child and present with a ceiling that is related to their intellectual age level capacity. They will learn more slowly than other children and there will be some things that they cannot learn. The definition of "intellectual disability" under IDEA:

> "...significantly subaverage general intellectual functioning, existing concurrently with deficits in adaptive behavior and manifested during the developmental period, that adversely affects a child's educational performance."

Early intervention is available as a system of services to help infants and toddlers with disabilities (until their 3rd birthday) as mandated by IDEA in the form of an IFSP which is used to emphasize the unique needs of the child and family. These children need support in learning basic adaptive life skills to be facilitated by educators and caregivers:

- Social communicating
- Caring for basic personal needs of hygiene and grooming (dressing, bathing, going to the bathroom)
- Health behaviors
- Safety behaviors
- Home/family life skills (cleaning, setting the table, preparing food/meals)
- Social skills (manners, conversation rules, group dynamics and getting along with others in a group, following the rules of playing a game, etc.)
- Basic education skills of reading, writing, math
- Development of workplace skills

To learn more about early intervention services:

http://www.nichcy.org/state-organization-search-by-state

http://www.nichcy.org/babies/overview/

http://www.nichcy.org/schoolage/

DIVORCE CHALLENGES AND NEEDS OF CHILDREN

Several issues to be considered in working with a family system where the parents of a young child are divorced are discussed below. The risk for a child being used to gratify the

229

emotional needs of a parent or used as a weapon against the other parent increases in a divorce situation. There needs to be direct education about how such behavior is detrimental to the child and, if necessary, a referral for conjoint therapy is made with specific requests for intervention being a part of the referral process.

However, the above issues are not the only ones that can cause distress to a young child. Being split between two homes can be confusing. Additionally, confusion and general distress can be amplified when the parents bring new partners into their life and these people become a part of the child's family system. This highlights the importance of the parents to make every effort to be aware of how their child is impacted by the choices they make and what they need to do to help their child to make effective adjustments to the changes in their life. Below is a vignette of some of the issues which may be encountered and what can be done to help the child.

A couple who had been married for 15 years divorced after the first birthday of their second child. Their first child is 13. Both children are girls. The older daughter chose to reside with her mother after her father remarried. The parents share 50-50 custody of the 3 year old. The mother and father of the child have different philosophies of parenting and discipline. The father states that the mother is too lenient and the mother feels that the father is too strict. The father is concerned that because the mother is more lenient that his younger daughter will choose to be at her mother's home. He has asked advice about what he can do to minimize confusion for his daughter and ensure that she enjoys his home even though his home has stricter rules.

The parents are reinforced for being sensitive to blended family issues and how the child is affected by differences between her parent's homes. They are told that while children are generally resilient, they thrive when there is consistency between the two homes and parents practice good communication for co-parenting. What is most important is that both homes offer a structure of age-appropriate rules for guidance, learning, and safety. When parents take the time to set boundaries with appropriate expectations and limitations and are consistent, children know that parents care and they feel secure and loved. Some recommendations for consistency include:

- Encourage the child to bring a special stuffed toy from one home to another, thus creating their own selected piece of comfort and consistency
- Both homes should have the child's favorite story time books and other favorite picture books
- Both homes should strive to maintain similar daily routines and schedules
  - Create family routines of sharing, nurturing and exploring
  - Be mutually respectful and supportive of each other's home
- Both homes should display the child's artwork and photos
- If divergence of differences is resulting in negativity or conflict
  - Recognize and acknowledge the differences
  - If necessary seek counseling for co-parenting and conflict resolution
- Ultimately, the only control each person can assert is over their own interpretation of words and events and how they choose to deal with them
- Self-responsibility and doing what is right – even when it is difficult

BUILDING RESILIENCE IN CHILDREN

The focal population identified for treatment in this book would greatly benefit from enriching life experiences with building and reinforcing the development of resilience. It is a combination of appropriate caregiver protectiveness combined with the development of resilience that provides for more effective ways of thinking about the challenges and adversities that they are confronted with (the framing of their daily life experiences). Children need to know that there is always an adult in their life who believes in them and loves them unconditionally. Resilience is a basic human capacity. Caregivers promote resilience in children through their words, actions, and the environment they provide. This foundation encourages children to become increasingly autonomous, independent, responsible, empathic, and altruistic (unselfish, humane, philanthropic). Embedded in this process is teaching children to communicate with others, solve problems, and successfully handle negative thoughts, feelings and behaviors. Children themselves become increasingly active in promoting their own resilience, thus demonstrating a positive feedback loop. Children need these abilities and sources of support to face the common and uncommon experiences of life. Everyone travels their own unique path in life. Living life effectively requires thought and reflection about who we are and why, what we learn from difficult experiences, and recognizing that while we all have our own "specialness" it does not set us apart as more or less important. Resilient children are hopeful and possess high self-worth. They learn to set realistic goals and expectations. Resilient children are aware of their relative strengths and weaknesses. They develop effective interpersonal skills with peers and adults and are able to seek out assistance and nurturance in appropriate ways. They focus on what they have control over or can assert an influence over while letting go of the factors which are outside of their sphere of control and influence. Additionally, children live up to or down to the expectations of caregivers. Ginsburg (2006) sets forth the "7-Cs" of resilience. The following offers a resource of caregiver guidelines for building the resilience of children in their lives.

The 7-Cs of Resilience

- Competence – is the feeling of knowing one has the ability to effectively manage a situation. Caregivers facilitate competence by
  - Helping a child to identify and focus on individual strengths
  - Linking and focusing identified mistakes on specific incidents to understand one's own actions and learn from them
  - Empowering a child to make decisions
  - Proceeding carefully that the desire to protect a child doesn't mistakenly send the message that it is believed that they lack the competence to deal with their life experiences
  - Recognizing and accepting the competencies of siblings/others individually and avoid comparisons
- Confidence – belief in one's own abilities is based upon confidence. Confidence is built by
  - Focusing on the best assets in a child so that they are able to see it
  - Clearly, expressing the best qualities (honesty, integrity, fairness, persistence, kindness, etc.)
  - Recognizing when they have done well
  - Praising honesty about specific achievement (don't dilute praise, give it when it is earned to maintain being authentic/genuine)
  - Not pushing a child to take on more than they can effectively or realistically handle
- Connection – close ties to family and community results in a solid sense of security which contributes to the development of strong values and prevents alternative destructive choices in trying to gain love and attention. Connection is facilitated by
  - Creating a sense of physical safety and emotional security within the home
  - Allowing the expression of all emotions, which allows a child to seek support when circumstances are difficult/challenging
  - Addressing conflict in a family openly with the goal to resolve conflicts/problems
  - Creating family time to share activities/games/ reading/ideas/etc.
  - Fostering healthy relationships that reinforce positive messages
- Character – the development of core morals and values (right from wrong/good from bad) and to demonstrate a caring/empathic attitude toward others (the golden rule). Character is strengthened by
  - Demonstrating how behaviors affect others

- ○ Helping a child recognize themselves as a caring person
- ○ Demonstrating the importance of community
- ○ Encouraging the development of spirituality
- ○ Avoiding racist/hateful statements and stereotyping
- Contribution – helping children to see that they make the world a better place. Understanding the importance of their contribution provides a source of purpose and motivation. Support a child by teaching them how to contribute by
  - ○ Communicating to a child that many people in their world are similar in that they lack all that they need (everyone is challenged in some way)
  - ○ Reinforcing the importance of being helpful, caring and generous
  - ○ Creating opportunities for a child to contribute. It is a self-reinforcing experience of feeling good about what one had done
- Coping – learning to cope effectively with stress and adversity helps prepare a child to overcome life's challenges. Lessons of positive coping is derived from
  - ○ Modeling positive coping strategies on a consistent basis
  - ○ Guiding a child to develop positive and effective coping strategies
  - ○ Understanding that often risky behaviors are attempts to alleviate the stress /pain/ disappointments in a child's daily life
  - ○ Not condemning a child's negative behaviors which could act to increase feelings of shame instead of learning from experiences and improving their skill set
- Control – when a child realizes that they can control the outcome of their decisions they have an increased ability to recover quickly or bounce back from a difficult situation. The understanding that they can make a difference promotes their feelings of competence and confidence. Feelings of control are facilitated by
  - ○ Helping a child to understand that life experiences are not all random and that many things that happen are the consequence of another person's choices and actions
  - ○ Learning that discipline is about teaching (not punishing or controlling), and discipline is valued for learning the consequences associated to actions

POSITIVE PARENTING

The CDC provides developmental factsheets which offer a brief summary of age-related milestones and accompanying parenting skills. The parenting information is a progression which highlights the type of parent activities which promotes child development caregiver skill building:

- Infants (0–1 years) http://www.cdc.gov/ncbddd/child/infants.htm
  - ○ Talk to your baby. Hearing the caregiver voice is soothing
  - ○ When a baby makes sounds, answer by reflecting what they have said and add words to it. This promotes and reinforces the development of using language/talking
  - ○ Sing to your baby
  - ○ Play music to foster a love of music. Also music is mathematical so listening to music may play a positive role for later math skills
  - ○ Praise your baby and give them a lot of love and affection
  - ○ Enjoy special cuddling time and holding your baby. When a baby is nurtured they feel cared for and secure
  - ○ Choose the right time to play. The best time to play with a baby is when they are alert and relaxed. If they are getting tired or fussy it is time for a break
  - ○ Parenting is hard work. Therefore, it is important that caregivers take care of themselves physically, mentally, and emotionally. If a parent is well rested and emotionally balanced they are going to enjoy their time with baby more as demonstrated by being positive and loving
- Toddlers (1–2 years) http://www.cdc.gov/ncbddd/child/toddler1.htm
  - ○ Keep reading to your toddler

232

- ○ Ask them to find objects for you, to name parts of their body/objects
- ○ Play matching games like shape sorting and simple puzzles
- ○ Encourage exploring and trying new things
- ○ Help to develop toddler's language by talking to them and expanding words (e.g., they say blank, you say "yes, blanket". They say baba you say "yes, bottle")
- ○ Promote a child's growing independence by encouraging them to dress and feed themselves
- ○ Encourage interest, curiosity and ability to recognize common objects by taking field trips to the park, bus/train ride, walking in the neighborhood and identifying things (like all the different types of trees or flowering plants)
- Toddlers (2–3 years) http://www.cdc.gov/ncbddd/child/toddler2.htm
  - ○ Set up a routine reading time (foster the love of books and reading)
  - ○ Encourage a child to use their imagination and engage in pretend play
  - ○ Play follow the leader
  - ○ Help a child to explore their surroundings (go for a walk/wagon ride) and explore new environments (going to the library, planetarium, etc.)
  - ○ Encourage the child to say their name and age
  - ○ Teach a child simple songs and nursery rhymes
- Preschoolers (3–5 years) http://www.cdc.gov/ncbddd/child/preschooler.htm
  - ○ Continue a reading ritual, and nurture a love for books and reading by fun anticipated trips to the library
  - ○ Let a child help with simple chores and thank for their help (this is also practice being a good family member)
  - ○ Facilitate continued language development by speaking to them in complete sentences using adult language
  - ○ Be clear and consistent with discipline. Model the behavior that is expected of the child
  - ○ Facilitate healthy mood management. When a child is upset guide them through the steps to solve problems

Offer a child a limited number of simple choices (what to wear, play, eat for a snack, book to read)

Resources

Barkley, R. (2000). *Taking charge of ADHD: The complete authoritative guide for parents* (revised ed.). New York: Guilford Press.

Casenhiser, D., Breinbauer, C., & Greenspan, S. I. (2007). Evaluating Greenspan's social emotional Growth Scale/chart as a screening for autism. Presented at the ICDL 11th Annual International conference: Critical Factors for Optimal Outcomes for Children with Autism and Special Needs. Tyson Corner, VA: November 2007.

Chatoor, I., Schaffer, S., Dickson, L., & Egan, J. (1984). Nonorganic failure to thrive: A developmental perspective. *Pediatric Ann, 13*, 829–843.

Chatoor, I., Schaeffer, S., Dickson, L., Schaefer, S., & Egan, J. (1985). A developmental classification of feeding disorders associated with failure to thrive: Diagnosis and treatment. In D. Drotar (Ed.), *New directions in failure tot hrive:R esearcha ndc linicalp ractice(pp. 235–238).* New York: Plenum.

DeGangi, G. A. (2000). *Pediatric disorders in regulation of affect and behavior.* San Diego: Academic Press.

Dunn-Buron, K., & Curtis, M. (2003). *The incredible 5-point scale.* Autism asperber Publishing Company.

Ginsburg, K. (2006). A parent's guide to building resilience in children and teens: Giving your child roots and wings. *American Academy of Pediatrics.*

Greenspan, S. I. (2002). *The secure child: Helping our children feel safe and confident in a changing world.* Perseus Books. www.perseusbookgroup.com

Johnson, C., Myers, S., & The Council on Children with Disabilities, (2007). Identification and evaluation of children with autism spectrum disorders. *Pediatrics, 120,* 1183–1215.

Karp, H. (2005). *The happiest baby on the block.* Bantam.

Katz, L. G., & McClellan, D. E. (1997). Fostering children's social competence: *The teacher's role.* Washington DC: NAEYC.

Mahler, M., Pine, F., & Bergman, A. (1975). *The psychological birth of the human infant.* New York: Basic Books.

Mulligan, S. (1996). An analysis of score patterns of children with attention disorders on the sensory integration and praxis tests. *American Journal of Occupational Therapy, 50*(8), 647–654.

Parush, S., Sohmer, H., Seinberg, A., & Kaitz, M. (1997). Somatosensory functioning in children with attention deficit hyperactivity disorder. *Developmental Medicine & Child Neurology, 39*(7), 3464–3468.

Schore, A. N. (2002). Dysregulation of the right brain: A fundamental mechanism of traumatic attachment and the pathogenesis of posttraumatic stress disorder. *Australian and New Zealand Journal of Psychiatry, 36*(1), 9–30.

Schore, A. N. (2005). Attachment, affect regulation, and the developing right brain: Linking developmental neuroscience to pediatrics. *Pediatric Review, 26*, 204–217.

Sprectley, M, & Boyd, R. (2009). Efficacy of applied behavioral intervention in preschool children with autism for improving cognitive, language, and adaptive behavior: a systematic review and meta-analysis. *Journal Pediaterics, 154*(3), 338–344.

Thompson, R. A., Lewis, M. D., & Calkins, S. D. (2008). Reassessing emotion regulation. *Child Devel Perspect, 2*(3), 124–131.

Williamson, G. G., & Anzalone, M. E. (2001). *Sensory integration and self-regulation infants and toddlers: Helping very young children interact with their environment.* Washington DC: ZERO to THREE National Center for Infants, Toddlers and Families.

Wolraich, M. L., Drotar, D. D., Dworkin, P. H., & Perrin, E. C. (2008). *Developmental-behavioral pediatrics. Evidence and practice.* Philidephia: Mosby, Inc..

Zerzan, J. (2007). Feeding relationship during the first year of life. Page reviewed: 3/16/2007. <http://depts.washington.edu/growing/Feed/Relation.htm>.

Further Reading

American Academy of Pediatrics, (2004). In S. P. Shelov, & R. E. Hannemann (Eds.), *Caring for your baby and young child: Birth to age 5* (4th ed.). New York: Bantam Books.

Armstrong, K., Previtera, N., & McCallum, R. N. (2000). Medicalizing normality? Management of irritability in infants. *Journal of Paediatrics and Child Health, 36*, 301–305.

Attachment and Reactive Attachment Disorders <http://helpguide.org/mental/parenting_bonding_reactive_attachment_disorders.htm>.

Ayers, A. J. (2005). *Sensory integration and the child: Understanding hidden sensory challenges.* Los Angeles: WPS.

Barkoukis, A., Reiss, N. S., & Dombeck, M. (2008). Separation anxiety disorder and assessment. Updated Feb 4, 2008. <http://www.mentalhelp.net/poc/view_doc.php?type=doc&id-14509&cn=37>.

Bronson, M. (2000). *Self-Regulation in early childhood: Nature vs nurture.* New York: Guilford Press.

California Department of Education (CDE). (2005). Desired results developmental profile (DRDP). Sacramento: <http://www.cde.ca.gov/sp/cd/ci/desiredresults.asp>.

California Department of Education, Social-Emotional Development Domain; California Infant/toddler Learning & Development Foundations. 916-322-6233 itfoundations@cde.ca.gov Last Reviewed: Wed. February 24, 2010.

California Department of Education <http://www.cde.ca.gov/sp/se/fp/documents/ecii>.

Chatoor, I., & Surles, J. (2004). Eating disorders in mid-childhood. *Primary Psychiatry, 11*(4), 34–39.

Chatoor, I., Hirsch, R., & Persinger, M. (1997). Facilitating internal regulation of eating: A treatment model for infantile anorexia. *Infants Young Child, 9*(4), 12–22.

Cohen, J., Ngozi, O., Clothier, S., & Poppe, J. (2005). Helping young children succeed: Strategies to promote early childhood social and emotional development. National Conference of State Legislatures. A project of NCLS and ZERO TO THREE.

Denham, S., & Weissberg, R. (2003). Social-emotional learning in early childhood: What we know and where we go from here. In E. Chesebrough (Ed.), *A blueprint for the promotion of prosocial behavior in early childhood.* New York: Kluwer Academic/Plenum Publishers.

Don, N., McMahon, C., & Rossiter, C. (2002). Effectiveness of an individualized multidisciplinary programme for managing unsettled infants. *Journal of Pediatric Child Health, 38*, 563–567.

Dunn, J. (1994). Changing minds and changing relationships. In C. Lewis, & P. Mitchell (Eds.), *Children's early understanding of mind: Origins and development.* Hillsdale, NJ: Lawrence Erlbaum Associates.

Ferber, R. (1985). *Solve your child's sleep problem.* New York: Simon & Schuster.

Fisher, A. G., Murray, E. A., & Bundy, C. (1991). *Sensory integration: Theory and practice.* Philadelphia: FA Davis Company.

Forbes, E., Cohn, J., Allen, N., & Lewinsohn, P. (2004). Infant affect during parent–infant interaction at 3 and 6 months: Differences between mothers and fathers and influence of parent history of depression. *Infancy, 5*(1), 62–84.

Ganz, J. S. (2002). *Including SI for parents: Sensory integration strategies at home and at school.* Prospect, Ct: Biographical Publishing Company.

Garcia-Winter, M. (2007). *Thinking bout you thinking about me* (2nd ed.). Jessica Kingsley Publishers.

Greenspan, S. I. (2001). The basic course on the grenspan floortime approach. <www.stanleygreenspan.com> ICDL Training Videotapes on the DIR Model and Floortime Techniques www.icdl.com/

Greenspan, S. I. (1997). Developmentally based psychotherapy. Available from publisher. Madison, CT: International Universities Press 800-835-3487.

Greenspan, S. I., & Lourie, R. S. (1981). Developmental structuralist approach to classification of adaptive and pathologic personality organizations: Infancy and early childhood. *American Journal of Psychiatry, 138,* 725–735.

Greenspan, S. I., & Weider, S. (1993). Regulatory disorders. In C. H. Zeanah (Ed.), *Handbook of infant mental health (pp. 280–290).* New York: Guilford Press.

Greenspan, S. I., & Weider, S. (1997). *The child with special needs: Encouraging intellectual and emotional growth.* New York: Addison Wesley.

Greenspan, S. I., Wieder, S., & Simons, R. (1998). *The child with special needs.* Reading, MA: Merloyd Laurence.

Greenspan, S. I. (2002). The affect diathesis hypothesis. The role of emotions in core deficit in autism and the development of intelligence and social skills. *Journal of Developmental and Learning, 5,* 1.

Kraniwitz, C. S. (1998). *The out of sync child: Recognizing and coping with sensory integration dysfunction.* New York: Skylight Press Books.

Lagattuta, K. H., & Thompson, R. A. (2007). The development of self-conscious emotions: Cognitive processes and social influences. In J. L. Tracy, R. W. Robins, & J. P. Tangney (Eds.), *The self-conscious emotions: Theory and research.* New York: Guilford Press.

Lamb, M. E., Bornstein, M. H., & Teti, D. (2002). *Development in infancy: An introduction* (4th ed.). Mahwah, NJ: Lawrence Erlbaum Associates.

Lerner, C., & Ciervo, L. A. (2003). *Healthy minds: Nurturing children's development from 0–36 months.* Washington, DC: Zero to Three Press.

Messinger, D., & Fogel, A. (2007). The interactive development of social smiling. In R. V. (2007). Kail (Ed.), *Advances in child development and behavior* (vol. 35). Burlington, MA: Elsevier.

Miller, L. C., Anzalone, M. E., Lane, S. J., Cermak, S. A., & Osten, T. E. (2007). Concept evolution in sensory integration: A proposed nosology for diagnosis. *American Journal of Occupational Therapy, 61,* 2.

National Information Center for Children and Youth with Disabilities (NICHCY), for a copy of the Parent Guide for EI.

National Scientific Council on the Developing Child. (2004). Children's emotional development is built into the architecture of their brains. Working Paper No. 2. <http://developingchild.net> outside source/accessed 01.10.11.

NECTAC for state examples of IFSP forms and guidance <http://www.nectac.org/topics/families/stateifsp.asp>.

NHS choices. Last reviewed 4/8/10. Dyspraxia-treatment. <http://www.nhs.uk/Conditions/Dyspraxia-(childhood)/Pages/Treatment.aspx>.

Pediatric Therapy Network. (2009). www.pediatrictherapynetwork/research/ptnresearch.cfm.

Peirano, P., Algarin, C., & Uauy, R. (2003). Sleep-wake states and other regulatory mechanisms throughout early human development. *Journal of Pediatrics, 143*(4), 70–79.

Raver, C. (2002). Emotions matter: Making the case for for the role of young children's emotional development for early school readiness. SRCD Social Policy Report, 16(3).

Reebye, P., & Stalker, A. (2007). Regulation disorders of sensory processing in infants and young children. *BC Medical Journal, 49*(4), 194–200.

Reite, M., Weissberg, M., & Ruddy, J. (2009). Clinical manual for evaluation and treatment of sleep disorders. Health and Fitness.

Saarni, C., et al. (2006). Emotional development: Action, communication, and understanding. In N. Eisenberg (Ed.), *Handbook of child psychology* (6th ed.), vol. 3, *social, emotional, and personality development.* Hoboken, NJ: John Wiley and Sons.

Shonkoff, J. P. (2004). *Science, policy and the developing child: Closing the gap between what we know and what we do.* Washington, DC: Ounce of Prevention Fund. <http://ounceofprevention.org/downloads/publications/shonkoffweb.pdf> accessed 01.10.11

Siegel, L. M. (2007). *The complete IEP guide: How to advocate for your special ed child* (5th ed.). Berkeley CA: Nolo.

Siegel, L. M. (2007). *IEP guide: Learning disabilities* (3rd ed.). Berkeley CA: Nolo.

Thompson, R. A. (2006). The development of the person: Social understanding, relationships, self, conscience. In N. Eisenberg (Ed.), *Handbook of child psychology* (6th ed.), vol 3, *Social, emotional, and personality development.* Hoboken, NJ: John Wiley and Sons.

Thompson, R. A., & Goodvin, R. (2005). The individual child: Temperament, emotion, self and personality. In M. H. Bornstein, & M. E. Lamb (Eds.), *Developmental science: An advanced textbook* (5th ed.). Mahwah, NJ: Lawrence Erlbaum Associates.

Versfeld, P. Developmental coordination disorder and dyspraxia. <http://www.skillsforaction.com/?q=node/16>.

Ward, T. M. (2007). Caring for children with sleep problems. *Journal of Pediatric Nursing, 22*(4), 283–296.

Weller, E. B., & Weller R. A. (2000). Trauma and the development of eating disorders. Updated 5/17/2000 <http://www.medscape.org/viewarticle/420318>.

Wingert, P., & Brant, M. (2005). Reading your baby's mind. Newsweek, Aug. 15, 32–39.

Zeanah, C. H., Scheeringa, M., Boris, N. W., Heller, S. S., Smyke, A. T., & Trapani, J. (2004). Reactive attachment disorder in maltreated toddlers. *Child Abuse Neglect, 28*, 877–888.

CHAPTER 4

Resources

BUSINESS FORMS AND INTERVIEW FORMAT
Business Forms
PATIENT REGISTRATION

Client Information Form

Filled out by:_____ Date:_____

Child's Name:_____ Child's Date of Birth:_____ Age:_____

Sex: Male   Female   Child's Ethnic Group/Race:_____

Child's Address:_____

Child's Health Insurance: None   Medicaid   Private Insurance   Other:_____

Person(s) With Legal Custody of Child

1. Name:_____ Relationship to Child:_____

   Address: _____

   Home Phone:_____ Cell Phone:_____ Work Phone:_____

   Birth Date:_____ Age:_____ Highest Education Completed:_____

   Ethnicity:_____

   Occupation:_____ Employer:_____

   Work Schedule:_____ Okay to contact at work? Yes   No   If so, when?_____

2. Name:_____ Relationship to Child:_____

   Address: _____

   Home Phone:_____ Cell Phone:_____ Work Phone:_____

   Birth Date:_____ Age:_____ Highest Education Completed:_____

   Ethnicity:_____

   Occupation:_____ Employer:_____

   Work Schedule:_____ Okay to contact at work? Yes   No   If so, when?_____

Is the child adopted?   Yes   No

Who does the child live with on a regular basis?_____

FIGURE 4.1

Therapist's Guide to Pediatric Affect and Behavior Regulation. DOI: http://dx.doi.org/10.1016/B978-0-12-386884-8.00004-5

Other Adults and Children Living in the Child's Home

Below list all other adults and children living with the child (include step siblings, foster children, related adults and unrelated adults):

Name	Age	Gender	Relationship to Child

Child's Full Or Half-Siblings That Do Not Live In The Same House With The Child

Name	Age	Gender	Relationship to Child

Contact Person for Appointments

Name:_____ Relationship to Child:_____

Address:_____

Home Phone:_____ Cell Phone:_____ Work Phone:_____

* If the Child's Birth Parents Do Not Have Legal Custody:

Mother's Name:_____ Date of Birth:_____

Address:_____

Occupation:_____ Employer:_____

Reason for not having custody of child: _____

How often does she see the child?_____

If deceased, when?_____ Cause of death? _____

Fathers's Name:_____ Date of Birth:_____

Address:_____

Occupation:_____ Employer:_____

Reason for not having custody of child: _____

How often does she see the child?_____

If deceased, when?_____ Cause of death? _____

FIGURE 4.1 (Continued)

238

Presenting Concerns About Child

What concerns do you have about the child? _____

_____

What are the child's strengths? _____

_____

What are you wanting to happen for the child? _____

_____

Child's Pre-School/School History (If yes, describe)

1. Identified learning problems? No Yes _____

_____

2. Behavior problems? No Yes _____

_____

3. Identified suicidal problems? No Yes _____

_____

4. Are they receiving special help (special education, tutor help in school plan, speech pathologist, occupational therapist, school psychologist, counselor, etc.)? No Yes _____

_____

5. Other school problems? No Yes _____

_____

FIGURE 4.1   (Continued)

Child's Medical History

Child's physician/pediatrician:_____ Phone:_____

Address:_____

Date of last doctor visit: _____ Reason:_____ Outcome:_____

Does the child take medication for behavioral/emotional problems?

Name of Medication	Dose	Purpose	Effect	Prescribing Doctor

Does the child take medication for other reasons (illness, allergies, disability)?

240

Name of Medication	Dose	Purpose	Effect	Prescribing Doctor

If the child has allergies – to what (please describe food, pets, etc.)?

_____

_____

_____

Are there concerns about the child's health? No Yes   Describe_____

_____

_____

FIGURE 4.1   (Continued)

<u>Pregnancy and Newborn Stages</u> (If yes, please describe)

1. Medical problems during mother's pregnancy with this child (bleeding, high blood pressure, infections, diabetes, convulsions, extra small weight gain, injuries, etc.)?   No Yes

If yes:_____

2. Did the mother take medications during the pregnancy?   No Yes

If yes:_____

3. Did the mother smoke during the pregnancy?   No Yes

If yes:_____

4. Did the mother drink alcohol during the pregnancy?   No Yes

If yes:_____

5. Did the mother use drugs during the pregnancy?   No Yes

If yes:_____

6. Did the mother experience high stress during the pregnancy (marital problems, domestic violence, financial problems, job problems, problems with other relationships)?   No Yes

If yes:_____

7. Were there any problems with labor delivery (prolonged labor, bleeding, breech birth, forceps used, C-section, etc.)?   No Yes

If yes:_____

8. Was the child born prematurely?   No Yes

If yes:_____

9. Did the child have any problems as a newborn (born blue, jaundice, birth defects, seizures, infections, injuries, feeding, or sleep problems)?   No Yes

If yes:_____

10. Was the child difficult to care for as a baby?   No Yes

If yes:_____

FIGURE 4.1   (Continued)

<u>Developmental Delays</u>

1. Have any developmental problems been identified? No Yes

If yes:_____

2. Was the child slow or have problems with any of the following (If yes, describe)

- Walking alone   No Yes _____
- Speaking   No Yes _____
- Bowel training   No Yes _____
- Bladder training   No Yes _____
- Staying dry at night   No Yes _____
- Tying shoes   No Yes _____
- Riding bike   No Yes _____
- Reading   No Yes _____
- Writing   No Yes _____

3. Child's Temperament

- Is the child overactive?   No Yes _____
- Does the child have trouble paying attention?   No Yes _____
- Does the child have trouble staying with one activity?   No Yes _____
- Does the child go from happy to sad quickly (without any obvious cause)?   No Yes _____
- Does the child get frustrated easily?   No Yes _____
- Does the child get upset by changes?   No Yes _____
- Are the child's emotional responses unpredictable?   No Yes _____
- Does it take the child a long time to warm up to new people and/or new situations?   No Yes _____
- Does the child overreact to physical pain?   No Yes _____
- Does the child react strongly to other things?   No Yes _____

<u>Child's Early Behavior</u>

Has the child demonstrated any problems with the following (If yes, explain):

- Discipline   No Yes _____
- Temper   No Yes _____
- Fighting   No Yes _____
- Moods   No Yes _____
- Relationships with others   No Yes _____
- Other behaviors   No Yes _____

FIGURE 4.1 (Continued)

Family History

Has any relative of the child had any of the following problems?

- Neurological disease (seizures, spills, etc.)?   No Yes _____
- Chronic disease (diabetes, thyroid, heart disease, stroke)?   No Yes _____
- Mental illness (schizophrenia, bipolar disorder, depression, anxiety, etc.)?   No Yes _____
- Mental retardation?   No Yes _____
- Learning problems?   No Yes _____
- Behavior problems?   No Yes _____
- Excessive use of alcohol?   No Yes _____
- Drug problems/drug addiction?   No Yes _____
- Trouble with the law?   No Yes _____
- Trouble holding a job?   No Yes _____
- Suicidal behavior?   No Yes _____
- Violent behavior?   No Yes _____
- Other problems?   No Yes _____

Has anyone in the child's family seen a psychologist, psychiatrist or other mental health provider?

_____

_____

Current Living Situation

Are any of the following a part of the child's current living situation? (If yes, explain)

- Marital/relationship problems between the child's major caregivers?   No Yes _____
- Problems with a sibling or other people in the home?   No Yes _____
- Problem with work?   No Yes _____
- Financial problems?   No Yes _____
- Recent major changes or stressors in the child's living situation or family?   No Yes _____
- Violence in the home or neighborhood?   No Yes _____
- Alcohol or drug problems in the home or neighborhood?   No Yes _____
- Other problems?   No Yes _____

Please write down anything else that you think is important to this evaluation:

_____

_____

_____

_____

FIGURE 4.1 (Continued)

243

CLINICAL INTAKE FORM
For Children
Intake packet to be filled out prior to appointment and returned to office

Child Information Form:

Name_____   Date _____

Date of Birth_____   Referred by_____

Grade_____ School_____   District_____

Person Completing Form:_____   Relationship to Child:_____

Mother (or Guardian)

Name_____

Street Address_____

City _____

State_____ Zip_____

Home Phone _____

Cell/Work Phone_____

Date of Birth _____

Marital Status _____

Education_____

Occupation_____

Employer _____

Father (or Guardian)

Name_____

Street Address_____

City_____

State_____ Zip_____

Home Phone _____

Cell/Work Phone _____

Date of Birth _____

Members of Household:

Name_____ Age_____ Sex_____ Relationship_____

Name_____ Age_____ Sex_____ Relationship_____

Name_____ Age_____ Sex_____ Relationship_____

Name_____ Age_____ Sex_____ Relationship_____

Ethnicity: (check all that apply)   ___Caucasian   ___Hispanic/Latino(a)   ___African American

___Native American   ___Asian   _____Other

Is the Child currently on medication?

Drug_____Dose_____Purpose_____Prescribed by_____

Reason for currently seeking services:_____

_____

Previous therapy/evaluation: Yes/No If yes where/when_____

_____

FIGURE 4.2

Referral Questions:

Describe the reasons for referral. Please include specific behaviors or problems that you would like help with.

_____

_____

_____

_____

_____

_____

_____

_____

_____

_____

_____

_____

245

What Services or interventions have been previously performed (if any)?

_____

_____

_____

_____

FIGURE 4.2 (Continued)

Family History:

Please indicate any family members on either side who have had any of the following:

MEDICAL PROBLEMS	MOTHER'S SIDE	FATHER'S SIDE
Mental Retardation		
Learning Disabilities/Problems		
Hyperactivity/Attention problems		
Speech/Language problems		
Seizures		
Headaches		
Genetic Disorders		
Miscarriages		
Multiple Sclerosis		
Tourette's Syndrome		
Thyroid problems		
Other medical problems		

PSYCHIATRIC PROBLEMS	MOTHER'S SIDE	FATHER'S SIDE
Depression/Suicide		
Bipolar (Manic-Depression)		
Anxiety Disorder		
Panic Attacks		
Obsessive-Compulsive Disorder		
Phobias and Fears		
Attention Deficit/Hyperactivity		
Autism Spectrum Disorder		
Schizophrenia		
Hallucinations		
Alcohol/Drug Abuse (Specify)		
"Nervous Breakdowns"		
Other		

FIGURE 4.2 (Continued)

Pregnancy, Delivery and Birth:

During pregnancy, mother…(check all that apply and describe)
- o   Drank alcohol or used drugs_____
- o   Smoked_____
- o   Suffered any illness, infection, trauma, fevers _____

_____
- o   Had toxemia _____
- o   Experienced vaginal bleeding/spotting_____
- o   Almost miscarried_____
- o   Took medication (which?) _____
- o   Had other significant events occur _____

_____

During labor and delivery, mother and/or baby…(check all that apply and describe)
- o   Went into early labor _____
- o   Suffered fetal distress_____
- o   Had induced labor_____
- o   Suffered complications (breach birth, cord around neck, lack of oxygen, C-section, forceps, required oxygen, etc.)_____

_____

_____
- o   Required special care (ICU, incubator, etc.)_____

_____

Length of pregnancy_____ weeks   Baby's APGAR score: _____
Baby's weight_____ lbs   oz   Baby's length _____

After birth did the baby have problems with…(describe)
- o   Breathing_____
- o   Jaundice_____
- o   Sucking or feeding _____
- o   Food, milk or other allergies_____
- o   Other problems_____

Describe the child's personality, mood and temperament as an infant and toddler:

_____

_____

_____

FIGURE 4.2   (Continued)

Developmental History:

At what age did the child:

Crawl:_____   Sit up:_____   Walk alone:_____

Say first word:_____   Speak in sentences:_____

Become potty trained:_____

Please indicate if the child suffered any of these problems as an infant or young child and describe:

- Delayed development or growth_____
- Ear infections, tube placement _____
- Head banging _____
- Repetitive or unusual movements_____
- Restlessness or over activity_____
- Attention problems_____
- Aggression (hitting, biting, kicking)_____
- Difficulty making or keeping friends_____
- Shunned by peers _____
- Defiance, resistance to authority_____

Describe the child's current friendships:

_____

_____

_____

What type of discipline is used with the child? Is it effective?

_____

_____

_____

FIGURE 4.2   (Continued)

What type of rewards are used with the child? Are they effective?

_____

_____

_____

School History:

Child began school at age _____

Describe the child's preschool/kindergarten experience?

_____

_____

_____

Medical History:

When the child was last tested for:

Vision_____   Does the child wear/need glasses or contacts?_____

Hearing_____   Does the child wear/need hearing aids? _____

List any medications prescribed for the child, dosages and reason for the medication:

<u>Medication</u>   <u>Dosage</u>   <u>Reason</u>

_____

_____

_____

Please indicate and describe the child's current and past health problems:

<u>Age and Duration</u>   <u>Treatment</u>

- Headaches_____
- Seizures_____
- Head injury_____
- Loss of consciousness_____
- Meningitis_____
- Encephalitis_____

FIGURE 4.2   (Continued)

- Brain tumor_____
- Paralysis _____
- High fever_____
- Fainting spells_____
- Coma_____
- HIV infection/AIDS_____
- Near drowning _____
- Electric Shock_____
- Drug/alcohol exposure _____
- Psychiatric hospitalization _____
- Psychological counseling _____
- Other_____

If the child has suffered head injury, please describe the incident:

_____

_____

_____

Date of the incident:_____

Did the child suffer loss of consciousness?_____   How long?_____

Did the child have amnesia of events before the incident?_____   After? _____

Did the child remember the incident itself? _____

Was the child treated by a doctor?_____   Hospitalized?_____

Describe the length and course of the hospitalization:_____

_____

Indicate the neurodiagnostic procedures performed:

	Date	Doctor/Hospital	Result (if known)
CT or brain scan			
MRI of brain			
EEG			
Lumbar puncture (spinal tap)			

FIGURE 4.2   (Continued)

- Other (PET, SPECT, etc.)_____

Physician(s) currently caring for the child?

_____

_____

Please indicate and describe whether your child currently or in the past has experienced or complained of the symptoms listed below. Please indicate whether the problem has been resolved or is ongoing.

Physical Symptoms:

- Sensitivity to noise _____
- Sensitivity to light_____
- Ringing in the ears _____
- Dizziness_____
- Nausea/vomiting_____
- Blurred vision _____
- Double vision _____
- Hearing problems _____
- Problems with taste or smell_____
- Numbness or tingling in extremities_____
- Sleep problems _____
- Fatigue _____

Psychological Symptoms:

- Depression_____
- Mood swings_____
- Irritability _____
- Anger_____
- Aggression _____
- Low frustration tolerance _____
- Can't handle stress _____
- Anxiety_____

FIGURE 4.2   (Continued)

- Hates to be in crowds _____
- Social withdrawal/social problems_____
- Difficulty with change _____

Cognitive Symptoms:

Memory

- Poor short-term memory_____
- Poor long-term memory _____

Reasoning

- Reasoning problems _____
- Takes things too literally_____
- Difficulty understanding consequences of actions_____

Language

- Problems understanding what others say _____
- Says "what" a lot_____
- Needs frequent repetition to understand_____
- Does not listen_____
- Can't follow a 3-step command _____
- Trouble expressing self verbally_____
- Talks too much/too little_____
- Problems finding the right word to say_____
- Stutters_____

Visuospatial

- Gets lost frequently_____
- Has trouble with directions_____
- Trouble with visual tasks (puzzles, games, etc.)_____
- Poor drawing ability _____
- Poor penmanship_____

Other

- Attention problems_____
- No concept of time_____

FIGURE 4.2 (Continued)

- Clumsy, poor motor skills_____
- Drop in school performance (which subjects?)_____

Strengths/Interests:

Please describe the child's strengths:

_____
_____
_____
_____

Please describe the child's interests:

_____
_____
_____
_____

Additional Information:

Please provide any other information or describe any other concerns which have not been covered in this questionnaire.

_____
_____
_____
_____

253

FIGURE 4.2 (Continued)

Videotape Agreement

Name of Child

Name(s) of Parent/Guardian

I _____, as parent/guardian of _____
authorize permission to videotape my child for the purpose of professional education,
supervision, and treatment as part of the service agreement.

The video agreement states:

1. The client consents to the use of videotape to be taken in the office of the EASSC during the course of individual treatment.
2. The videotape will be used solely in the interest of the advancement of mental health and educational services for the purpose of professional education, supervision, treatment and research. The videotape will not be used for any other purpose.
3. The doctor agrees not to use, or permit the use of the name of the child named above in connection with any direct or indirect use of exhibition of the videotape for any use other than set forth in the service agreement.
4. The doctor is the sole owner of all rights in and to the videotape.
5. There shall be no financial compensation for the use of such videotape.

_____   _____

Parent/Guardian signature   Date

_____   _____

Clinician signature   Supervisor signature

FIGURE 4.2   (Continued)

Psychological Services/Psychotherapy/Interventions

Psychological interventions, including psychotherapy, are not easy to describe in a few general statements. Effective treatment depends upon the particular problems you and/or your child may be experiencing, as well as personality factors and establishing a good therapist-client relationship. Psychotherapy also calls for active effort on you/your child's part. For therapy to be most successful, you/your child will have to work on the things we talk about during the sessions and at home. Psychological treatment includes potential for some risk as well as benefits. Since therapy may involve discussing unpleasant aspects of you/your child's life, you may experience uncomfortable feelings which may be temporarily discomforting. On the other hand, psychological treatment has been known to produce many benefits such as reduction in distress, solutions to specific problems, and better relationships. There can be no guarantees of what you will experience. Every effort will be made to minimize risks by providing well-supervised and trained therapists and by frequent evaluations of client progress/status.

The first few sessions will involve an evaluation of you/your child's needs. By the end of this evaluation period, your therapist will be able to offer you an initial impression of your needs and a plan for what treatment might include, if you and/or your child decide to continue with therapy. If you ever have any questions about procedures, you should discuss them whenever they arise.

Psychological Services – psychological/neuropsychological/psychoeducational evaluations

Evaluations are designed to provide benefits such as an accurate description of client, cognitive, intellectual and psychological strengths and weaknesses, treatment planning, school and vocational planning. However, as with psychotherapy, evaluations include potential for risks as well as benefits, as previously described. Evaluations may involve several appointments of several hours each, and generally consist of interviews with the client, parent(s), administration of tests and/or questionnaires, and, when indicated, interviews with school personnel, physicians or other individuals who can provide helpful information to aid in the evaluation. The parent's written consent will be necessary to authorize these contacts. Following the completion of the

FIGURE 4.2 (Continued)

evaluation, a session will be held with you (and your child, if appropriate, for child clients) and your clinician to discuss the results. It may take several weeks for your clinician to produce a written report of the evaluation. **If a report must be written by a certain date, please discuss this with your clinician well in advance.** Every effort will be made to make sure that reports are written and disseminated in a timely manner.

Confidentiality

*The following information may change from state to state. It is the therapist's responsibility to assure that they present and protect information in accordance with the laws and ethics/standards of practice from their own state and jurisdictions.

State law protects the privacy of communications between a client and psychologist. Every effort will be made to keep your evaluation and treatment strictly confidential. In most situations, the clinic will only release information about you/your child's treatment to others if you sign a written authorization form that meets certain legal requirements.

256

In the following situation, no authorization is required:

On occasion, your clinician may find it helpful to consult with another health or mental health professional. During such a consultation, every effort is made to avoid revealing the identity of the client. The other professional is legally bound to keep the information confidential. If you don't object, it is our policy to tell you about such consultations only if it is important to you/your child and your therapist working together. All consultations are noted in the client's clinic record.

FIGURE 4.2   (Continued)

Limits of Confidentiality

There are unusual situations where the therapist may be required or permitted to disclose information without your authorization. These include:

a) If the clinic has knowledge, evidence, or reasonable concern regarding the abuse or neglect of a child, elderly person, or disabled person, it is required to file a report with the appropriate agency. Once such a report is filed, we may be required to provide additional information.

b) If a client communicates an explicit threat of serious physical harm to a clearly identifiable victim or victims, and has the apparent intent and ability to carry out such a threat, the clinic may be required to take protective actions. These actions may include notifying the potential victim, contacting the police, and/or seeking hospitalization for the client.

c) If we believe that there is an imminent risk that a client will physically harm himself or herself, we will also take protective actions.

d) Although courts have recognized a therapist-client privilege, there may be circumstances in which a court would order the therapist to disclose personal health or treatment information. We also may be required to provide information about court-ordered evaluations or treatments. If you are involved in, or contemplating litigation, you should consult with an attorney to determine whether a court would be likely to order the clinic to disclose information.

e) The therapist is required to provide information requested by a legal guardian of a minor child, including a non-custodial parent.

f) If a government agency is requesting information for health oversight activities or to prevent terrorism (Patriot Act), the therapist may be required to provide it.

g) If a client files a complaint or lawsuit against the clinic or professional staff, the clinic may disclose relevant information regarding the client in order to defend itself. If any of these situations were to arise, the clinic would make every effort to fully discuss it with you before taking action, and would limit disclosure to what is necessary.

FIGURE 4.2   (Continued)

While this written summary of exceptions to confidentiality should prove helpful in informing you about potential problems, it is important that you discuss any questions you have with us now or in the future. The laws governing confidentiality can be quite complex. In situations where specific advice is required, formal legal advice may be needed.

Emergency Care and Crisis Situations

The office is open Monday – Friday from 8am-5pm. If you have a crisis during this time frame we will have you come to the office, or we may refer you to a facility that will be better prepared to deal with a specific identified situation.

If it is after hours or during the weekend and you cannot reach us and are having an emergency, contact a local hospital emergency room or other community resources directly such as:

(Psychiatric Phone Information)

_____

258

Professional Records and Client Rights

The laws and standards of the psychology profession require that the clinic keep Protected Health Information (PIH) about you in your clinical record. Generally, you may examine and/or receive a copy of your clinical record, if you request it in writing. There are a few exceptions to the access: 1) the unusual circumstances described above, 2) when the record makes reference to another person (other than a health care provider) and we believe that access is reasonably likely to cause substantial harm to that person, or 3) where information has been supplied confidentially by others. Also, the clinic will not release copyrighted test information or raw data without a subpoena. Because these are professional records, they can be misinterpreted. For this reason, it is recommended that you initially review them in the presence of your child's therapist, or have them forwarded to another mental health professional so you can discuss the contents. In most circumstances, it is allowed to charge a copying fee for reproducing your child's records. If

FIGURE 4.2 (Continued)

the clinic refuses your request for access to your child's records, you have the right to a review of this decision (except for information supplied confidentially by others) which the therapist will discuss with you upon request.

HIPAA provides you with several new or expanded rights with regard to your child's clinical records and disclosures of protected health information. These rights include requesting that the clinic amend your record; requesting restrictions on what information from your clinical records is disclosed to others; requesting an accounting of most disclosures of protected health information that you have neither consented to nor authorized; determining the location to which protected information disclosures were sent; having any complaints you make about clinic policies and procedures recorded in your records; and the right to a paper copy of this Agreement, the attached Notice form, and our privacy policies and procedures. Your child's therapist will be happy to discuss any of these rights with you.

Summary of Client Responsibilities

As a client, you agree to:

1. Keep regular appointments and actively participate in your treatment.
2. Attempt any therapeutic assignments you/your child agree to perform.
3. Make a commitment to living and using clinic and community resources to solve difficulties. You/your child will be asked to agree to disclose to the therapist feelings of being in crisis and/or suicidal, to work with the therapist to develop a crisis plan, and to give the clinic discretion regarding needed disclosures in a crisis situation.
4. Not to come to the clinic under the influence of alcohol or other drugs. If you/your child appear intoxicated, the clinician will cancel the cession and request that the intoxicated person refrain from driving. Failure to do so will require a DUI report.
5. Never bring a weapon of any sort to the clinic.
6. Ask your therapist questions right away if you are uncertain about your child's evaluation, therapeutic process or any clinic policy.
7. Pay agreed-upon evaluation and treatment fees or make arrangements to do so.

FIGURE 4.2   (Continued)

8. If the client is a child, a parent or adult must remain in the waiting room in case of emergency.

Informed Consent

Your signature below indicates that you have read this agreement and agree to its terms.

These matters have been explained to you and you fully and freely give consent for your child to receive clinic evaluation and/or treatment services.

_____

Name of Client(s) please print

_____   _____

Signature of Client(s) and/or Minor Child   Date

_____   _____

Signature of Legal Representative of Minor Child   Date

_____   _____

Witnessed by   Date

FIGURE 4.2   (Continued)

Comprehensive Clinical Intake

(Therapist/Business Name)

Therapist(s) Name(s)
Therapist(s) Name(s)
Therapist(s) Name(s)

Street Address
City, State Zip
Phone Number
Fax Number
Email

GENERAL INFORMATION

1. For you convenience, you may download a map to our office from our website. Our office is located (description of where to find therapist office).

2. It is your responsibility to contact your insurance company to open your case for preauthorization for treatment and confirm benefits for "**Outpatient Mental Health**" services before your first appointment. Be sure to state that this is for "outpatient mental health" benefits, otherwise the insurance personnel may quote you the benefits for major medical services instead.

3. Please arrive 10 minutes prior to the first appointment with your paperwork completely filled out (prior to your arrival), along with your insurance card(s) and any other paperwork requested by our office.

4. If a child is being brought to this office for treatment, be sure to bring a copy of the child custody order issued by the court for our records.

5. It is our office policy that you provide us with payment in full at the time of the first visit, unless you are part of an HMO/PPO that provides us with a specific co-pay amount which you are required to pay at the time of service. Otherwise, please contact our office in advance of your appointment to be told the exact amount you will need to pay at the time of your first visit. We will bill your insurance and, if they pay for your services, we will apply your initial payment towards your account.

6. If you have any questions, please feel free to contact our office at (office contact number).

REGARDING EVALUATION REFERRALS

You have been referred to this office for an evaluation in order to determine the cause of your current problems, whether that be ADHD, some type of learning disorder, neurological problems, or a psychological disorder. For this reason, you have been given a very detailed history and symptom checklist to fill out which will assist (therapist name) in identifying what areas require further evaluation. While there may be some information that you do not know, please do your best to provide as much information as you can.

Because (therapist name) receives a large number of referrals for evaluation, he/she is usually not able to provide ongoing counseling or treatment. Therefore, if his/her evaluation reveals the need for treatment, he/she may need to refer you to another qualified therapist to assist you.

For those individuals that are identified as having ADHD, he/she will work with your primary care physician to accurately determine the correct medication and dosage. He will discuss this process with you in detail at your first meeting.

FIGURE 4.3

OFFICE POLICIES

(Therapist name) would like to welcome you to his/her practice and is pleased to have you as a patient. We are providing you with this informational letter to help you understand how this office operates. Every effort will be made to treat you with courtesy and respect. Please read this information carefully and write down any questions that you might have so that you can discuss them with (therapist name) or his/her staff.

APPOINTMENTS

Patients are seen only by appointment. Before your first visit with (therapist name), please complete all of the forms which have been sent to you and be sure to bring them with you to your first appointment.

You will not be seen by the doctor unless all forms are filled out prior to your visit.

This will allow the office staff and (therapist name) to serve you in the most time efficient manner possible. If this information cannot be completed prior to your appointment, please arrive one hour early in order to complete the forms. If they are already completed, **please arrive 15 minutes before your first appointment** so that the staff can prepare your chart.

Upon arrival at the office for any appointment, always announce yourself to the receptionist so that (therapist name) can be informed that you have arrived.

Initial interviews and follow-up therapy visits will last about 45 minutes. Other types of evaluation and testing may involve greater amounts of time. This will be discussed with you by (therapist name).

CANCELLATIONS

When you schedule an appointment, that time is reserved specifically for you. Appointment reminder cards are provided whenever subsequent appointments are scheduled at the office. It is the patient's responsibility to remember and keep scheduled appointments. A minimum of 24 hours notice is required if you are canceling or re-scheduling an appointment.

You will be charged ($_____) for missed appointments and appointments which are canceled with less than 24 hours notice. In the case of evaluations where multiple hours of testing have been scheduled, you will be charged ($_____/hr).

EMERGENCIES

If you need to contact (therapist name) between sessions, please leave a message with the office or have him/her paged at (phone number), and your call will be returned as soon as possible. If an emergency situation arises, please indicate that, "this is an emergency" when leaving your message. Calls made between 5:00 p.m. and 9:00 a.m. should be of an urgent or emergency nature only. In the event that (therapist name) is unavailable due to illness, vacation, or other circumstances, emergency calls will be forwarded to the doctor that has agreed to handle crisis calls for him/her. In the event that (therapist name) or the doctor on call is unable to be reached, then emergency evaluations can be obtained at (name of behavioral health center, address, phone number). For children and adolescents, call the (pediatric unit). Otherwise, you should call "9-1-1" to access emergency medical services.

FIGURE 4.3   (Continued)

CONFIDENTIALITY AND RELEASE OF INFORMATION

Information disclosed within sessions and the written records pertaining to those sessions are confidential and will not be released to anyone without the written consent of the patient or the parent/guardian, in the case of minors and/or dependent adults, except where (therapist name) is mandated by (state) law to report otherwise confidential information. Circumstances which are required by law to be reported are:

1. Patient's who pose an imminent threat of danger to themselves or others.
2. Instances of suspected abuse or neglect of a child (physical, sexual, and/or emotional abuse).
3. Instances of suspected abuse or neglect of a dependent adult.

Disclosure may also be required pursuant to a legal proceeding. If you place your mental status at issue in litigation initiated by you, the defendant may have the right to obtain the psychotherapy records and/or testimony from (therapist name).

In couple and family therapy, or when different family members are seen individually, confidentiality and privilege do not apply between the couple or among family members. (Therapist name) will use his clinical judgment when revealing such information.

Disclosure of confidential information may be required by your health insurance or workman's compensation carrier, or HMO/PPO/MCO/EAP in order to process your claims. Only the minimum necessary information will be communicated to the carrier. (Therapist name) has no knowledge or responsibility for any actions which result from a third party misusing or re-releasing such information without his/her expressed consent.

As a patient, you have the right to review or receive a summary of your records at any time (with notice of 5 or more working days), except in limited legal or emergency circumstances or when (therapist name) assesses that releasing such information might be harmful in any way. In such circumstances (therapist name) may provide the records to a qualified mental health professional of your choice and that individual may then choose to review the information with you if it is deemed clinically appropriate. You will be charged an appropriate fee for any preparation time which is required to comply with an information request.

All other requests to release information regarding your treatment and your condition must be authorized in writing specifically allowing the release of psychiatric records. (Therapist name) will provide you with a Release of Information form or you may chose to place your request in writing. There will be no charge for releasing records to other treating medical or mental health professionals. For all other requests to copy records, there will be a minimum charge of $15.00 to cover the expenses of photocopying, postage and handling.

PSYCHOLOGICAL AND NEUROPSYCHOLOGICAL SERVICES

Psychotherapy is not easily described in general statements. It varies depending on the personality of both the therapist and the patient and the particular problems which the patient brings. There are a number of different approaches which can be utilized to address the problems you hope to address. It is not like visiting a medical doctor, in that psychotherapy requires a very active effort on your part. In order to be most successful, you will have to work on things that you and (therapist name) talk about both during your sessions and at home.

Psychotherapy has both benefits and risks. Risks sometimes include experiencing uncomfortable feelings such as sadness, guilt, anxiety, anger, frustration, loneliness and helplessness. Psychotherapy often requires discussing unpleasant aspects

FIGURE 4.3 (Continued)

of your life. Psychotherapy has also been shown to have benefits for people who undertake it. Therapy often leads to a significant reduction in feelings of distress, better relationships and resolution of specific problems. But there are no guarantees about what will happen.

If you are being seen only for a neuropsychological assessment, you should be aware that the evaluation process can include some tests that are challenging and designed to exceed the limits of your cognitive abilities. Very rarely will you be able to tell if the errors you make represent poor performance. Many times people think they have done poorly on a test only to find out later that their performance was very good. (Therapist name) wants to obtain your best performance because this is the only way to identify your true strengths and weaknesses. Therefore you should report to the person administering the tests and notify them of any medications taken that day. Problems with fatigue, pain, anxiety, nervousness, frustration, anger and depression could affect your performance and you should communicate any such experiences at the time it is happening so that these problems can be addressed. If necessary, testing will be discontinued for the day in order to avoid having your performance affected by these experiences.

Your first session will involve an evaluation of your needs, although additional sessions are sometimes needed. By the end of the evaluation, (therapist name) will be able to offer you some initial impressions of what your work will include and an initial treatment plan to follow, if you decide to continue. You should evaluate this information along with your own assessment about whether you feel comfortable working with (therapist name). Therapy and/or testing involves a large commitment of time, money and energy, so you should be careful about the clinician you select. If you have any questions about (therapist name) procedures, you should discuss them whenever they arise. If your doubts persist, he will be happy to help you to secure and appropriate consultation with another mental health professional.

<u>FINANCIAL AGREEMENT & OFFICE BILLING/INSURANCE POLICIES</u>

1. I understand that professional services are rendered and charged to the patient and not to the insurance company. Not all issues/conditions/problems which are the focus of psychotherapy or an evaluation are reimbursed by insurance companies. **It is my responsibility to verify the specifics of my coverage. I am responsible for payment for any services or charges not covered by my insurances.** I understand that this office does not assume responsibility for claim denials, claim disputes, or for insurance payment of my account.

2. I agree to pay all deductibles, co-payments, and/or co-insurance amounts not paid by my insurance(s). These will be paid at the time services are rendered, unless other arrangements have been made. Under no circumstances does this office accept liens as payment on an account.

3. I understand that if my insurance(s) require a referral from my primary care physician, (therapist name) must have verification of the referral **prior** to my first appointment. I will bring my insurance information or insurance card(s) to my first appointment so that the office can properly identify my program(s).

4. If my sessions are to be billed to **Worker's Compensation**, I will provide the name of my carrier, the address where the billing is to be sent, my claim/case number, the name and phone number of my case worker, and a copy of the "Employee's Claim for Worker's Compensation Benefits" (DWC Form 1).

5. I authorize the release of information concerning my treatment or the treatment of my dependent(s) to my insurance company(s), including that an insurance company representative may review the clinical record.

FIGURE 4.3 (Continued)

6. I authorize direct payment by my insurance company(s) to (therapist name) Ph.D. and (company name).

7. I accept ultimate responsibility for payment for the services that I or my dependent(s) receive, whether or not my insurance(s) cover these services. This includes, but is not limited to fees for: clinical services or treatment, failed appointments and/or appointments not cancelled with 24 hours notice, report/letter writing, time spent in court or talking to attorneys on my behalf or the behalf of my dependent(s), telephone conversations longer than 5 minutes, site visits, reading records, longer sessions, travel time, etc.

8. I understand that I will receive a statement if I have an outstanding balance on my account and I am to pay any portion that is my responsibility within 15 days of receipt of a statement. A finance charge of 1% per month may be added to my account if payment is overdue.

9. I understand that there will be a $15.00 service fee for any checks returned by my bank due to non-sufficient funds, closed accounts, etc. I agree to accept full responsibility for such fees. The amount of the returned check, plus the service fee, must be paid within 10 days of written notice.

10. I will notify the Office Manager if any problem arises regarding my ability to make timely payments. If my account is overdue (unpaid) and there is no agreement on a payment plan, I understand that this office can use legal means (court, collection agency, etc.) to obtain payment.

11. I am aware of (therapist name) office policy requiring 24 hours notice to cancel an appointment. I understand that I may notify the office staff or the answering service of the intention to cancel an appointment. I further acknowledge that I will be charged $_____/hour for any appointment which I or my dependent(s) fail to keep without providing 24 hours notice.

My signature below signifies that I have read, understood, and agree to the above terms of the office policies, this financial agreement and office billing/insurance policies.

_____
Patient Name (Printed)

_____
Responsible Party (Printed)
(If patient is a minor or dependent adult)

_____
Signature of Responsible Party

____/____/_____
Date

FIGURE 4.3 (Continued)

(Therapist/Business Name)

Therapist(s) Name(s)
Therapist(s) Name(s)
Therapist(s) Name(s)

Street Address
City, State Zip
Phone Number
Fax Number
Email

PAYMENT AGREEMENT/AUTHORIZATION TO BILL INSURANCE

Name of Patient: _____
Please print name

"If Minor" Responsible Party Name: _____
Please print name

Our office policy states that if (therapist name) is not a participating, contracted provider with your health plan, then payment in full is due at the time of service.

Please read the following declaration then sign and date below where indicated.

I request that payment of authorize medical services furnished to me or my minor child be made by my insurance company, on mine or my minor child's behalf, to the provider of service indicated above. I authorize the medical provider listed above. I authorize the medical provider listed above and his agents to release any information concerning my medical care to my insurance company and any of its agents for the sole purpose of determining benefits payable on my medical related charges.

I understand my signature on this form authorizes my insurance company to make payment directly to the provider referenced above and that I am authorizing my provider to release all medical information necessary to adjudicate my medical claims. If other health insurance coverage is indicated in Item 9 of the Expo-1500 claim form, or elsewhere on other approved claim forms, or electronically submitted claims, my signature authorizes release of my medical information to that insurance company or agency as well. In HMO, PPO, or IPA assigned insurance, where the physician or supplier referenced above is a participating provider, my provider agrees to accept the allowable charge determination of my insurance carrier as the full charge, and the patient is responsible only for deductibles, coinsurance, in any non-convert services. Deductibles and coinsurance are based upon the charge to termination of my insurance carrier. If the provider is not a participating provider, then I, as the patient or responsible party understand the charges in full or my responsibility AND ARE PAYABLE AT THE TIME OF EACH SERVICE.

I understand that if (therapist name) is not a participating provider, I will pay for services in full at the time of service. This policy applies to secondary and subsequent plans as well.

***I understand this to be a lifetime beneficiary insurance authorization, unless I cancel this authorization and writing.

_____   _____
Signature of Insured or Responsible Party (Minor)   Date

FIGURE 4.3 (Continued)

266

(Therapist/Business Name)

Therapist(s) Name(s)
Therapist(s) Name(s)
Therapist(s) Name(s)

Street Address
City, State Zip
Phone Number
Fax Number
Email

CUSTODY ORDER VERIFICATION

_____

Minor Patient Name

In cases where the patient is a minor and the patient's parents are separated or divorced or legal guardianship exists, we require that you furnish us with a photocopy of your complete Custody Order as it relates to your minor child. (There will be a $25 charge to copy your custody order if you arrive without a copy.) The Order must include the custody arrangement and healthcare responsibilities of each party.

The custody order will provide your doctor with information as to the status of the legal custody of the minor, as well as any specific language that may impact a parent or guardian's right to consent to mental health treatment.

Joint Legal Custody can be awarded separate from Joint Physical Custody. Joint Legal Custody means that either parent acting alone may consent to mental health treatment unless the order of Joint Legal Custody has language to the contrary. Orders specifically requiring shared medical decision making responsibilities (barring emergencies) will require the consent of both parents.

If you need help determining your rights to obtain and authorize mental health treatment for your child, please contact your legal representative.

_____

Your signature below certifies that you have read and understand the requirements as they relate to furnishing our office with a copy of your Custody Order and authorizing mental health services for your minor child in the event of separation, divorce or legal guardianship;

☐　Check here if there is no record of any Custody Order for this patient and sign and date below:

_____　　　_____

Signature of Parent/Legal Guardian　　　　　　　　　　Date

☐　Check here if you have furnished our office with a copy of the patient's current Custody Order and sign and date below:

_____　　　_____

Signature of Parent/Legal Guardian　　　　　　　　　　Date

FIGURE 4.3　(Continued)

267

PATIENT AND BILLING DATA

PATIENT

Name:_____ Sex: M F

Last   First   MI

Address:_____ City:_____ State:_____ Zip Code:_____

Home Phone:_____ Cell Phone:_____ Work Phone:_____ Ext._____

Your Title: (Please check one) Mr._____ Mrs._____ Ms._____ Other:_____ Date of Birth____/____/_____

What is your relationship to the Responsible Party?

Self _____ Spouse _____ Daughter _____ Son _____ Other (specify) _____

Who referred you to this office? _____

Occupation:_____ Employer:_____

Marital Status: Single_____ Married_____ Separated_____ Divorced_____ Widowed_____

Social Security #:_____/____/_____ Driver's License #:_____

If patient is a minor, he/she resides with:

Mother_____ Father_____ Both Parents_____ Other (please specify)_____

****

ACCOUNT RESPONSIBLE (Person who will pay the balance after insurance pays)

Self_____ Spouse_____ Parent_____ Other (please specify)_____

Name:_____

Last   First   MI

Address:_____ City:_____ State:_____ Zip Code:_____

Home Phone:_____ Cell Phone:_____ Work
Phone:_____ Ext._____

Your Title: (Please check one) Mr._____ Mrs._____ Ms._____ Other:_____ Date of Birth:____/____/_____

****

Primary Care Physician:_____ Phone:_____

In case of emergency, contact:_____

Their relationship to you:_____

Their home phone:_____ Work Phone:_____

Is your condition work related? Yes_____ No_____

****

FIGURE 4.3 (Continued)

If referred by Attorney or litigation is pending:

Name of Attorney:_____

Address: _____ City:_____ State:_____ Zip:_____

Phone:_____

****

PRIMARY INSURANCE COMPANY

Name:_____

Mailing Address (for mental health claims):_____

City:_____ State:_____ Zip Code:_____

Attention:_____ Phone:_____

INSURED (The person who is the policy holder)

Name:_____
　　　　　　　Last　　　　　　　　　　First　　　　　　　　　　MI

Address:_____ City:_____ State:_____

Zip Code:_____ Home Phone:_____ Cell Phone:_____ Work Phone:_____Ext._____

Patient's relationship to insured?

Self_____　Spouse_____　Daughter_____　Son_____　Other (specify)_____

Insured Date of Birth:____/____/_____　Sex:　M　F　Employer:_____

ID/SS#_____　Effective date of insurance:_____

Group Claim #:_____　Group Name:_____

****

SECONDARY INSURANCE COMPANY

Name:_____

Mailing Address (for mental health claims):_____

City:_____ State:_____ Zip Code:_____

Attention:_____ Phone:_____

FIGURE 4.3　(Continued)

INSURED (The person who is the policy holder)

Name:_____

Last   First   MI

Address:_____ City:_____ State:_____

Zip Code:_____ Home Phone:_____ Cell Phone:_____ Work

Phone:_____ Ext.____

Patient's relationship to insured?

Self____ Spouse____ Daughter____ Son____ Other (specify)_____

Insured Date of Birth:____/____/_____ Sex: M F Employer:_____

ID/SS#_____ Effective date of insurance:_____

Group Claim #:_____ Group Name:_____

RELEASE OF INFORMATION:

Patient Name:_____

I hereby provide authorization for (therapist name) to exchange information regarding the medical and psychological condition, and drug and alcohol treatment of the patient named above with:

_____
(Name of Patient's Personal Physician)

Signature:_____ Date:____/____/_____

CONSENT FOR TREATMENT

I hereby provide consent for (therapist name) to provide psychological evaluation and treatment to myself, my minor child, or dependent.

Signature:_____ Date:____/____/_____

FIGURE 4.3 (Continued)

(Therapist/Business Name)

Therapist(s) Name(s)
Therapist(s) Name(s)
Therapist(s) Name(s)

Street Address
City, State Zip
Phone Number
Fax Number
Email

Child Psychological History

Date:_____

Name of person filling out form_____ Relationship to patient_____

Patient Name:_____ Sex:_____ Age:_____ Date of Birth:_____

Social Security #_____ School:_____ Grade:_____ Teacher:_____

Home Address:_____

Home Phone:_____ Parent's Work Phone:_____

Referred By_____ Reason For Referral:_____

Litigation Pending?_____ Attorney:_____ Phone:_____

History of Present Problem

How long ago did the problem(s) begin:_____

Please describe the problems that you would like help with:

_____

_____

_____

_____

_____

_____

_____

_____

_____

_____

_____

_____

FIGURE 4.3   (Continued)

Doctors Notes

FIGURE 4.3   (Continued)

Psychiatric History

Place a check for each symptom that applies.

☐ Suicidal thoughts	☐ Homicidal thoughts
☐ Depression/sadness	☐ Anxiety/nervousness
☐ Recurrent/intrusive thoughts	☐ Nightmares
☐ Loss of appetite	☐ Recurrent/intrusive disturbing recollections or dreams
☐ Weight loss	☐ Overwhelming need to perform certain behaviors/rituals
☐ Overeating	☐ Excessive fears or phobias
☐ Weight gain	☐ Significant concerns with physical problems
☐ Difficulty sleeping	☐ Poor frustration tolerance
☐ Apathy	☐ Explosive anger
☐ Fatigue	☐ Rapid mood changes
☐ Loss of interest in almost all activities	☐ Euphoria (feel on top of the world)
☐ Feeling worthless	☐ Racing thoughts
☐ Feelings of hopelessness	☐ Decreased need for sleep
☐ Poor self esteem	☐ Aggressive
☐ Sexual problems	☐ Visual or auditory hallucinations
☐ Anorexia or Bulimia	☐ Stomach aches
☐ Unmotivated	☐ Bizarre behavior
☐ Dependent	☐ Shy and withdrawn
☐ Quiet	☐ Self-mutilates
☐ Resists change	☐ Self-stimulates
☐ Wetting bed or clothes	☐ Exhibits sexually inappropriate behavior
☐ Bowel movements in underwear	☐ Risk-taking
☐ Emotional	☐ Is cruel to other people
☐ Immature	☐ Swears a lot
☐ Is very fidgety	☐ Steals things without people knowing on several occasions
☐ Can't remain seated	
☐ Can't wait his/her turn when playing with others	☐ Often runs away from home and stays away overnight
☐ Answers before s/he hears the whole question	☐ Easily lies to others
☐ Rarely follows other's instructions	☐ Firesetting
☐ Destroys other people's property	☐ Doesn't go to school
☐ Is cruel to animals	☐ Breaks into other people's property
☐ Starts fights with others	☐ When fighting, has used a weapon
☐ Other unusual behavior:_____	

Indicate which stressors the child is experiencing currently (within last 6 months) or in the past.

Now	Past		Now	Past		Now	Past	
___	___	Death of family member	___	___	Illness of family member	___	___	Illness of friend
___	___	Personal injury/illness	___	___	Parents separated	___	___	Parents divorced
___	___	Conflicts with family	___	___	Conflicts with friends	___	___	Conflicts at school
___	___	Academic difficulties	___	___	Change in residence	___	___	Legal problems
___	___	Sexual assault	___	___	Incest/sexual abuse	___	___	Physical abuse
___	___	Verbal/emotional abuse	___	___	Other Problems: _____			

FIGURE 4.3 (Continued)

Is s/he currently receiving therapy?_____ From who?_____
When did s/he start therapy?_____ For what problem(s)?_____
_____

List current psychiatric medications and dosages:_____

Has s/he received therapy in the past?_____ From who?_____
When (Start and finish):_____ For what problem(s)?_____
_____

List pas psychiatric medications: _____

Has s/he been hospitalized for psychological problems?_____ When?_____
Where was s/he hospitalized?_____
Has s/he ever attempted suicide?_____ When?_____ How?_____

DOCTORS NOTES

FIGURE 4.3 (Continued)

Birth and Developmental History

Place of Birth:_____ Were parents married at time of birth?_____

Was mother under a doctor's care during the pregnancy?_____ Was the child adopted?_____ If so, at what age?_____

Circle any illnesses during pregnancy:

Anemia	Toxemia	Herpes	Measles	German measles	Bleeding
Kidney disease	Heart disease	Hypertension	Abdominal trauma	Infection	Diabetes

Medications taken during pregnancy:_____

Were drugs or alcohol taken during pregnancy? Yes_____ No_____ If yes, specify:_____

Was there significant emotional stress during pregnancy? Yes_____ No_____ If yes, specify:_____

Was the birth: On time _____   Premature _____ (By how long _____)   Late_____ (By how long _____)

Was labor: Spontaneous _____   Induced _____   Duration of labor _____(Hours)   Cesarean required? _____

Was the presentation: Normal _____   Breach _____   Transverse (Crosswise) _____   Posterior first _____

Did the baby experience any of these problems: Fetal distress _____   Prolapsed cord _____   Low placenta (Placenta previa) _____

Premature separation of the placenta (Abruption placenta) _____   Cord wrapped around neck _____

Any other problems that mother or child had:_____

Was general anesthesia used? _____ Were forceps used? _____ Were there breathing problems? _____

Color at birth: Normal _____   Blue_____   Yellow_____   Was oxygen used (How long)?_____ APGAR Score _____

Birth weight:_____   Length:_____

Circle those that apply to the first few weeks after birth:

Excessive sleeping	Laziness	Irritability	Excessive crying	Stiffness	Limpness
Tremors	Twitching	Feeding difficulties	Vomiting	Jaundice	Other_____

Transfusions required?_____ Medication required? (For what)_____

Surgery required? (For what)_____

Give approximate ages that developmental milestones were achieved:

Head control_____   Rolled over_____   Sat alone_____   Walked_____   Run_____

Said first word_____   Used sentences_____   Self feeding w/ utensils_____   Toilet trained_____

Dress self_____   Tie shoes_____   Color within lines_____

Circle any problems that occurred in later development:

Hearing	Speaking	Stuttering	Reading	Writing	Spelling	Arithmetic	Behavior	Hyperactivity
Attention difficulties	Seizures	Coordination						

List family members with developmental or learning problems:_____

FIGURE 4.3   (Continued)

275

DOCTORS NOTES

276

FIGURE 4.3   (Continued)

Medical History

Please check all the conditions that have been diagnosed.

____AIDS, ARC or HIV+	____Diabetes	____Immune system disease	____Poisoning
____Allergies	____Enzyme deficiency	____Jaundice	____Polio
____Arthritis	____Encephalitis	____Kidney problems	____Parkinson's Disease
____Asthma	____Ear Infections	____Liver disorder	____Rheumatic Fever
____Abscessed ears	____Fever (104 or higher)	____Lung disease	____Radiation exposure
____Arteriosclerosis	____Genetic disorder	____Lead poisoning	____Scarlet fever
____Bleeding disorder	____Head injury/concussion	____Leukemia	____Senility (Dementia)
____Blood disorder	____Heart problems	____Metabolic disorder	____Stroke or TIA
____Broken bones	____Hereditary disorder	____Meningitis	____Tuberculosis
____Brain disease	____Headaches	____Measles	____Tumor
____Cerebral palsy	____Hearing problems	____Mumps	____Thyroid disease
____Colds (excessive)	____Huntington's disease	____Malnutrition	____Venereal disease
____Chicken pox	____Hypertension	____Multiple sclerosis	____Vision problems
____Hormone problems	____Oxygen deprivation	____Carbon monoxide poisoning	____Pneumonia
____Cancer	____Hazardous substance exposure		____Whooping cough

Other medical/physical problems_____

Has your child ever been diagnosed with epilepsy or a seizure disorder? Yes_____ No_____ If yes, check the one you have been diagnosed with.

PARTIAL

____Simple partial (Jacksonian)
____Complex partial (Psychomotor)
____Partial evolving into generalized

GENERALIZED

____Absence (Petit mal)
____Myoclonic
____Clonic
____Tonic
____Tonic-clonic (Grand mal)
____Atonic

____UNCLASSIFIED TYPE

List any medications currently being taken (over-the-counter or prescription), and the dosage.

Medication and dosage

1)_____ 4)_____
2)_____ 5)_____
3)_____ 6)_____

List any medications your child is ALLERGIC or sensitive to:_____

Past Hospitalizations (When, where and for what):

_____
_____
_____
_____
_____

Outpatient Surgeries (When, where and for what):

FIGURE 4.3 (Continued)

_____
_____
_____

Name of family physician: _____

Address: _____

Phone: _____ Date of your last medical check-up: _____

Medical Testing

Check all medical tests that recently have been done and report any abnormal findings:

	Check here if normal	**Abnormal findings**
____Angiography	____	_____
____Blood work	____	_____
____Brain scan	____	_____
____CT scan	____	_____
____EEG	____	_____
____Lumbar puncture or spinal tap	____	_____
____Magnetic Resonance Imaging (MRI)	____	_____
____Neurological office exam	____	_____
____PET scan	____	_____
____Physicians office exam	____	_____
____Skull x-ray	____	_____
____Ultrasound	____	_____
____Other testing:_____	____	_____

DOCTORS NOTES

FIGURE 4.3 (Continued)

Family History

Father's Name_____ Age_____ Health Problems_____

Education_____ Occupation_____ Employer_____

Mother's Name_____ Age_____ Health Problems_____

Education_____ Occupation_____ Employer_____

Date of parent's marriage_____ Years married_____ Current marital problems?_____ If separated, give date _____

If divorced, date_____ Previous marriages? (Father)_____ (Mother)_____

Subsequent marriages? (Father)_____ (Mother)_____

If divorced, current custody arrangement _____

Please provide information regarding step-parents if parents are divorced:

Name	Age	Education	Occupation	Date married	# Years
_____	___	_____	_____	_____	_____
_____	___	_____	_____	_____	_____
_____	___	_____	_____	_____	_____
_____	___	_____	_____	_____	_____

Names and ages of brothers and sisters (Include step-brothers and step-sisters):

_____
_____
_____

List anyone else who has lived in the home during your child's life: _____

List names of any family members (e.g., Immediate and distant relatives) with any of the following problems:

Alcohol/drug abuse_____

Criminal history _____

Emotional/behavioral problems _____

Medical problems (e.g., Heart disease, Cancer, Seizures)_____

Learning/developmental problems _____

279

```
DOCTORS NOTES




```

FIGURE 4.3   (Continued)

Social History

How long has s/he lived in current home? _____ Apartment or home? _____ How long in this town? _____

How many changes in residence in child's lifetime?_____ Ages moves occurred?_____

What towns has s/he lived in the past?_____

How many friends does your child have in your neighborhood? _____ First name of best friend in neighborhood: _____

How often does s/he play with neighborhood friends? _____ Any conflict problems (What type)? _____

What are his/her most frequent play activities? _____

How many friends does s/he have at school? _____ First name of best friend at school: _____

Is your child well liked/accepted at school?_____ Any conflict problems (What type)? _____

Does s/he have a girlfriend/boyfriend? _____ First name:_____ Involved how long? _____

Is this relationship stable? _____ Type of problems (if any): _____

How many girlfriends/boyfriends in the past? _____ Starting at what age: _____ Is s/he currently sexually active? _____

When did s/he first become sexually active? _____ Currently using birth control (What type)? _____

Any aborted pregnancies/miscarriages? _____ Any children outside of marriage? _____ Names/Ages:_____

List clubs and organizations that s/he is involved in:_____

_____

Is your child involved in a church? _____ Denomination:_____ Attend how often? _____

What time/activities do you share with your child?_____

Please describe your last vacation (when & where): _____

DOCTORS NOTES

Educational History

Current grade (Or highest grade/degree completed): _____ Current school: _____

Past schools attended (List in order): _____

_____

Hardest subject(s):_____ Favorite subject(s):_____

Grades earned in elementary school:_____ Junior High G.P.A _____ High School G.P.A _____

Grades repeated: _____ Learning problems (what subjects): _____

Special education placement (Type):_____ During which grades:_____

Extracurricular activities (Music, Sports, Clubs, etc.) _____

Expulsions/suspensions/conduct problems (Type of problem and date):_____

Additional schooling or non-academic training:_____

FIGURE 4.3 (Continued)

DOCTORS NOTES

Occupational History

Present employer:_____ Position:_____
Length of employment:_____ Hours worked per week_____ Current responsibilities_____

List previous employment (Include dates and type of work):
_____
_____
_____
_____

Have you ever been terminated from a job (Please explain):_____
At any time on the job were you ever exposed to dangerous chemicals or substances (e.g., Mercury, Lead, Radiation, Solvents, Pesticides, Chemicals, etc.)? Yes _____ No _____ If yes, explain:_____

DOCTORS NOTES

Legal History

Present legal problems (Describe):_____
Past arrest (For what?):_____
Convictions (For what?): _____
Time served in juvenile hall, jail or prison (Give dates and locations):_____
_____

DOCTORS NOTES

FIGURE 4.3   (Continued)

Child/Teen General Symptom Checklist

Parents please rate your child or teen on each of the symptoms listed below using the following scale. If possible, to give us the most complete picture, have the child or teen rate him/herself as well. **For young children it may not be practical to have them fill out the questionnaire.** Use your best judgment and do the best you can.

0	1	2	3	4	NA
Never	Rarely	Occasionally	Frequently	Very Frequently	Not Applicable/Not Known

Ch/Tn	Parent	
_____	_____	1. Depressed or sad mood
_____	_____	2. Not as much interest in things that are usually fun
_____	_____	3. Significant recent weight or appetite changes
_____	_____	4. Recurrent thoughts of death or suicide
_____	_____	5. Sleep changes, lack of sleep or marked increased in sleep
_____	_____	6. Low energy or feelings of tiredness
_____	_____	7. Feelings of being worthless, helpless, hopeless or guilty
_____	_____	8. Plays alone or appears socially withdrawn
_____	_____	9. Cries easily
_____	_____	10. Negative thinking
_____	_____	11. Periods of an elevated, high or irritable mood
_____	_____	12. Periods of a very high self esteem or big thinking
_____	_____	13. Periods of decreased need for sleep without feeling tired
_____	_____	14. More talkative than usual or feel pressure to keep talking
_____	_____	15. Fast thoughts or frequent jumping from one subject to another
_____	_____	16. Easily distracted by irrelevant things
_____	_____	17. Marked increase in activity level
_____	_____	18. Cyclic periods of angry, mean or violent behavior
_____	_____	19. Periods of time where you feel intensely anxious or nervous
_____	_____	20. Periods of trouble breathing of feeling smothered
_____	_____	21. Periods of feeling dizzy, faint or unsteady on your feet
_____	_____	22. Periods of heart pounding, fast heart rate or chest pain
_____	_____	23. Periods of trembling, shaking or sweating
_____	_____	24. Periods of nausea, abdominal upset or choking
_____	_____	25. Intense fear of dying
_____	_____	26. Lacks confidence in abilities
_____	_____	27. Needs lots of reassurance
_____	_____	28. Needs to be perfect
_____	_____	29. Seems fearful and anxious
_____	_____	30. Seems shy or timid
_____	_____	31. Easily embarrassed
_____	_____	32. Sensitive to criticism
_____	_____	33. Bites fingernails or chews clothing

282

FIGURE 4.3 (Continued)

_____	_____	34. Persistent refusal to go to school
_____	_____	35. Excessive fear of interacting with other children or adults
_____	_____	36. Persistent, excessive fear (heights, closed spaces, specific animals, etc.) please list _____
		_____
_____	_____	37. Excessive anxiety concerning separation from home or from those to whom the child is attached
_____	_____	38. Recurrent bothersome thoughts, ideas or images which you try to ignore
_____	_____	39. Trouble getting "stuck" on certain thoughts, or having the same thought over and over
_____	_____	40. Excessive or senseless worrying
_____	_____	41. Others complain that you worry too much or get "stuck" on the same thoughts
_____	_____	42. Compulsive behaviors that you must do or you feel very anxious, such as excessive hand washing, cleaning, checking locks, or counting or spelling
_____	_____	43. Needing to have things done a certain way or you become very upset
_____	_____	44. Recurrent and upsetting thoughts of a past traumatic event (molest, accident, fire, etc.), please list
		_____
_____	_____	45. Recurrent distressing dreams of a past upsetting event
_____	_____	46. Feelings of reliving a past upsetting event
_____	_____	47. Spend effort avoiding thoughts or feelings related to a past trauma
_____	_____	48. Feeling that your future is shortened
_____	_____	49. Startle easily
_____	_____	50. Feel like you're always watching for bad things to happen
_____	_____	51. Refusal to maintain body weight above a level most people consider healthy
_____	_____	52. Intense fear of gaining weight or becoming fat even though underweight
_____	_____	53. Feelings of being fat, even though you're underweight
_____	_____	54. Recurrent episodes of eating large amounts of food
_____	_____	55. A feeling of lack of control over eating behavior
_____	_____	56. Engage in activities to eliminate excess food, such as self induced vomiting, laxatives, strict dieting or strenuous exercise
_____	_____	57. Persistent worry with body shape and weight
_____	_____	58. Involuntary physical movements or motor tics (eye blinking, shoulder shrugging, head jerking or picking)
		How long have motor tics been present?_____ How often?_____ Describe_____
_____	_____	59. Involuntary vocal sounds or verbal tics (coughing, puffing, blowing, whistling swearing)
		How long have verbal tics been present?_____ How often?_____ Describe_____
_____	_____	60. Repetitive, seemingly driven motor behavior (hand shaking or waving, body rocking, head banging, mouthing of objects, self-biting, picking at skin or bodily orifices, hitting own body) that interferes with normal activities or results in self inflicted bodily injury that requires medical treatment (or would result in an injury if preventive measures were not used)
_____	_____	61. Passage of feces in inappropriate places (clothing or floor)
_____	_____	62. Bed wetting. If present, how often?_____

FIGURE 4.3 (Continued)

_____ _____ 63. Failure to speak in specific social situations (e.g., at school) despite speaking in other situations

_____ _____ 64. Delusional or bizarre thoughts (thoughts you know others would think are false)

_____ _____ 65. Visual hallucination, seeing objects or images are not really present

_____ _____ 66. Hearing voices that are not really present

_____ _____ 67. Odd behaviors

_____ _____ 68. Poor personal hygiene or grooming

_____ _____ 69. Inappropriate mood for the situation (i.e., laughing at sad events)

_____ _____ 70. Frequent feelings that someone or something is out to hurt you

_____ _____ 71. Problems with social relatedness before the age of 5, either by failing to respond appropriately to others or becoming indiscriminately attached to others

_____ _____ 72. Multiple changes in caregivers before the age of 5

_____ _____ 73. Steals

_____ _____ 74. Bullies, threatens, or intimidates others

_____ _____ 75. Initiates physical fights

_____ _____ 76. Cruel to animals

_____ _____ 77. Force others into things they do not want to do (sexually or criminally)

_____ _____ 78. Sets fires

_____ _____ 79. Destroys property

_____ _____ 80. Break in to others home, school, car or place of business

_____ _____ 81. Lies

_____ _____ 82. Stays out at night despite parental prohibitions

_____ _____ 83. Runs away overnight

_____ _____ 84. Cuts school

_____ _____ 85. Doesn't seem sorry for hurting others

_____ _____ 86. Negative, hostile, or defiant behavior

_____ _____ 87. Loses temper

_____ _____ 88. Argues with adults

_____ _____ 89. Actively defies or refuses to comply with adults' requests or rules

_____ _____ 90. Deliberately annoys people

_____ _____ 91. Blames others for his or her mistakes or misbehavior

_____ _____ 92. Touchy or easily annoyed by others

_____ _____ 93. Angry and resentful

_____ _____ 94. Spiteful or vindictive

_____ _____ 95. Impairment in communication as manifested by at least one of the following: (Check those that apply)

    _____ Delay in, or total lack of, the development of spoken language (not accompanied by an attempt to compensate through alternative modes of communication such as gesture or mime)

    _____ In individuals with adequate speech, marked impairment in the ability to initiate or sustain a conversation with others

FIGURE 4.3 (Continued)

_____ Repetitive use of language or odd language

_____ Lack of varied, spontaneous make-believe play or social imitative play appropriate to developmental level

_____ _____ 96. Impairment in social interaction, with at least two of the following: (Check those that apply)

_____ Marked impairment in use of multiple nonverbal behaviors such as eye-to-eye gaze, facial expression, body postures, and gestures to regulate social interaction

_____ Failure to develop peer relationships appropriate to developmental level

_____ Lack of spontaneous seeking to share enjoyment, interests, or achievements with other people (e.g., by a lack of showing, bringing, or pointing out objects of interest)

_____ Lack of social or emotional reciprocity

_____ _____ 97. Repetitive patterns of behavior, interests, and activities, as manifested by at least one of the following: (Check those that apply)

_____ Preoccupation with an area of that is abnormal either in intensity or focus

_____ Rigid adherence to specific, nonfunctional routines or rituals

_____ Repetitive motor mannerisms (e.g., hand or finger flapping or twisting, or complex whole-body movements)

_____ Persistent preoccupation with parts of objects

_____ _____ 98. Stutters

_____ _____ 99. Feel tired during the day
_____ _____ 100. Feel cold when others feel fine or they are warm
_____ _____ 101. Often feel warm when others feel fine or they are cold
_____ _____ 102. Problems with brittle or dry hair
_____ _____ 103. Problems with dry skin
_____ _____ 104. Problems with sweating
_____ _____ 105. Problems with chronic anxiety or tension

_____ _____ 106. Has difficulty learning math facts
_____ _____ 107. Poor math grades or test scores
_____ _____ 108. Has difficulty with abstract concepts and reasoning
_____ _____ 109. Has difficulty remembering
_____ _____ 110. Makes spelling errors in written assignments
_____ _____ 111. Needs words repeated when taking spelling tests
_____ _____ 112. Poor spelling grades or test scores
_____ _____ 113. Has difficulty reading or spelling phonetically
_____ _____ 114. Has difficulty sounding out unknown words
_____ _____ 115. Poor reading grades or test scores
_____ _____ 116 Avoids reading
_____ _____ 117. Reading is slow or choppy
_____ _____ 118. Complains about eye strain or fatigue
_____ _____ 119. Squints, blinks or rubs eyes when reading
_____ _____ 120. Skips words or lines when reading
_____ _____ 121. Poor reading comprehension
_____ _____ 122. Reverses letters or words
_____ _____ 123. Has difficulty hearing
_____ _____ 124. Has poor handwriting
_____ _____ 125. Has poor coordination
_____ _____ 126. Has difficulty writing a paper
_____ _____ 127. Makes grammatical errors
_____ _____ 128. Has poor vocabulary

FIGURE 4.3 (Continued)

Child Brain System Checklist

Parents please rate your child on each of the symptoms listed below using the following scale. If possible, to give us the most complete picture, have the child or teen rate him/herself as well. **<u>For young children it may not be practical to have them fill out the questionnaire.</u>** Use you r best judgment and do the best you can.

0 Never	1 Rarely	2 Occasionally	3 Frequently	4 Very Frequently	NA Not Applicable/Not Known

Ch/Tn	Parent	
_____	_____	1. Fails to give close attention to details or makes careless mistakes
_____	_____	2. Trouble sustaining attention in routine situations (i.e., homework, chores, paperwork)
_____	_____	3. Trouble listening
_____	_____	4. Fails to finish things
_____	_____	5. Poor organization for time or space (such as backpack, room, desk, paperwork)
_____	_____	6. Avoids, dislikes, or is reluctant to engage in tasks that require sustained mental effort
_____	_____	7. Loses things
_____	_____	8. Easily distracted
_____	_____	9. Forgetful
_____	_____	10. Poor planning skills
_____	_____	11. Lack clear goals or forward thinking
_____	_____	12. Difficulty expressing feelings
_____	_____	13. Difficulty expressing empathy for others
_____	_____	14. Excessive daydreaming
_____	_____	15. Feeling bored
_____	_____	16. Feeling apathetic or unmotivated
_____	_____	17. Feeling tired, sluggish or slow moving
_____	_____	18. Feeling spacey or "in a fog"

Ch/Tn	Parent	
_____	_____	19. Fidgety, restless or trouble sitting still
_____	_____	20. Difficulty remaining seated in situations where remaining seated is expected
_____	_____	21. Runs about or climbs excessively in situations in which it is inappropriate
_____	_____	22. Difficulty playing quietly
_____	_____	23. "On the go" or acts as if "driven by a motor"
_____	_____	24. Talks excessively
_____	_____	25. Blurts out answers before questions have been completed
_____	_____	26. Difficulty awaiting turn
_____	_____	27. Interrupts or intrudes on others, e.g., butts into conversations or games)
_____	_____	28. Impulsive (saying or doing things without thinking first)

Ch/Tn	Parent	
_____	_____	29. Excessive or senseless worrying
_____	_____	30. Upset when things do not go your way
_____	_____	31. Upset when things are out of place
_____	_____	32. Tendency to be oppositional or argumentative
_____	_____	33. Tendency to have repetitive negative thoughts
_____	_____	34. Tendency toward compulsive behaviors

FIGURE 4.3 (Continued)

_____ _____ 35. Intense dislike for change

_____ _____ 36. Tendency to hold grudges

_____ _____ 37. Trouble shifting attention from subject to subject

_____ _____ 38. Trouble shifting behavior from task to task

_____ _____ 39. Difficulties seeing options in situations

_____ _____ 40. Tendency to hold on to own opinion and not listen to others

_____ _____ 41. Tendency to get locked into a course of action, whether or not it is good

_____ _____ 42. Needing to have things done a certain way or you become very upset

_____ _____ 43. Others complain that you worry too much

_____ _____ 44. Tend to say no without first thinking about question

_____ _____ 45. Tendency to predict fear

_____ _____ 46. Frequent feelings of sadness

_____ _____ 47. Moodiness

_____ _____ 48. Negativity

_____ _____ 49. Low energy

_____ _____ 50. Irritability

_____ _____ 51. Decreased interest in others

_____ _____ 52. Decreased interest in things that are usually fun or pleasurable

_____ _____ 53. Feelings of hopelessness about the future

_____ _____ 54. Feelings of helplessness or powerlessness

_____ _____ 55. Feeling dissatisfied or bored

_____ _____ 56. Excessive guilt

_____ _____ 57. Suicidal feelings

_____ _____ 58. Crying spells

_____ _____ 59. Lowered interest in things usually considered fun

_____ _____ 60. Sleep changes (too much or too little)

_____ _____ 61. Appetite changes (too much or too little)

_____ _____ 62. Chronic low self-esteem

_____ _____ 63. Negative sensitivity to smells/odors

_____ _____ 64. Frequent feelings of nervousness or anxiety

_____ _____ 65. Panic attacks

_____ _____ 66. Symptoms of heightened muscle tension (headaches, sore muscles, hand tremor)

_____ _____ 67. Periods of heart pounding, rapid heart rate or chest pain

_____ _____ 68. Periods of trouble breathing or feeling smothered

_____ _____ 69. Periods of feeling dizzy, faint or unsteady on your feet

_____ _____ 70. Periods of nausea or abdominal upset

_____ _____ 71. Periods of sweating, hot or cold flashes

_____ _____ 72. Tendency to predict the worst

_____ _____ 73. Fear of dying or doing something crazy

_____ _____ 74. Avoid places for fear of having an anxiety attack

_____ _____ 75. Conflict avoidance

_____ _____ 76. Excessive fear of being judged or scrutinized by others

FIGURE 4.3 (Continued)

_____ _____ 77. Persistent phobias

_____ _____ 78. Low motivation

_____ _____ 79. Excessive motivation

_____ _____ 80. Tics (motor or vocal)

_____ _____ 81. Poor handwriting

_____ _____ 82. Quick startle

_____ _____ 83. Tendency to freeze in anxiety provoking situations

_____ _____ 84. Lacks confidence in their abilities

_____ _____ 85. Seems shy or timid

_____ _____ 86. Easily embarrassed

_____ _____ 87. Sensitive to criticism

_____ _____ 88. Bites fingernails or picks skin

_____ _____ 89. Short fuse or periods of extreme irritability

_____ _____ 90. Periods of rage with little provocation

_____ _____ 91. Often misinterprets comments as negative when they are not

_____ _____ 92. Irritability tends to build, then explodes, then recedes, often tired after a rage

_____ _____ 93. Periods of spaciness or confusion

_____ _____ 94. Periods of panic and/or fear for no specific reason

_____ _____ 95. Visual or auditory changes, such as seeing shadows or hearing muffled sounds

_____ _____ 96. Frequent periods of déjà vu (feelings of being somewhere you have never been)

_____ _____ 97. Sensitivity or mild paranoia

_____ _____ 98. Headaches or abdominal pain of certain origin

_____ _____ 99. History of a head injury or family history of violence or explosiveness

_____ _____ 100. Dark thoughts, may involve suicidal or homicidal thoughts

_____ _____ 101. Periods of forgetfulness or memory problems

Bradley A. Schuyler, Ph.D.
Schuyler Psychological Associates

FIGURE 4.3   (Continued)

ADDITIONAL BUSINESS RELATED FORMS

Many of the following forms are associated with the IFSP/IEP process. They have been included because of their potential of being effectively adapted to varying environments providing intervention to young children and their families.

Assessment Plan

Student Name_____ D.O.B._____ C.A._____ Grade_____
School_____ Track_____ Date_____ Address_____
Phone_____ Pupil's Language_____ ❏EL ❏FEP
REASON FOR ASSESSMENT/AREAS OF CONCERN _____

For initial referrals only

Student Referred by _____ Date Referred _____

School years interventions were provided in general education_____

The following assessments are proposed to assist in determining your child's educational needs. All assessments will be given by appropriately qualified personnel. The assessment will be in the areas checked below and may include pupil observation in a group setting, classroom work samples, district or statewide group assessments, individualized testing, teacher interview(s) and an interview with you. It also may include a review of reports you have authorized us to request or that already exist in current records. Assessments will be non-discriminatory, and alternative means of assessment may be used in situations when standardized assessments are inappropriate. Within 60 days of receipt of this signed assessment plan, an Individualized Educational Program (IEP) team meeting will be held. You will be invited to attend and review assessment results and participate in determining your child's educational needs and eligibility for special education services.

❏ **PRE-ACADEMIC/ACADEMIC ACHIEVEMENT:**   ❏ Special Education   ❏ Teacher
❏ Psychologist   ❏ Other:_____
Purpose: To determine current reading, writing, and math skills or preacademic skills such as matching or sorting.

❏ **SOCIAL/EMOTIONAL BEHAVIOR:**   ❏ Psychologist   ❏ Infant/Preschool Specialist
❏Other:_____
Purpose: To evaluate how the student handles feelings and emotions and how he/she gets along with other people.

❏ **SELF HELP/ADAPTIVE SKILLS:**   ❏ Psychologist   ❏ Other:_____
Purpose: To evaluate how the student functions in daily life activities.

❏ **PSYCHO-MOTOR DEVELOPMENT:**   ❏ Psychologist   ❏ Infant/Preschool Specialist
❏ Other:_____
Purpose: To determine how well an individual coordinates body movements in both small and large muscle activities or to evaluate visual perceptual skills.

❏ **LANGUAGE/SPEECH/COMMUNICATION DEVELOPMENT:**   ❏ Speech-Language
❏ Pathologist   ❏ Infant/Preschool Specialist   ❏ Other:_____
Purpose: To determine an individual's ability to understand, relate to, and use language and speech clearly and appropriately.

❏ **INTELLECTUAL DEVELOPMENT:**   ❏ Psychologist   ❏ Infant/Preschool Specialist
❏ Other:_____
Purpose: To determine how well individuals remember what they have seen and heard, how well they can use that information to solve problems, and to assist in predicting the student's learning rate. Verbal and performance instruments may be used as appropriate.

❏ **HEALTH ASSESSMENT:**   ❏ School Nurse   ❏ Infant/Preschool Specialist
❏ Other:_____
Purpose: To evaluate developmental patterns and current health status as they relate to school functioning.

FIGURE 4.4

❑ **VOCATIONAL/PREVOCATIONAL**: ❑ Special Education Teacher ❑ Psychologist
❑ Other:_____
Purpose: To determine the individual's interest and or aptitude as it relates to future job and life skill areas.

❑ **OTHER**:_____

Responsible Personnel:_____

If you have any questions contact:

_____   _____
                      Name/Title   Date

Phone: (_____)_____

PARENTAL CONSENT FOR PUPIL ASSESSMENT

I understand the purpose of the proposed Assessment Plan and have received a copy of my Parent Rights. I authorize the use of a suitable interpreter or prerecorded tests in my child's primary language as appropriate. I further understand that no individualized education program will result from this assessment without my consent. The box checked below indicates my decision.

❑ **Yes**, I give permission to conduct the assessment as described above and will make my child available for the assessment. I understand that assessment cannot begin until a copy of this form has been signed and returned. I ❑do ❑do not give permission to the school district to bill the LEA Medi-Cal Billing Option Program for this assessment, if applicable. (Income from this program is used by the district to offset costs of providing special education services and will not affect your child's individual benefits.)

❑ **No**, permission is denied.

❑ Please consider the following Independent Educational Evaluation reports as part of the assessment process:_____

Please sign and return, keeping one copy for your records.

_____
Parent/Legal Guardian/Adult Student/Person Acting as Parent (Specify)

_____
Telephone Number

_____
Date

For more information about special education and your rights contact your district special education office or visit the Ventura County SELPA website at www.venturacountyselpa.com

Copy to: ❑District Office   ❑Cumulative File   ❑Case Manager   ❑Parent/Adult Student
              ❑Related Services

Ventura County Special Education Local Plan Area (SELPA)   CSS SE-1165(10/10)

FIGURE 4.4   (Continued)

Functional Analysis Assessment

As required by the Hughes Bill of 1990

Date of Report_____

Examiner(s)_____

IDENTIFYING INFORMATION

Student_____ Date of Birth_____ Age_____ ❏M ❏F

Grade_____ School/Program_____ District_____

REASON FOR REFERRAL

_____

_____

_____

BACKGROUND INFORMATION/PERTINENT INFORMATION FROM FILE REVIEW

Relevant health and medical information (including current medications)_____

_____

Results of previous assessment (including eligibility for Special Education Services)_____

_____

Previous behavioral interventions and results_____

_____

Results of interviews with "significant others"_____

_____

OPERATIONAL DEFINITION OF PROBLEM BEHAVIOR

_____

_____

OBSERVATION OF STUDENT/BEHAVIOR

Dates and times of day student was observed_____

FIGURE 4.5

Settings in which the student was observed _____

Who observed the student?_____

Was the behavior graphed?_____

Frequency, duration, and intensity of targeted inappropriate behaviors_____

_____

ANALYSIS OF TARGETED BEHAVIOR(S)

Antecedent event(s)/setting variables. The following antecedents have been observed to occur before or in the presence of target behaviors:

Ecological analysis of setting(s) in which the targeted behavior(s) occur most frequently. Factors which should be considered include, but are not limited to, the following: physical setting, social setting, activities and nature of instruction, scheduling, quality of communication between individual, staff and other students, degree of independence, degree of participation, amount of quality of social interaction, degree of choice and variety of activities.

Current consequences of the targeted behavior(s):_____

_____

Based on the data collected, it appears that the target behavior(s) function to: _____

_____

Alternative positive replacement behavior(s): _____

_____

Operational definition of alternative behavior(s):_____

_____

Antecedents of alternative behavior(s): _____

_____

Current consequences of alternative behavior(s):_____

_____

Conclusion: Positive Behavioral Intervention Plan Necessity (Both criteria must be met):
❑ Student exhibits a serious behavior problem.
❑ This behavior problem significantly interferes with the implementation of the goals and objectives of the student's IEP.

FIGURE 4.5   (Continued)

Conclusion: BICM recommendations for IEP team consideration (Choose one finding):

❏Develop a positive behavior intervention plan based on the *Functional Analysis Assessment.* (The complete positive behavior intervention plan includes 4 sections: 1) *Determination of Need for a Functional Analysis Assessment*; 2) *This form, the Functional Analysis Assessment, which documents data collection procedures, the BICM, and subsequent IEP team recommendations*; 3*) the Behavior Support Plan developed by the IEP*; 4) *The Positive Behavior Intervention Plan, which documents the additional requirements during the implementation.*)

❏No *Positive Behavior Intervention Plan* (PBIP) required. Develop a *Behavior Support Plan.*

❏No plan required. Rationale:

Signature_____ Position_____ Date_____

Signature_____ Position_____ Date_____

FIGURE 4.5   (Continued)

Functional Behavior Assessment
Checklist for Teachers and Staff

Completed by_____ Date of Report_____

IDENTIFYING INFORMATION

Student_____ Date of Birth_____ Grade_____ ❑M ❑F

STUDENT STRENGTHS – Please identify the student's strengths. Some possible strengths include: academic interests, social skills, hobbies, sports, etc.

NATURE AND SCOPE OF THE BEHAVIOR – To gain a better understanding of the nature and scope of the problem behavior please check the most relevant item(s). Then use the space at the bottom of each section to provide a brief description of the problem behavior, predictors, and consequences.

PROBLEM BEHAVIOR – *Description of behavior of concern that has been occurring.*

❑Tardy	❑Inappropriate language	❑Disrupts Class Activities	❑Theft
❑Inattentive	❑Fighting/Physical Aggression	❑Insubordination/Disrespectful	❑Vandalism
❑Sleeping	❑Verbally Harasses	❑Work Not Completed	❑Others

What does the behavior look like (be specific)?

PREDICTOR(S) & SETTING EVENT(S) – *Person(s), place, or time where the behavior is most likely to occur.*

Location	Person(s)	Time	Academic Concerns	Setting Event(s)
❑In Class	❑Peer(s)	❑Before School	❑All Classes	❑Use of medication
❑Hall	❑Teacher(s)	❑Morning	❑Reading	❑Physical Health
❑Cafeteria	❑Staff	❑Lunch	❑	❑Illegal Drug Use
❑Bus	❑	❑Home Room	❑	❑Conflict at Home
❑	❑	❑Afternoon	❑	❑

Is there a specific activity that is difficult for the student?

CONSEQUENCES – *What typically happens after the behavior of concerns occurs?*

Obtain Attention	Escape/Avoid Demand or Situation	Current Strategies
❑Peer Attention	❑Escape Difficulty/Activity	❑Change Seating
❑Adult Attention	❑Adult Attention	❑Contact Parent
❑Activity	❑Negative Peer Attention	❑Send to Office
❑	❑	❑
❑	❑	❑

What strategies have been effective?

After an incident what does the student obtain (e.g. attention) or avoid (e.g. difficult task)?

FIGURE 4.6

Functional Behavior Assessment

Complete an FBA for each behavior that is interfering with the student's behavior or that of others.

IDENTIFYING INFORMATION

Student_____ Birth date_____ Age_____ ❑M ❑F
Grade_____ School_____District_____
Staff Participating in Assessment_____ Date of Assessment_____

TARGET BEHAVIOR # Describe specifically what the behavior looks like. If there is more than 1 behavior, complete an additional form.	
IDENTIFY AND DESCRIBE THE DATA SOURCES USED TO ANALYZE THESE BEHAVIORS.	❑Interview ❑Observation ❑Review of Records (health, discipline, etc.)
DESCRIBE THE FREQUENCY, INTENSITY, AND DURATION OF THE BEHAVIOR. When does the behavior occur? How often? How long does it last? Description should be based upon data collection and/or record review.	
WHAT ARE THE PREDICTORS/TRIGGERS FOR EACH BEHAVIOR? Describe the situations in which the behavior is likely to occur (people, time, place, subject, etc.)	
WHAT ARE THE CONSEQUENCES THE STUDENT ACHIEVES BY THE BEHAVIOR? Describe what happens after the behavior occurs and/or what the student get/avoid or protest.	
WHAT IS THE FUNCTION OF THE BEHAVIOR? Is it to obtain, avoid, or protest?	
WHY IS THIS THE PROBABLY FUNCTION OF THE BEHAVIOR?	
WHAT ALTERATIONS TO THE ENVIRONMENT, INSTRUCTION, OR INTERACTIONS COULD PREVENT THE BEHAVIOR FROM REOCCURRING?	

FIGURE 4.7

IDENTIFY FUNCTIONALLY EQUIVALENT REPLACEMENT BEHAVIORS. Describe what the student should do INSTEAD of the problem behavior.	
DESCRIBE CURRENT METHODS OF REINFORCEMENT AND RECOMMEND ANY CHANGES IN REINFORCEMENT.	
WHAT GOALS, SERVICES, ETC. ARE YOU RECOMMENDING?	Goals numbered Other recommendations

Completed by_____ Date_____

FIGURE 4.7 (Continued)

Behavior Support Plan

For behavior interfering with the student's learning or the learning of his/her peers.
Complete a Behavior Support Plan for each target behavior identified.

Student:_____ Date:_____

IDENTIFICATION

1. The behavior impeding learning is *(Description of what the behavior looks like)*: _____
   _____
   _____

2. It impedes learning because: _____

3. The need for a Behavior Support Plan is: ❑Early ❑Intervention ❑Moderate ❑Serious
   ❑Extreme

4. Frequency or intensity or duration of behavior: ❑Reported by_____
   ❑And/or Observed by_____

PREVENTION: PART 1 – ENVIRONMENTAL FACTORS AND NECESSARY CHANGES

5. What are the predictors for the behavior? *(Situations in which the behavior is likely to occur: people, time, place, subject, etc.)* _____
   _____

6. What supports the student using the problem behavior? *(What is missing in the environment/curriculum or what is the environment/curriculum that needs changing?)*_____
   _____

Remove student's need to use the behavior

7. What environmental changes, structures, and supports are needed to remove the student's need to use the behavior? *(Changes in Time/Space/Materials/Interactions to remove likelihood of behavior)*_____
   _____
   _____

   Who will establish?_____
   Who will monitor? _____
   Frequency? _____

ALTERNATIVES: PART 2 - FUNCTIONAL FACTORS AND NEW BEHAVIORS TO TEACH AND SUPPORT

8. Team believes the behaviors occur because *(Function of behavior in terms of getting, protest, or avoiding something)*:_____
   _____

Accept a replacement behavior that meets same need

9. What team believes the student should do **INSTEAD** of the problem behavior? *(How should the student escape/protest/avoid or get his/her need met in an acceptable way?)*_____
   _____

10. What teaching strategies/necessary curriculum materials are needed? *(List successive teaching steps for student to learn replacement behavior(s) and/or curriculum materials needed)*_____
    _____

11. What are reinforcement procedures to use for establishing, maintaining, and generalizing the replacement behavior(s)?_____
    _____

FIGURE 4.8

Selection of reinforce based on:
❑Reinforcer for using replacement behavior
❑Reinforcer for general increase in positive behavior(s)
By whom:_____ Frequency?_____

EFFECTIVE REACTION: PART 3 – REACTIVE STRATEGIES

12. What strategies will be employed if the problem behavior occurs again?_____
_____
_____
_____

1. Prompt student to switch to the replacement behavior.
2. Describe how staff should handle the problem behavior if it occurs again.
3. Positive discussion with student after behavior ends.
   Optional?
4. Any necessary further classroom or school consequences.
   Personnel?

OUTCOME: PART 4 – BEHAVIORAL GOALS

Use the following charts as a guide and transfer the information to a Marin SELPA Annual Goal form:
13. Behavioral Goal(s)

Required: Functionally Equivalent Replacement Behavior (FERB) Goal

By Whom	Who	Will do X behavior	For the purpose of Y	Instead of Z behavior	For the purpose of Y	Under what conditional conditions	At what level of proficiency	As measured by whom and how

Option 1: Increase General Positive or Decrease Problem Behavior

By When	Who	Will do what, or will not do what	At what level of proficiency	Under what conditional conditions	As measured by whom and how

Option 2: Increase General Positive or Decrease Problem Behavior

By When	Who	Will do what, or will not do what	At what level of proficiency	Under what conditional conditions	As measured by whom and how

The above behavioral goal(s) are to: ❑increase use of replacement behavior and may also include:
❑Reduce frequency of problem behavior
❑Develop mew general skills that remove student's need to use the problem behavior

Observation and Analysis conclusion:
Are curriculum accommodations or modifications also necessary?   ❑Yes ❑No
Where described:_____
Are environmental supports/changes necessary?   ❑Yes ❑No
Is reinforcement of replacement behavior alone enough (no new teaching is necessary)?   ❑Yes ❑No
Are both teaching of new replacement behavior AND reinforcement needed?   ❑Yes ❑No

FIGURE 4.8 (Continued)

This BSP to be coordinated with other agency's service plans? ❑Yes ❑No

Person responsible for contact between agencies:_____

COMMUNICATION: PART 5 – COMMUNICATION PROVISIONS

Manner and content of communication _____

_____

_____

_____

_____

1. Who	2. Under what conditions? (contingent/continuous)	3. Delivery method?	4. Expected Frequency?	5. Content?	6. How will this be a two-way communication?

1. Who	2. Under what conditions? (contingent/continuous)	3. Delivery method?	4. Expected Frequency?	5. Content?	6. How will this be a two-way communication?

1. Who	2. Under what conditions? (contingent/continuous)	3. Delivery method?	4. Expected Frequency?	5. Content?	6. How will this be a two-way communication?

PARTICPATION: PART 6 – PARTICIPANTS IN PLAN DEVELOPMENT

❑Student

❑Parent/Guardian

❑Parent/Guardian

❑Educator and Title

❑Educator and Title

❑Administrator

❑Other

FIGURE 4.8 (Continued)

299

CHILD SYMPTOM CHECKLIST

Child   Parent

_____   _____   1. Fails to give close attention to details or makes careless mistakes

_____   _____   2. Trouble sustaining attention in routine situations (i.e., homework, chores, paperwork)

_____   _____   3. Trouble listening

_____   _____   4. Fails to finish things

_____   _____   5. Poor organization for time or space (such as backpack, room, desk, paperwork)

_____   _____   6. Avoids, dislikes, or is reluctant to engage in tasks that require sustained mental effort

_____   _____   7. Loses things

_____   _____   8. Easily distracted

_____   _____   9. Forgetful

_____   _____   10. Poor planning skills

_____   _____   11. Lack clear goals or forward tinking

_____   _____   12. Difficulty expressing feelings

_____   _____   13. Difficulty expressing empathy for others

_____   _____   14. Excessive daydreaming

_____   _____   15. Feeling bored

_____   _____   16. Feeling apathetic or unmotivated

_____   _____   17. Feeling tired, sluggish or slow moving

_____   _____   18. Feeling spacey or "in a fog"

_____   _____   19. Fidgety, restless or trouble sitting still

_____   _____   20. Difficulty remaining seated in situations where remaining seated is expected

_____   _____   21. Runs about or climbs excessively in situations in which it is inappropriate

_____   _____   22. Difficulty playing quietly

_____   _____   23. "On the go" or acts as if "driven by a motor"

_____   _____   24. Talks excessively

_____   _____   25. Blurts out answers before questions have been completed

_____   _____   26. Difficulty awaiting turn

_____   _____   27. Interrupts or intrudes on others, e.g., butts into conversations or games)

_____   _____   28. Impulsive (saying or doing things without thinking first)

_____   _____   29. Excessive or senseless worrying

_____   _____   30. Upset when things do not go your way

_____   _____   31. Upset when things are out of place

_____   _____   32. Tendency to be oppositional or argumentative

_____   _____   33. Tendency to have repetitive negative thoughts

_____   _____   34. Tendency toward compulsive behaviors

_____   _____   35. Intense dislike for change

_____   _____   36. Tendency to hold grudges

_____   _____   37. Trouble shifting attention from subject to subject

_____   _____   38. Trouble shifting behavior from task to task

_____   _____   39. Difficulties seeing options in situations

_____   _____   40. Tendency to hold on to own opinion and not listen to others

_____   _____   41. Tendnecy to get locked into a course of action, whether or not it is good

_____   _____   42. Needing to have things done a certain way or you become very upset

_____   _____   43. Others complain that you worry too much

300

FIGURE 4.9

_____   _____   44. Tend to say no without first thinking about question

_____   _____   45. Tendency to predict fear

_____   _____   46. Frequent feelings of sadness

_____   _____   47. Moodiness

_____   _____   48. Negativity

_____   _____   49. Low energy

_____   _____   50. Irritability

_____   _____   51. Decreased interest in others

_____   _____   52. Decreased interest in things that are usually fun or pleasurable

_____   _____   53. Feelings of hopelessness about the future

_____   _____   54. Feelings of helplessness or powerlessness

_____   _____   55. Feeling dissatisfied or bored

_____   _____   56. Excessive guilt

_____   _____   57. Suicidal feelings

_____   _____   58. Crying spells

_____   _____   59. Lowered interest in things usually considered fun

_____   _____   60. Sleep changes (too much or too little)

_____   _____   61. Appetite chages (too much or too little)

_____   _____   62. Chronic low self-esteem

_____   _____   63. Negative sensitivity to smells/odors

_____   _____   64. Frequent feelings of nervousness or anxiety

_____   _____   65. Panic attacks

_____   _____   66. Symptoms of heightened muscle tension (headaches, sore muscles, hand tremor)

_____   _____   67. Periods of heart pounding, rapid heart rate or chest pain

_____   _____   68. Periods of trouble breathing or feeling smothered

_____   _____   69. Periods of feeling dizzy, faint or unsteady on your feet

_____   _____   70. Periods of nausea or abdominal upset

_____   _____   71. Periods of sweating, hot or cold flashes

_____   _____   72. Tendency to predict the worst

_____   _____   73. Fear of dying or doing something crazy

_____   _____   74. Avoid places for fear of having an anxiety attack

_____   _____   75. Conflict avoidance

_____   _____   76. Excessive fear of being judged or scrutinized by others

_____   _____   77. Persistent phobias

_____   _____   78. Low motivation

_____   _____   79. Excessive motivation

_____   _____   80. Tics (motor or vocal)

_____   _____   81. Poor handwriting

_____   _____   82. Quick startle

_____   _____   83. Tendency to freeze in anxiety provoking situations

_____   _____   84. Lacks confidence in their abilities

_____   _____   85. Seems shy or timid

_____   _____   86. Easily embarrassed

_____   _____   87. Sensitive to criticism

_____   _____   88. Bites fingernails or picks skin

FIGURE 4.9 (Continued)

_____	_____	89. Short fuse or periods of extreme irritability
_____	_____	90. Periods of rage with little provocation
_____	_____	91. Often misinterprets comments as negative when they are not
_____	_____	92. Irritability tends to build, then explodes, then recedes, often tired after a rage
_____	_____	93. Periods of spaciness or confusion
_____	_____	94. Periods of panic and/or fear for no specific reason
_____	_____	95. Visual or auditory changes, such as seeing shadows or hearing muffled sounds
_____	_____	96. Frequent periods of déjà vu (feelings of being somewhere you have never been)
_____	_____	97. Sensitivity or mild paranoia
_____	_____	98. Headaches or abdominal pain of certain origin
_____	_____	99. History of a head injury or family history of violence or explosiveness
_____	_____	100. Dark thoughts, may involve suicidal or homicidal thoughts
_____	_____	101. Periods of forgetfulness or memory problems

FIGURE 4.9   (Continued)

Positive Behavioral Intervention Plan

For a complete PBIP for a "serious behavior" include the Behavior Support Plan and this form

Student:_____ Date:_____

The behavior meets the definition of "serious behavior" for which other interventions specified in the IEP have been ineffective. This serious behavior as defined in the California Education Code is:
Assaultive
Self-injurious
Serious property damage
Other pervasive maladaptive behavior

Date when a Behavior Intervention Case Manager (BICM) was determined to be required:_____

Behavior Intervention Case Manager appointed:_____

A Functional Analysis Assessment was conducted on:_____

SPECIFIED DATA COLLECTION DURING BEHAVIOR INTERVENTION PLAN IMPLEMEMNTATION

A. Schedules for recording the frequency of the use of the interventions
    How often:_____
    By whom: _____
    Method of recording:_____
B. Schedules for recording frequency of targeted problem behaviors
    How often:_____
    By whom: _____
    Method of recording:_____
C. Schedules for recording frequency of replacement behaviors
    How often:_____
    By whom: _____
    Method of recording:_____
D. Criteria for discontinuing the use of interventions:
    If ineffective, discontinuation criteria and next steps:
    If _____ (condition), then _____ (next steps).
    If alternative interventions required, discontinuation criteria and next steps:
    If _____ (condition), then _____ (next steps).

EVALUATION OF PROGRAM EFFECTIVENESS – PERSONNEL, FREQUENCY, METHOD, DATA TO EVALUATE

A. Designated frequency of scheduled intervals to evaluate the Behavior Support Plan determined by IEP Team:

    _____
    _____
    _____

FIGURE 4.10

303

B. Program Effectiveness conducted between/by: (teacher, BICM, parent(s), other(s)) Specify:

_____

_____

_____

C. Designated method of conducting program effectiveness review:
- Meetings at (location/times):_____
- Telephone conferences (times):_____
- Email:_____
- Other:_____

D. Date to evaluate: measures of frequency, duration, and intensity of targeted behavior to be evaluated by comparison with baseline.

MODIFICATIONS WITHOUT IEP TEAM MEETING

Minor modifications may be made by BICM or qualified designee if parent is notified of the need and reviews evaluation data prior to changes.

A. Parent notified of right to question any modification through IEP procedures

B. Anticipated changes include increasing and decreasing (Check all that apply)

❑Frequency of reinforcement
❑Prompting of alternative behavior
❑Frequency of teaching new behavior
❑Environmental structure

OTHER SETTING RECEIVING COPIES OF THIS PLAN

A. Notification only setting(s):_____

B. Implement across setting(s): _____

Personnel responsible for implementing in other sites include:_____

_____

_____

_____

_____

_____

_____

FIGURE 4.10   (Continued)

COMMONLY USED IFSP FORMS

Family's IFSP
(Individualized Family Service Plan)

Child's Name:

Date of Birth: Gender:

Address:

```
Photo
Optional
```

Phone: Home: _____ 's Work:
_____ 's Work:

Change of Address:

Primary Language:

Parent / Caregiver: Relationship:

Parent / Caregiver: Relationship:

Parent / Caregiver: Relationship:

Service Coordinator: Date Assigned:

Service Coordinator: Date Assigned:

Service Coordinator: Date Assigned:

IFSP Duration: From: To: Review Date(s):_____

305

The IFSP is a working document that outlines the Early Intervention services to be provided. The plan is developed collaboratively between families and professionals based on the findings of a multidisciplinary assessment and evaluation. The IFSP should be developed within 45 days of referral. It should be reviewed every six months and revised each time eligibility is re-determined. It can be reviewed more frequently, and changes can be made at any time the family and program agrees it is necessary.

Universal IFSP Form
Revised January 2008

Massachusetts Department of Public Health
Early Intervention Services

FIGURE 4.11

Child's Name:
Date of Birth:

FAMILY PAGE

Every family is different and has its own priorities, concerns, and resources. This is your family's opportunity to tell other members of the team about your child and family, and your involvement with other community providers. The information on this page is confidential and will not be shared without your permission. This page should be completed each time eligibility is re-determined.

How would you describe your child and your family? What do you see as the strength as well as the concerns and priorities of both your child and your family?

Are there any other medical or community services that your family is receiving that you would like the Early Intervention staff to know about?

Information Given By: Date:

Universal IFSP Form
Revised January 2008

Massachusetts Department of Public Health
Early Intervention Services

FIGURE 4.12

Child's Name:
Date of Birth:

DEVELOPMENTAL PROFILE

The child's developmental Profile (pg. 3&4) summarizes the assessment and evaluation results and information gathered about your child's health and development. It may or may not include developmental levels depending on the desires of your family and other team members. This section is designed to be shared with insurance companies, physicians, schools, and others as designated by the parent(s)/guardian(s).

Date of Assessment and evaluation: Age of Child: mos.
Parent/Caregiver Name(s):

Eligibility Evaluation Instruments Used:
- ☐ Early Intervention Developmental Profile (Michigan)
- ☐ Battelle Developmental Inventory – 2nd Edition

Other Assessment and evaluation Input:
- ☐ Parent/Caregiver Report
- ☐ Clinical Observation
- ☐ Other:

Participants and Disciplines:

307

MEDICAL HISTORY/HEALTH STATUS:

VISUAL AND HEARING STATUS:

SUMMARY AND RECOMMENDATIONS:

FIGURE 4.13

Child's Name:
Date of Birth:
DEVELOPMENTAL PROFILE (Cont.)

Date of Assessment and Evaluation: Child's Age: mos.

Social Emotional/Personal Social/Interaction: Dev. Level:	Cognition: Dev. Level:
Motor Development including Gross Motor and Fine Motor: Dev. Level:	**Adaptive/Self Care:** Dev. Level:
Communication including Expressive and Receptive: Dev. Level:	

Universal IFSP Form
Revised January 2008

Massachusetts Department of Public Health
Early Intervention Services

FIGURE 4.13   (Continued)

Child's Name:
Date of Birth:

OUTCOMES AND STRATEGIES

*This page outlines the specific **measurable results, outcomes and strategies** that have been developed with the family as part of the Early Intervention Team based on the concerns identified through the assessment and evaluation process and family priorities. The Service Coordinator should discuss with the family what they hope to achieve through their Early Intervention experience.*

Start Date:	Desired Family Outcomes and Strategies

Universal IFSP Form
Revised January 2008

Massachusetts Department of Public Health
Early Intervention Services

FIGURE 4.14

Child's Name:
Date of Birth:

SERVICE DELIVERY PLAN

*This page identifies the **Early Intervention Services** to be provided to the child and family and may include home visits, community child groups and EI only child groups, parent groups, transportation, specialty services, etc. The provider of each service should be identified by discipline; and the location should include natural settings such as home, child care settings, playgroups, and other community sites. Changes in specific Early Intervention services, frequency, or location requires prior notification and parent/guardian signature and are recorded on IFSP Review pages, and updated below. EI services are supported by the Department of Public Health through state and federal funds; Medicaid; private health insurance and fees for some families based on family size and income.*

Start Date:	Type of Service/Location/Frequency/Duration/Service Provider/Discipline	End Date:

In what natural environments (where and with whom) will services be provided? How will collaboration with individuals in these environments occur?

Individualized clinical justification on the IFSP for services that do not occur in a natural setting (as determined by the parent and IFSP team) must include the following: An explanation of why the IFSP team determined that the outcomes could not be met in the child's natural settings, an explanation of why the IFSP team determined that the outcomes could not be met in the child's natural settings, and explanation of how services provided in this setting will support the child's ability to function to his/her natural environment, and a transition plan with timelines.

Universal IFSP Form
Revised January 2008

Massachusetts Department of Public Health
Early Intervention Services

FIGURE 4.15

Child's Name:
Date of Birth:

TRANSITION PLAN

EI services are available to eligible children until a child turns three, or until a child is determined ineligible. This page outlines the **Transition Plan** process when Early Intervention services end. Planning may begin at any time, but no later than when your child is 2 years 6 months of age. The process includes activities and tasks performed by the family and EI staff and should include a review of options for families, information for parents regarding the process of transition, support available to parents, information to be sent to the LEA and/or other community providers, and the specific plan for how the child will successfully transition to the next setting.

Start Date:	Transition Activities/Strategies
	☐ Provide explanation to family that transition planning activities occur for all children beginning at any time but no later than 30 minutes, and will be further discussed when appropriate.
	☐ Identify the options available to the child and family in the community. (For example, public school, Head Start, child care, preschools, library story hour. Family Networks, parent-child programs, recreational activities etc.) What are the steps to further explore these options? Who will be responsible for these steps?
	☐ Review training or informational opportunities available to parents on transitions and further futures placements. These may include trainings and/or informational opportunities with school representatives offered through EI, the local Parent Advisory Council (PAC), Federation for Children with Special Needs Parent Training and information Center, Family Networks, etc.
	☐ Explore support options available to parents. These may include working with your service Coordinator, Family TIES, PAC, parent-to-parent programs, public benefits or respite programs or other local, state and national resources.

Universal IFSP Form
Revised January 2008

Massachusetts Department of Public Health
Early Intervention Services

FIGURE 4.16

Start Date:	Transition Activities/Strategies
	☐ Describe the steps to prepare the child for a transition. What will support the child's adjustment or transition to a new program? (For example, visiting a new classroom or community setting, providing information to the new program, providing parents with information about early childhood development or community resources, etc.
	☐ Convene a transition planning conference. A transition planning conference is a meeting to review the child's services, discuss possible program options with community providers, if applicable, and establish transition activities.
	☐ Transition Plan not completed for the following reason(s):

Universal IFSP Form
Revised January 2008

Massachusetts Department of Public Health
Early Intervention Services

FIGURE 4.16   (Continued)

Child's Name:
Date of Birth:

TRANSITION PLAN

There are specific activities and timelines to be followed when your child may be eligible for special education or related services according to Part C of the IDEA (34 CFR 303.148). This page outlines the steps and procedures that the EI program must follow.

Start Date:	Transition Activities/Strategies

	☐ Date of notification to Local Education Agency (LEA):_____ EI programs are required by IDEA to release minimal personally identifiable information as a way to notify your local school system or child's potential eligibility for special education or related services.
	
	 OR
	☐ Parent has chosen to Opt Out. No personally identifiable information will be the LEA until consent is obtained to release information.
	
	Referral to the LEA: With a parent's written consent, a referral must be made at least six months before the child's 3rd birthday (MA Special Education Regulations (603 CMR 28.00m section 28.04 (1)(4) and the MDPH Early Intervention Operational Standards.)
	
	       ☐ Date LEA Referral was made:_____
	Notes:
	
	Determine the information that will support the child's transition. Written consent must be given before the EI program releases any information to the school system (for example, information from your child's IFSP, evaluations/assessments, etc.)
	      ☐ IFSP (specify sections of IFSP to send):_____
	      ☐ Evaluations or Assessments
	      ☐ Other Information:_____
	Notes:
	
	Convene a transition planning conference: A transition planning conference is a meeting to review the child's services, discuss possible program options with the LEA and establish transition activities. With parent's permission, the LEA is notified and invited to this meeting.
	
	Date Invitation sent to LEA_____
	Date of Transition Planning Conference _____ (*known as the 90 day meeting with Local Education Agency (LEA). New federal language notes this meeting may occur up to 9 months before a child's third birthday.*)
	
	Did the LEA attend the Transition Planning Conference? ☐ Yes ☐ No
	Notes:

313

Universal IFSP Form
Revised January 2008

Massachusetts Department of Public Health
Early Intervention Services

FIGURE 4.16 (Continued)

Review Date:_____   **Child's Name:**
☐**Six-Month Review**   ☐**NCSEAM Family Survey**   **Date of Birth:**
                        IFSP Review Page

The IFSP is a working document that should be reviewed every six months, and revised each time eligibility is re-determined. It can be reviewed more frequently, and changes can be made at any time that the family and program agree it is necessary. Changes to Outcomes and Services will be updated on the appropriate pages within the IFSP document.

Summary of Discussion:

Review of child's developmental progress; Outcomes; Changes in Services; etc:

☐   I/We have received the **Individualized Service Plan Meeting Notice** for an IFSP review meeting.

☐   I/We have been informed of and received a copy of my family rights.

☐   I/We have participated in the development of this IFSP and:

☐   I/We agree to the services described in this plan.

☐   I/We would like to have an IFSP Meeting with other team members to review the IFSP.

☐   I/We agree to the services in this plan with the following exceptions:

> Parents must give written consent before early intervention services can begin. Parents may choose to give consent to some changes in service and not others. Your consent means that you have been made aware of any changes and that you agree to them. The IFSP services that a parent(s) agrees to must be provided.

314

Parent Signature:_____   EI Staff Signature(s):_____

Parent Signature:_____   _____

Child's Name:
Date of Birth:

SIGNATURE PAGE

*This **Signature Page** must be completed in order to **begin** EI services. Participants in the development of the IFSP may include community representatives, extended family members, and others invited by the family. Once the IFSP document is signed please send/deliver a copy to the family. Please ensure the parent identifies that they have been given rights **and** accept services.*

Parents must give written consent before early intervention services can begin. If the parents do not give consent for any early intervention service or if they withdraw consent after first giving it, that service will not be provided. The early intervention services that parents agree to by signing below must be provided.

❑ I/We have been informed of and received a statement of our rights during the IFSP development process and I/We understand that any services I/We accept will be provided.

❑ I/We have received the **Individualized Family Service Plan Meeting Notice** for the IFSP meeting.

I/We have participated in the development of our IFSP and:

❑ I/We accept the services described in this plan.

❑ I/We accept the services in this plan with the following exceptions:

Comments:

315

Signatures

Parent/Guardian_____   Date_____

Parent/Guardian_____   Date_____

Other Team Members:

Service Coordinator_____   Date_____

Other Team Member _____   Date_____

Other Team Member _____   Date_____

Other Team Member _____   Date_____

Director (Optional)_____   Date_____

Universal IFSP Form
Revised January 2008

Massachusetts Department of Public Health
Early Intervention Services

FIGURE 4.18

Interview Format

THE INTERVIEW PROCESS

The National Guideline Clearinghouse sets forth an outline recommendation to be considered for the assessment of a child. In their recommendation, they list the professional and government health organizations that participated in defining the necessary parameters of assessment and the assessment process.

This parameter was reviewed at the Member Forum at the Annual Meeting of the American Academy of Child and Adolescent Psychiatry (AACAP) in October 2005. From July 2006 through September 2006, this parameter was reviewed by a Consensus Group convened by the Work Group on Quality Issues.

This practice parameter was approved by the AACAP Council on October 11, 2005.

Recommendations by The National Guideline Clearinghouse

Major Recommendations

Principle 1. The psychiatric assessment of a Child or Adolescent Must Include Both Historical and Current Information about the Family and Its Functioning, Typically Gathered from the Child and Primary Caretaker(s).

Structured Guide to Eliciting Family History

Demographic data should document family moves, changes in family composition, socioeconomic circumstances, family illness, legal difficulties, and altered family structure.

The family's historical report should be supplemented by ancillary sources of data. These sources can include history from other professionals who have evaluated or treated family members, as well as information from schools, local social service agencies, the courts, and child welfare agencies. These sources often provide a broader perspective of family functioning by providing information that the family either sees as unimportant or is unable or unwilling to communicate clearly to the clinician. Parents must give their consent for clinicians to gather history from these sources, with an adolescent's assent also prudent practice.

Gathering family history by interviewing ex-spouses, common-law partners, and stepparents also raises legal issues. The clinician may receive history from any individual regarding a child but should divulge information about the child only to those who have a legal right or permission to receive it.

The following is a guide to the areas that should be covered in gathering a detailed family history. These are questions the clinician should consider and may, in some cases, directly ask the family or family members.

1. Family Demographics
   - This information should include names and ages of parents and siblings, parents' occupations, current composition of family/household (including nonbiological members), health and psychiatric status of family members, and custody status.

2. Clinical Symptomatology of the Child
   - What is the interactional context of the symptomatic behavior (e.g., oppositional behavior)? What are the typical sequences of family interaction associated with the problem?
   - Is there a characteristic family profile associated with the clinical problem being assessed (e.g., coercive, inconsistent parenting practices in conduct-disordered children)? If so, questions related to this profile should be pursued.
   - Is on particular person blamed for the problem? Does the family feel responsible for the clinical problem (e.g., a child's dependency), or do they perceive themselves as responding to something deviant within the child (e.g., a child's difficulty sustaining attention)?
   - Are there family interactions that precipitated the current problem, predisposed to the current problem, or maintain the current problem?
   - Do individual symptoms appear to maintain a family's preferred interactional pattern? What are the mechanisms?

3. Individual Parent History
   - How did each parent negotiate his or her formative developmental years? Are there specific events in the parent's family of origin that appear to have had particular impact (e.g., sexual abuse)? Has cumulative

316

FIGURE 4.19

developmental experience (e.g., having experienced harsh, punitive parenting) had an enduring effect on the parents' current parenting behaviors?

- Does the parent have a diagnosed mental disorder or a medical disorder that affects parenting? How does it affect parenting?
- What is the style of the parents' pervasive personality functioning? How does it affect parenting?
- Are there identifiable patterns in the occupational or marital functioning that suggest personality strengths or weaknesses?
- Is there a particular developmental stage of child development that is problematic for the parent?
- How does each parent respond to siblings of the identified patient?
- What is the parents' level of insight and self-observation?

4. Parent Relationship History
   - What attracted the mother and father to each other? What is the chronological history of their relationship?
   - What were the couple's early relationship (e.g., premarital) expectations of each other? How have these been modified?
   - Were there previous marriages of relationships? Were children the result of the relationships? What ere the factors in termination of these relationships? Do such factors affect the current marriage? In what way do ex-spouses affect the current marriages?
   - What are the current areas of satisfaction and dissatisfaction with respect to vocation, finances, sexual relationship, and parenting?
   - What is the legal status of the parents' relationship?

5. History of Family as a Unit
   - How has the family negotiated the anticipated events of each family developmental stage: birth of first child, young children, adolescents, and launching young adults?
   - What are the unanticipated or unique challenges that this family has faced (e.g., unemployment, family illness)? Has the family responded in an adaptive or maladaptive manner?
   - How has the family's socioeconomic status affected their children? Is it related to clinical presentation?
   - How has the family's cultural and religious perspective affected their children? Is it related to clinical presentation?
   - Are there specific events of significance (e.g., family moves, remarriages)?
   - Is the family isolated from the larger community or is it interrelated to other groups?
   - Is there a current theme or challenge that dominates the family's attention? How is this related to the symptomatic child?

Principle 2. The Family Assessment of a Child or Adolescent Must Include an Observation of the Child's Interaction with Caretaker(s).

History taking occurs simultaneously with ongoing observation of parent-child interaction.

Clinicians should be attuned to any interactive process that contravenes known principles of healthy child development.

Structured Guide to Assessment of Basic Elements of Family Functioning

The following is a guide to four elements of basic family functioning, areas that should be covered in a comprehensive family assessment. It is structured in the format of questions the clinician should consider and, in some cases, may ask the family. The following dates are gathered through family members' historical report and clinician observation of family interaction.

1. Family Structure: Family structure refers to the typical organizational and transactional patterns and hierarchies that exist between the individuals or subsystems within the family. Important components of the family structure are its adaptability or flexibility, its level of cohesiveness, and the nature of its subsystems (e.g., spousal, parental and sibling) and the boundaries between them.
   - Adaptability: Healthy family function denotes a flexible structure in which transactional patterns are stable but can shift when circumstances dictate that change is needed. Clinical families may be too chaotic, with patterns and individual family roles constantly changing, or too rigid, where the family is unable to change typical ways of interacting as life's circumstances demand change. (Here, and in subsequent text, the term

FIGURE 4.19 (Continued)

317

clinical family denotes families whose problems in a specific area of functioning are associated with a clinical disorder in one of their children.)

- Cohesion: Healthy family functioning is indicated by a balance between connectedness and separateness. Clinical families may be either too emotionally close (enmeshment) or too emotionally distant (disengaged).
- Boundaries and subsystems: Healthy family functioning is indicated by emotional boundaries between individuals and subsystems that are permeable but clear, whereas in clinical families, boundaries may be rigid, diffused, or misaligned.

2. Family Communication: Family communication refers to the verbal and behavioral interactions by which family members impart information to each other about their individual needs and their perceptions of, and feelings about, others in the family. Components of family communication to be considered are clarity, directness, emotional expression, and problem solving.

- Clarity: Healthy family functioning is indicated by communication that is clear, direct, and consistent, with affective responses congruent to the message conveyed. Clinical families tend to communicate ambiguously and indirectly about both minor transactions and those with major importance, with affective expression that is muted, inappropriate, or incongruent.
- Emotional expression: Healthy family communication is characterized by affect that is congruent with the message conveyed. Clinical families may block the expression of feelings and do not express affect congruent with life experiences.
- Problem solving: Healthy family functioning identifies that problems exist, negotiates differences or conflicts, emphasizes positive reciprocal interactions among members, and uses new information in modifying behavior and/or perspective. Clinical families tend to have multiple individual perceptions of the problem, are unable to sacrifice toward common family goals, and are unable to perform the tasks necessary to assist family coping. Clinical families may be ineffective at problem solving and may have parent(s) who are poorly communicating, authoritarian, or indecisive.

3. Family Belief: The third area of observation, perhaps the most difficult to assess in initial interviews, is of family belief systems or shared constructions of reality. This refers to the observation that families have a type of memory function that goes beyond that of the beliefs and memories of each of its members. Clinical observations should attempt to ascertain beliefs termed "family myths" and "family legacies." This concept refers to ideas that guide decisions and actions in the family and help contribute to repetitive patterns of interaction that families demonstrate across generations. Healthy family beliefs and empower family continuity and adaptation (e.g., a family tradition of heroism and bravery). Clinical families may have beliefs that foster adaptation (e.g., men always leave their partners; adolescents are rebellious).

- What are the recurring themes in family life? Are there clusters of related problems such as alcohol-related problems, legal difficulties, or unquestioned beliefs or perceptions (e.g., men will abuse you and leave you; adolescent girls will be promiscuous).
- Are family roles rooted in family beliefs?
- Are there puzzling patterns of family interaction? Did they exist in previous generations?

4. Family Regulation of Child Development: In family health the developmental needs of children are met and their developmental tasks are mastered in the context of *family regulation*. The family must regulate the child's negotiation of these inevitable developmental tasks. Such regulation implies equilibrium between inhibiting and facilitating interactions between caretaker and child. The parents are attuned to their child's developmental needs and facilitate the emergence of the child's autonomous regulatory capacities. Family assessment should observe behaviors and gather history, which allows the clinician to clarify the nature and impact of regulatory processes. The following questions guide the clinician's task:

- Does the family have a balanced, empathic response to developmental needs of its children? This can be evaluated by the following review of basic developmental issues.
  - How does the family nurture and support?
  - How does the family set limits and teach internal self-control?
  - How does the family foster early socialization efforts?
  - How does the family facilitate achievement and success, including academic success?
  - How does the family facilitate independence/selfhood and individuation?

318

FIGURE 4.19 (Continued)

- Do parents regulate development in a coordinated pattern or is there a contrast in their efforts (e.g., one parent over involved with children and one parent under involved)?
- Is the family pattern of regulating developmental need characterized by overregulation (an excessive response to a child's developmental need that usurps the child's autonomous regulatory capacities), under regulation (a deficient response to a child's developmental need, which thus fails to support and nurture the child's emerging regulatory capacities), inappropriate (the family's responses are appropriate for an earlier developmental stage but are inappropriately applied to a child's developmental need in the current stage), irregular (the family that is consistent in on domain of function [e.g., feeding] but inconsistent in another [e.g., monitoring socialization]) or chaotic (no discernible pattern of family response to a child's developmental need) regulation?

Refer to Appendix B in the original guideline document for additional details on assessment of basic elements of family functioning.

Principle 3. The Family Interview Can Comprise Interviews with Individual Family Members, Groups of Members, or the Entire Family.

The family interview is the cornerstone of the family assessment. In addition to members of the immediate family, the interview should include those who interact with the child on a regular, sustained basis, in a manner that the clinician judges to be influential. This could include, for example, grandparents, other family members, or live-in partners.

It is important to keep legal issues in mind when planning interviews. Parents with legal custody should provide information to the clinician and can receive information about their child. However, the caregiver(s) with primary physical custody and children who have regular contact with the identified patient are usually those who attend interviews. A parent without primary physical custody should provide information and when the child visits this parent on a regular basis, a separate interview with that parent and child will provide a more comprehensive database.

319

Valuable information is obtained when data obtained from a family subunit interview are contrasted with data obtained from a whole family interview. The clinician must determine whether and in what sequence other family members should be interviewed and observed in interaction with the symptomatic child or adolescent. And individual interview with a child may supplement information gathered from an initial family interview, with its importance increasing coincident with a child's increasing age. An interview with a very young child is optional, and an interview with and adolescent is essential. Interviewing parents alone may provide an opportunity for the parents to freely discuss their relationship and provide differing views on their symptomatic child. Interviewing the child alone may allow the child to freely discuss conflicts that may not be easily divulged with parents present. This is particularly true with adolescents. Discrepant views of clinical problems often emerge more sharply in individual interviews and, once identified, may suggest family treatment as part of the treatment plan.

It is not uncommon for some family members to fail to attend, even when their presence has been requested. In this instance the clinician should interview all who actually attend but should be attentive to the absence of certain members and its meaning for the family. The absence of a member, most often a reluctant parent or adolescent, powerfully affects what happens in the session and is often an opportunity to understand some of the family difficulties associated with the child's presenting complaint.

The child or adolescent is invariably the identified patient, and interviewing other individuals regarding the child or adolescent's functioning raises the issue of confidentiality. Parents should be made aware of issues that are of concern to the younger child. As the child becomes an adolescent, this issue becomes more complicated and the adolescent's desire for confidence is respected unless an issue of dangerousness precludes maintaining confidentiality. Although interviewing individuals separately often helps them share their history more freely, confidentiality is maintained wherever possible.

FIGURE 4.19 (Continued)

The family interview is best conducted in a comfortable room large enough to accommodate the expected number of individuals. Furniture or objects potentially harmful to younger children should be removed. Games or activities for younger children should be present to facilitate rapport with them and decrease the likelihood of their behavioral disruption. It is important for the clinician to manage flexibly the simultaneous tasks of history taking and observing family interaction. At times, acute problems such as suicidal ideation or intense disagreement about an issue can prevent systematic gathering of background family history, effectively terminating some content data gathering while providing powerful experiential process data.

In the beginning of a family interview, each member is addressed in an informal manner that is consistent with his or her developmental level, with a goal of establishing rapport. One way that this is accomplished is by the clinician identifying family strengths and resources at the outset, best achieved through an informal interview style. The clinician then defines the problem by gathering relevant current and past history. While this is taking place, the clinician observes family interactions and facilitates the interactional stage with the use of probing questions. By asking family members about their individual responses, behaviors, and feelings, the clinician begins to understand how events have acquired specific meanings for each member and how these meanings differ.

It is not uncommon for conflict to emerge in the session while the clinician gathers history. At such points the antecedents and consequences of behavioral problems are not merely reported but demonstrated. A history of successful problem resolution should be reviewed, as well as discussing situations in which problems remain unresolved. A completion of the family interview includes the summation stage, in which the clinician formulates what he or she has observed, its relevance to the identified patient's problems, and the role, if any, family members may play in subsequent treatments. All of the family members should feel that they have been understood, and, whenever possible, the clinician should convey a sense of hope with respect to future family adjustment.

Principle 4. When the Clinical History Suggests Interactional Problems, the Family Members in Daily Contact with the Child Should Be Interviewed, with the Goal of Establishing An Understanding of the Family Context of Symptomatic Behaviors.

Because most families present to the clinic with a symptomatic child, it is prudent to begin a family assessment with a review child's symptomatology. Some problems present with an interactive focus: oppositional behavior, a child running away from home, a self-harm gesture after a family argument, or a child's refusal to eat. In these instances it is important to obtain a history of the sequence of events, behaviors, and family interactions associated with the clinical problem. The assessment goal is not only to describe the problematic behavior but also to understand the meaning and function of the behavior in relationship to the child's family. A given symptom, such as a temper tantrum, may have different meanings in different children and different families. To draw such distinctions, the family assessment must include a review of family circumstances and consequences of the problematic behavior. Questions should include a review of the family's past attempts at solving problems. In this sense, history taking, diagnostic formulation, and observation of the family occur concomitantly. During the assessment process the clinician must keep in mind the reciprocal nature of family influences. Although family interaction may be associated with symptoms in the child, the child's symptoms may provoke family responses.

Principle 5. The Family Interview Should Include Questioning Regarding Family Risk Factors for Specific Disorders.

The clinician should recognize that some disorders are associated with typical family or parenting styles, and this knowledge should inform history taking (e.g., coercive and inconsistent discipline in conduct-disordered youths, parental illness, and vulnerability in children with separation anxiety). A history of clinical symptomatology must include a review of which behavior management techniques parents have tried, either successfully or unsuccessfully. The clinician must always keep in mind that patterns of interaction may be primarily a response to a child with a biological vulnerability.

FIGURE 4.19   (Continued)

Principle 6. The Family Evaluation Should Provide Enough Data for a Clinician to Characterize Adequately the Family's Structure, Level of Communication, Belief System, and Regulatory Functioning.

Perhaps the most challenging aspect of family assessment is the systematic observation and categorization of the basic elements of family functioning. Four elements are described most frequently and subsume the most clinically relevant aspects of family function: structure, communication, belief systems, and regulatory processes. (See Principle 2 of this summary and Appendix B in the original guideline document for a full description of the elements.)

Principle 7. The Family Assessment is Enhanced by a Family Developmental History, a Marital/Relationship History, and Individual Parent History, Including a History of Psychiatric Disorders in Family Members.

A history of both parents should identify psychiatric and/or medical disorders that may be transmitted to their children, whether through experiential or genetic mechanisms. It is important to assess the parents' level of knowledge of child development and of the child's disorder and identify specific knowledge deficits of clinical significance. The overall goal of the parent history is to allow the clinician to achieve a full perspective of parental strengths and weaknesses.

See Principle 1 above and Appendix A in the original guideline document for interviewing guidelines.

Principle 8. For Complex Cases, the Clinician Should Consider Ancillary Techniques to Gather and Organize Relevant Data About Family Functioning.

Two helpful products of the family interview can be the family genogram and the family timeline. A genogram is a diagram made in conjunction with the family, or by the clinician alone, that identifies facts and relationship patterns of three or more generations of family members. Such a tool is essential in more complex family histories. The content of the genogram allows a family history to be seen in generational context beyond the presenting complaint and concerns of immediate family members. A timeline is a simple yet graphically useful instrument that maps a sequence of important events. The timeline provides a visual representation of the onset of psychiatric problems linked to clear precipitants and family context.

Because of the complexity of family assessment, a video record of family interactions can be useful for the clinician and, at times, for the family to view themselves. Video is often used in training settings but has limitations in other settings, largely due to the time-intensive nature of video review.

Principle 9. The Evaluation of the Family Requires the Clinician's Sensitive Awareness of Cultural Differences.

The family's cultural background directly affects its views of normative family structure, communication style, belief systems, and child development. The involvement of extended family members, style of emotional expression, and family values are examples of culturally influenced aspects of family function. It is important to understand the family's religion or world view/philosophy of life, especially when the presenting complaint involves issues directly related to these ideas.

Principle 10. A Comprehensive Family Assessment Should Lead to Treatment Interventions That Interrupt Family Functions That May Precipitate, Predispose, or Maintain Clinical Problems and Potentiate Family Functions That Promote Health and Optimize Disease Management.

Contemporary developmental psychopathology emphasizes risk and protective factors as etiologically relevant in the onset of psychopathology. The family is but one of these factors. When the family assessment is complete, it should be integrated with the other findings of the comprehensive psychiatric assessment. With the integrated data, the clinician can develop a formulation with respect to the reciprocal effects of family influence. The clinician must

FIGURE 4.19 (Continued)

321

have a clear understanding of the factors within the family that have affected the child and the aspects of the child's condition that have stressed the family. The complex judgment of determining the directional effects of family influence can be facilitated by considering certain aspects of the data gathered. Once complete, this case formulation guides the clinician in determining an approach to the family's role in treatment.

Areas of Family Assessment Related to Treatment Planning

- Family understanding of developmental norms
- Influence of parental psychiatric disorder
- Quality of parental commitment to the child's well-being
- Parental achievements apart from child rearing
- Family members and developmental task mastery
- Assessment of the heritability of the child or adolescent's disorder
- Level of parents; mutual support of each other
- Relationship of the child's behavior to environmental change

Clinical Algorithm(s)

None provided

Evidence Supporting the Recommendations

Type of Evidence Supporting the Recommendations

The type of supporting evidence is not specifically stated for each recommendation. Although empirical evidence may be available to support certain principles, principles are primarily based on expert opinion and clinical experience.

Benefits/Harms of Implementing the Guideline Recommendations

Potential Benefits

Appropriate assessment of the family of the child or adolescent with a psychiatric disorder

Potential Harms

Not Stated

Qualifying Statements

Qualifying Statements

American Academy of Child and Adolescent Psychiatry (AACAP) practice parameters are developed to assist clinicians in psychiatric decision making. These parameters are not intended to define the standard of care, nor should they be deemed inclusive of all proper methods of care or exclusive of others methods of care directed at obtaining the desired results. The ultimate judgment regarding the care of a particular patient must be made by the clinician in light of all of the circumstances presented by the patient and his or her family, the diagnostic and treatment options available, and available resources.

FIGURE 4.19 (Continued)

Implementation of the Guideline

Description of Implementation Strategy

An implementation strategy was not provided.

Institute of Medicine (IOM) National Healthcare Quality Report Categories

IOM Care Need

Getting Better
Living with Illness

IOM Domain

Effectiveness
Patient-centeredness

Identifying Information and Availability

Bibliographic Source(s)

Josephson A<, AACAP Work Group on Quality Issues. Practice parameter for the assessment of the family. J Am Acad Child Adolesc Psychiatry 2007 Jul;46(7):922-37. [550 references] PubMed.

Adaptation

Not applicable: The guideline was not adapted from another source.

Date Released

2007 Jul

Guideline Developer(s)

American Academy of Child and Adolescent Psychiatry – Medical Specialty Society

Source(s) of Funding

American Academy of Child and Adolescent Psychiatry

Guideline Committee

Work Group on Quality Issues

Composition of Group That Authored the Guideline

This parameter was developed by Allan M. Josephson, MD, principal author.

Work Group on Quality Issues Members: William Bernet, MD (Co-Chair); Oscar Bukstein, MD (Co-Chair); Heather J. Walter, MD (Co-Chair); Valerie Arnold, MD; Joseph Beitchman, MD; R. Scott Benson, MD; Allan Chrisman, MD; Tiffany Farchione, MD; Jogn Hamilton, MD; Helene Keable, MD; Joan Kinlan, MD; Jon McClellan, MD; David Rue, MD; Ulrich Schoettle, MD; Jon A. Shaw, MD; Saundra Stock, MD

AACAP Staff: Kristin Kroeger Ptakowski; Jennifer Medicus

FIGURE 4.19   (Continued)

323

Financial Disclosures/Conflicts of Interest

Dr. Bukstein receives or has received research support from, acted as a consultant to, and/or served on the speakers' bureaus of Cephalon, Forest Pharmaceuticals, McNeil Pediatrics, Shire, Eli Lilly, and Novartis. Drs. Josephson, Bernet, and Walter have no financial relationships to disclose.

Guideline Status

This is the current release of the guideline.

Guideline Availability

Electronic copies: Available in Portable Document Format (PDF) from the American Academy of Adolescent and Child Psychiatry (AACAP) Website.

Print copies: Available from AACAP, Communications Dept., 3615 Wisconsin Ave, NW, Washington, DC 20016. Additional information can be obtained through the AACAP Publication Store for Parameters and Guidelines.

Availability of Companion Documents

None available

Patient Resources

None available

NGC Status

This NGC summary was completed by ECRI on October 23, 2007.

Copyright Statement

324

Disclaimer

NGC Disclaimer

The National Guideline Clearinghouse™ (NGC) does not develop, produce, approve, or endorse the guidelines represented on this site.

FIGURE 4.19 (Continued)

Semi-Structured Parent Interview

Child's Name: _____ M/F: _____ Age: _____ DOB:_____
Parent/Guardian Name: _____ Relationship to child: _____
Interviewer's Name: _____ Credentials: _____

Purpose of Interview

This time is very important to the understanding of concerns which have initiated this process. The information that you have provided in this questionnaire provides the interviewer to clarify the child's functioning. It is appreciated that you consented to voluntarily have (child's name) be evaluated. During this interview, the interviewer will go through the responses to each question to hear more about your concerns. This interview is part of the evaluation of (child's name).

Confidentiality

All of the information provided in the evaluation of (child's name) will be summarized in a final written report. As previously stated, you have voluntarily agreed to participate in the evaluation of (child's name). The common practice of this review is to:
  1) Be respectful of your privacy, but not reporting information which is not relevant to this evaluation.
  2) To not include direct quotation of parental comments.
  3) At the end of the evaluation to discuss what information will and will not be included in this evaluation's summary report.

However, as a mandated reporter there are certain circumstances which require the disclosure of confidential information, which includes the reason to suspect child abuse or when a child poses a danger to themselves on someone else.

325

_____   _____
Parent Signature   Date

_____   _____
Interviewer's Signature   Date

FIGURE 4.20

I. Medical and Developmental History
    Before we proceed, I would like to talk about (child's name)'s medical and developmental history
    A) Medical History
        • Current medications for behavior problem(s)
        • Current medications for emotional problem(s)
        • Current medications for other problems
        • History of
            o Illness
            o Accidents
            o Operations
            o Medical Problems
        • Allergies? Yes   No   Uncertain
    B) Developmental History and Temperament
        • Developmental delays?   Yes   No   Uncertain
        • Problems in temperament?   Yes   No   Uncertain
        • Problems in early behavior?   Yes   No   Uncertain

II. Family Relations and Home Situations
    A) Who does (child's name) live with (if the parents are separated/divorced what are the custody arrangements and visitation with each family)?
        • Do they go to a daycare center (aside from family)?
        • How well does that work out?
    B) Home Environment
        • Is there anything about the living situation/home that is a problem for you or the family (additional persons residing in the home, work situation, financial problems, neighborhood violence or other problems)?
        • Are there any family members (or extended family member that the child has contact with) have any medical or mental health problems that may affect (child's name)?
        • Have there been any major changes recently in the living situation or family?

This is an appropriate section to probe where there are concerns of abuse/neglect, and whether there has even been possible abuse/neglect that was reported.
    C) Family Relations
        • How does (child's name) get along with family members? Who live in the home? (ask about each member of the family that resides at the home).
        • Who does (child's name) get along with best?
        • Who does (child's name) get along with least?
        • In general, do family members have difficulty getting along (a lot of conflict in the home)?
        • Do you have any difficulties getting along with members of the family (spouse/partner, relatives or other adults in the home)?
    D) Rules/Punishment
        • What are the rules/expectations about behavior in the home?
        • Who makes the rules?
        • How do you think (child's name) feels about the rules?
        • Are there any specific rules they have difficulty following?
        • What are the consequences/discipline/punishment procedures used in the home?
        • Who carries out the consequences/discipline/punishment?
        • Do children get spanked or physically punished for bad behavior?
        • Do you and your spouse/partner agree on how problem behaviors are handled?

FIGURE 4.20   (Continued)

- Have you ever talked with someone else about discipline/punishment (friend, relative, teacher, counselor, etc.)?
- Would you like help in learning to manage difficult behavior?

E) Chores/Rewards
- When (child's name) makes a good choice, what happens?
- Do you have any special rewards or treats for good behaviors/accomplishments?
- Does (child's name) ever do something good or special?
- Does (child's name) have any chores at home?
- Do they get an allowance or privileges? (If yes) what is required to get the allowance or privilege?

III. Presenting Concern(s)
- Please explain what concerns you most about (child's name).
- When did you first become concerned and why?
- How long has this problem been going on?

IV. Behavioral or Emotional Problems
A. Does (child's name) have a behavioral problem? Yes/No
- Does (child's name) have an emotional problem? Yes/No
- Be as detailed as possible about specifically what the problem(s) is, what they do. Please give examples.
- How long have they had this problem?
- How often does this problem occur?
- What are the specific circumstances under which the problem occurs?
- Be specific about when and where the problem generally occurs.
B. Prioritize the problems presented as well as prioritizing the necessary intervention and the order of their importance.
C. What precedes the identified priority problem? Ask these questions of each identified prioritized problem.
- What usually happens before the problem occurs?
- What do you think sets it off?
- Think carefully about everything that generally happens after the problem occurs.
  - What do you do to deal with the problem?
  - How are you feeling and reacting to the problem?
  - If (child's name) is at school/pre-school, daycare or other setting, what happens?
  - How does (child's name) feel/react when this happens?
D. Substitute Behaviors
- What would you like (child's name) to do instead of the problem behavior?
- What would be an acceptable change (substitute behavior)?

Prior to meeting, you (the parent) filled out a rating scale which was scored before prior meeting. I am going to share with you a summary (of all problems identified in the borderline or clinical range compared to a relative normative sample).

V. School Functioning
- How is (child's name) doing in school
- How many adults does (child's name) work with at school (teachers, speech pathologist, etc.)
- How do they get along with each of these adults?
- Is there anyone they are particularly close to out of these people?

327

FIGURE 4.20 (Continued)

VI. Learning Problem
- Do they have any identified learning problems
  - o   Yes   No   Uncertain
- If yes, what is it? (Elicit as much detail as possible.)
- How long has it been identified, and by whom?
- How is it being dealt with?

VII.   Special Help/School Services
- Does (child's name) receive any special help/special services in school?
  - o   Yes   No   Uncertain
- If yes, what kind of help (For instance, special education, IEP, remedial instruction, Title 1 services, 504 Plan, peer tutoring, individual aide, behavior plan, behavior specialist, guidance services, speech pathologist, school psychologist, etc.)
- How long have they needed special help?
- How long have they been receiving special help?
- Have they received special help in the past?
  - o   If yes, what?
- Do you think they are getting enough of the right kind of help?
- What else would you like done to help (child's name) at school?

VIII.   School Behavior Problem(s)
- Does (child's name) have behavior or emotional problems at school?
- If yes, what kind of problem(s)?
- What generally happens at school when this problem(s) arise?
- What has been done to address these problems?

Adopted from McConaughy 2005

FIGURE 4.20   (Continued)

THE INTAKE INTERVIEW

The interview method could be accomplished by a formal structured or semistructured instrument. However, when numerous family system issues are evident, it will likely be more beneficial to take the time to develop trust and positive regard demonstrated by the observer's genuine concern and interest. This will allow for a more cooperative clinical environment in which to explore the more intimate details of their daily lives, family background and other pertinent history. DeGangi (2000) offers an example outline of an assessment interview with the following considerations which should play a role in all clinical contacts with the perspective of meeting the client where they are which means being sensitive to wording, the type of information being sought, and the emotional cues being reflected during the interview. In other words, use common sense in this semistructured interview to adapt questions to the circumstance and response:

A. Referral
1. What is going on with your child that has brought you here?
2. Who referred you?
B. Chief Complaint or Presenting Problems
3. When did you first notice the problem? (When did it start?)
4. Have you noticed any changes in the problem since it started? If so, in what way(s) has it changed?
5. What is the problem like at its worst? What is/was that like for you? (While exploring this point it is important to acknowledge and validate the parental experience. This question is where parent level of functioning (depression/substance abuse) will be explored in association with potential child abuse/neglect.)
6. What have you tried that worked? What have you tried that hasn't worked or helped? (This question aids in the understanding of parental adaptability in responding to the challenges with the infant/child, as well as how responsive the infant/child has been to the efforts of the parents)
C. Current Functioning
7. Tell me about your child. What does he/she like to do when they are with you? What don't they like to play with? (Information associated with the child's choice of play offers knowledge/facts about how the child organizes themselves.)
8. What do you enjoy about your child? What do you like doing with them?
9. Tell me about an average day, starting with getting up in the morning. Be specific about each detail, i.e., behavior when getting up, what does the child eat and where, daily activities, nap/sleep schedule, how the child plays alone or with other children, what would cause variation in a typical day, etc.?
10. Is you child different when you take them places such as a store, friend's home, daycare, school? (Exploring potential of a child being overstimulated when out in the world, versus the regulatory disordered child who has difficult behavior at home but behaves well when out in the world.)
D. Developmental and Pregnancy History
11. I would like to know about your pregnancy. How did you feel during the pregnancy? During this time did you experience anything that was stressful (loss of a job, moving, loss of a loved one)?
12. Was this pregnancy planned or not? (Were there any fertility or health issues relevant to the pregnancy?)
13. What prenatal care was sought and received?
14. What were labor and delivery like?
15. What was your baby like when he/she was first born? (Was the baby alert, tracking the mother's voice, hyper-alert, constantly crying, etc.?)
16. What was your reaction to your baby when he/she was first born?

329

17. Many new mothers experience the "baby blues", did you? If so, how bad did it get? Were you treated by a doctor? If so, what was included in your treatment, what were you told, how did you get better and when?
18. Inquire about developmental milestones to determine appropriate time frames and accomplishments (sitting, walking, first words, first smile, use of gestures, etc.)
19. Did you breast feed your baby? Tell me about their eating and their growth. If it is or has been a problem, inquire regarding the following:
    a. What was meal time like, or what would you like meal time to be like?
    b. Did you or any other members of your family have problems with appetite, eating, or weight?
    c. How does it make you feel when your child doesn't eat?
    d. What did you do to help your child eat, or what have you tried to help your child eat? (Inquire regarding forced feeding, frequent meals, feeding environment, i.e., highchair or being held.)
20. Most children test limits. How do/did you handle discipline? Share with me a typical experience of when your child misbehaved. How did you handle it? Do you and your spouse/partner handle such things the same way or in different ways? Do the two of you set limits in a similar or different way? How were limits set in your home when you were a child and what did your mother and father do when you misbehaved?

E. Health History of Child
21. Has your child been healthy? Are there any allergies?
22. Any ear infections? How often?
23. Has your child had a problem with spitting up, regurgitating, or reflux?
24. What does your child eat during the day?
25. How often do you visit your pediatrician?
26. Is your child up to date on immunizations?
27. Is your child currently being treated for anything by their pediatrician?
28. Does your child have a history of any other health problems?

F. Diagnosis
29. Has your pediatrician given your child a diagnosis?
30. What do you think caused the problem?
31. What does your child remind you of?
32. Is there anyone in your family who had problems like your child?
33. What do you think will help with your child's problems?

The following questions are related to family functioning, history and expectations.

G. Family History
34. Who lives with you in your house?
35. Do you have family, friends, or other resources that you can depend on if your family has a crisis? Who lives nearby to help you?

*Ask both mother and father to answer the following questions:
36. Tell me about where you grew up. Where do you fall in your family birth order? How many brothers and sisters?
37. What was your childhood like (happy, sad, confusing, difficult times)? Were there any particular stresses or losses that you experienced growing up?
38. How long have you and your spouse been married? When did you first begin or plan to have children?
39. What does your family enjoy doing together?
40. Are there any particular stresses in your family right now that I should be aware of (i.e., loss of job, separations, etc.)?

H. Parental Expectations for Child
41. Did you have any fantasies or expectations about your child before they were born?
42. Did you have any experience with children before parenting this child?

43. What do you think your child will be like in 5 or 10 years from now?
44. For whom did you name your child?
45. Who does your child look like?
46. Does their personality remind you of anyone? How are they similar or different from their siblings?

I. Final History

There are some questions I need to ask of everyone. These are only to help me understand more about you and your child.

47. How much caffeine did you drink per day during the pregnancy? What prescription drugs did you take? What about non-prescription drugs? (Ask about specific drugs: alcohol, marijuana, cocaine, meth, crack, crank, heroin, etc.). For example, how much alcohol did you drink each day? Each week? How much (drug) did you use each day? Each week? How often did you use whatever drug of choice?
48. Did you or you spouse experience any physical abuse growing up? Sexual abuse?
49. Did anyone in your family have school-related problems? Emotional or behavioral problems? Anyone commit or attempt suicide? Any other medical/genetic problems?

FAMILY ASSESSMENT

Family assessments are based on a combination of observations, interviews, self-report measures and social history. Assessing the family is essential to determine the range of services that are needed for the family system, determining potential level of compliance (need for monitoring and support), to explore options and to make suggestions/recommendations. Therefore, to make sure there is an outcome of adequate information from the parents/caretakers acquired during the intake interview, the person conducting the interview needs to be able to answer the following questions when the interview is concluded (this is also in the assessment section):

- Are there safety and protection issues that must be addressed?
- What are the relative strengths and weaknesses of the family?
- What are the family's needs?
- Can the family meet the needs of the child?
- What are the resources available to the family (extended family, church, community, etc.)?
- Does this family have a functional hierarchical structure?
- Is the family enmeshed or disengaged?
- Are major mental health problems present in the family?
- Are there any substance abuse problems present in the family?
- Is there any evidence of personality disorder(s) present in the parents/caregivers?
- Is the family competent to provide for basic needs?
- Do the parents/caregivers have the ability to manage problem behaviors in age-appropriate ways without any safety risks?
- Is there any evidence of multigenerational patterns of abuse or neglect, substance abuse, etc?
- Parental/caretaker ability to empathize?
- Parental/caretaker ability to nurture?
- What resources have been helpful to this family system in the past?
- How does this family system cope with stress and crises?

Bibliography

DeGangi, G. A. (2000). *Pediatric disorders of regulatiion in affect and behavior*. San Diego: Academic Press.

Note: Page numbers followed by "*f*", "*t*" and "*b*" refers to figures, tables and Boxes respectively.

Printed and bound by CPI Group (UK) Ltd, Croydon, CR0 4YY

08/06/2025

01896877-0002